Artificial Intelligence Technology in Healthcare

Artificial Intelligence Technology in Healthcare: Security and Privacy Issues focuses on current issues with patients' privacy and data security including data breaches in healthcare organizations, unauthorized access to patients' information, and medical identity theft. It explains recent breakthroughs and problems in deep learning security and privacy issues, emphasizing current state-of-the-art methods, methodologies, implementation, attacks, and countermeasures. It examines the issues related to developing artificial intelligence (AI)-based security mechanisms which can gather or share data across several healthcare applications securely and privately.

Features:

- Combines multiple technologies (i.e., Internet of Things [IoT], Federated Computing, and AI) for managing and securing smart healthcare systems.
- Includes state-of-the-art machine learning, deep learning techniques for predictive analysis, and fog and edge computing-based real-time health monitoring.
- Covers how to diagnose critical diseases from medical imaging using advanced deep learning-based approaches.
- Focuses on latest research on privacy, security, and threat detection on COVID-19 through IoT.
- Illustrates initiatives for research in smart computing for advanced healthcare management systems.

This book is aimed at researchers and graduate students in bioengineering, artificial intelligence, and computer engineering.

Advances in Smart Healthcare Technologies

Editors: Chinmay Chakraborty and Joel J. P. C. Rodrigues

This book series focus on recent advances and different research areas in smart healthcare technologies including Internet of Medical Things (IoMedT), e-Health, personalized medicine, sensing, Big Data, telemedicine, etc. under the healthcare informatics umbrella. Overall focus is on bringing together the latest industrial and academic progress, research, and development efforts within the rapidly maturing health informatics ecosystem. It aims to offer valuable perceptions to researchers and engineers on how to design and develop novel healthcare systems and how to improve patient's information delivery care remotely. The potential for making faster advances in many scientific disciplines and improving the profitability and success of different enterprises is to be investigated.

Smart and Secure Internet of Healthcare Things

Nitin Gupta, Jagdeep Singh, Chinmay Chakraborty, Mamoun Alazab and Dinh-Thuan Do

Practical Artificial Intelligence for Internet of Medical Things

Emerging Trends, Issues, and Challenges

Edited by Ben Othman Soufiene, Chinmay Chakraborty, and Faris A. Almalki

Intelligent Internet of Things for Smart Healthcare Systems

Edited by Durgesh Srivastava, Neha Sharma, Deepak Sinwar, Jabar H. Yousif, and Hari Prabhat Gupta

Future Health Scenarios

AI and Digital Technologies in Global Healthcare Systems

Edited by Maria Jose Sousa, Francisco Guilherme Nunes, Generosa do Nascimento and Chinmay Chakraborty

Machine Learning and Deep Learning Techniques for Medical Image Recognition

Edited by Ben Othman Soufiene and Chinmay Chakraborty

Artificial Intelligence Technology in Healthcare

Security and Privacy Issues

Edited by Neha Sharma, Durgesh Srivastava, and Deepak Sinwar

For more information about this series, please visit: www.routledge.com/Advances-in-Smart-Healthcare-Technologies/book-series/CRCASHT

Artificial Intelligence Technology in Healthcare
Security and Privacy Issues

Edited by Neha Sharma, Durgesh Srivastava, and Deepak Sinwar

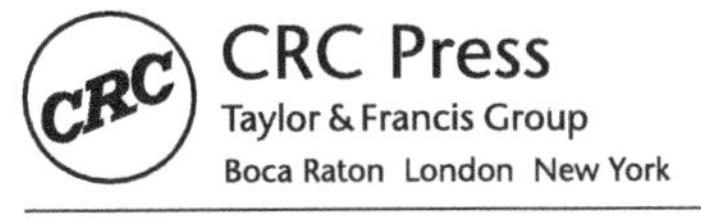

CRC Press
Taylor & Francis Group
Boca Raton London New York

CRC Press is an imprint of the
Taylor & Francis Group, an **informa** business

First edition published 2025
by CRC Press
2385 NW Executive Center Drive, Suite 320, Boca Raton FL 33431

and by CRC Press
4 Park Square, Milton Park, Abingdon, Oxon, OX14 4RN

CRC Press is an imprint of Taylor & Francis Group, LLC

Library of Congress Cataloging-in-Publication Data
Names: Sharma, Neha (Computer scientist), editor. | Srivastava, Durgesh (Computer scientist), editor. | Sinwar, Deepak, editor.
Title: Artificial intelligence technology in healthcare : security and privacy issues / edited by Neha Sharma, Durgesh Srivastava, and Deepak Sinwar.
Description: First edition. | Boca Raton, FL : CRC Press, 2024. |
Series: Advances in smart healthcare technologies | Includes bibliographical references and index.
Identifiers: LCCN 2024011696 (print) | LCCN 2024011697 (ebook) |
ISBN 9781032428390 (hardback) | ISBN 9781032456072 (paperback) |
ISBN 9781003377818 (ebook)
Subjects: LCSH: Artificial intelligence—Medical applications | Medical care—Information technology—Security measures. | Computer security. | Data protection.
Classification: LCC R859.7.A78 A787 2024 (print) | LCC R859.7.A78 (ebook) |
DDC 610.285—dc23/eng/20240621
LC record available at https://lccn.loc.gov/2024011696
LC ebook record available at https://lccn.loc.gov/2024011697

ISBN: 9781032428390 (hbk)
ISBN: 9781032456072 (pbk)
ISBN: 9781003377818 (ebk)

DOI: 10.1201/9781003377818

Typeset in Times
by codeMantra

Contents

Preface

In recent years, machine learning (ML) has raised expectations for artificial intelligence (AI) technology, particularly deep learning (DL), demonstrating exceptional performance in image identification, natural language processing, pattern matching, face recognition, and other areas. DL models have various advantages such as fast calculation of complicated problems, maximal application of unstructured data, decreased costs, and many more, but they also have some drawbacks such as opaqueness and computationally intensive. However, DL-based applications are utilized in day-to-day routines and work on massive amounts of data to attain higher accuracy; if these models lead to mistakes due to malicious actions, it will become onerous; thus, protecting the data from security breaches is a key worry.

This book focuses on the current issues with the patient's privacy and data security, but with climbing costs, there is an ever-growing concern about the ability of organization to protect against data breaches. The issues include the following: data breaches in healthcare organization are growing at a rapid rate, the use of mobile devices is putting the patient's data at risk, there is unauthorized access to patient's information, and medical identity theft poses a greater risk to patients. This book focuses on recent breakthroughs and problems in DL security and privacy issues, emphasizing current state-of-the-art methods, methodologies, implementation, attacks, and countermeasures. It is very important to examine the security concerns and related countermeasure approaches of AI models in healthcare. This book also examines the constraints that must be overcome when developing AI-based security mechanisms including federated learning and cloud computing, which are capable of gathering or sharing data across several healthcare applications securely and privately. A chapter-wise summary is mentioned as follows:

Chapter 1 discusses the use of AI in healthcare; it describes the ability of machines to mimic the human mind and a series of data processing techniques. AI has shown immense growth in healthcare and connects expert doctors to the medical system by allowing them frequent monitoring of the patient's health. The primary goal of AI is to offer better, more valuable, and cost-effective healthcare services by enhancing effectiveness and efficiency. This chapter is splintered into various sections. The first section is a brief introduction along with its subfields, and the second discusses its related work in medicine. It provides the additional discussion on the different steps of AI toward the different healthcare problems and challenges arising from current social structures, opportunities, and Healthcare 4.0.

Chapter 2 deals with AI's implications in healthcare and medical systems. AI has the capacity to improve patients' health, and it can not only aid in the development of pharmaceuticals but also improve the efficiency of the current ones. It deals with various applications of AI in healthcare and the recent advancements of AI in the medical industry like medical image processing, smart inhalers, and software like Fitbits. This chapter focuses on three major categories of AI, ML, DL, and NLP, which have a major impact on AI for healthcare. The growing expense of healthcare will remain controversial among healthcare stakeholders. However, there's still more improvement in AI, which, in turn, will improve the patient's conditions better. The implementation of AI in the clinical process and patient's clinical trial journey have been taken into consideration. This chapter further summarizes the potential for medical cost reduction and service quality improvement with help from the government.

Chapter 3 provides a complete review on the advancements of AI in healthcare. AI has cemented the cultural shift in every aspect of modern human life. People want to lead fulfilling lives, and maintaining good health is essential to this. Healthcare is one of the industries that tend to make use of AI to boost success rates. Healthcare AI is already beginning to replace traditional techniques. The healthcare industry incorporates numerous ML and DL algorithms. Many algorithms, including CNN, are employed to identify cancers. Early stroke detection uses Principle Component Analysis, Random Forest, and Decision Tree. K-NN and Support Vector Machine are effective algorithms designed to detect diabetes. AI uses ICA, genetic algorithms, and image processing to detect cancer and obesity. The fundamental objective of this chapter is to discuss the AI techniques for diagnosing diseases even under challenging circumstances and to identify them before they reach a critical stage. With AI in healthcare, it is anticipated that doctors would be able to treat patients more effectively and precisely in a shorter amount of time, increasing patient success rates.

Chapter 4 delves into the role of DL applications in modern healthcare services. The development and application of technologies are the cause for improvement in medical fields. Therefore, collection of data for processing and evaluation has become easier. DL is currently poised to displace ML due to its growing popularity and effectiveness. In the past ten years, DL has attracted an unprecedented amount of attention for its potential to analyze and diagnose biomedical and healthcare issues. Here the basic idea of DL is discussed, wide range of algorithms of DL that are utilized to study and diagnose various diseases and fields related to medical health care. DL is used in the treatment and prediction of various critical and severe illnesses including the fatal diseases and in detecting the frauds that happen in medical fields. This chapter discusses that the collaboration of medical professionals with DL would bring more advanced and effective treatment for both curable and incurable diseases.

Chapter 5 aims to provide an empirical evaluation of different learning models for the classification of fall dataset. This chapter focuses on different classification algorithms and finding and comparing their accuracy in identifying the fall of an elderly person, with accuracy. Falls are considered a very dangerous health problem in public, especially for elderly people. It can be life-threatening for people in fall risk groups, meaning the people of elderly age. For this study, a dataset which is based on the falls of elderly people has been used. There are seven different values of the vitals given for an elderly person which are related to the functioning of heart and brain along with the activity they were performing at that time. With the help of this data the outcome of that activity is being categorized in a fall or no fall scenario. The threshold value of each parameter being used for this classification has been obtained after intensive study from various medical records and sites. The experiment studies different algorithms for finding the best one, and the results show that the Random Forest Model accurately classifies with 99.1% accuracy as compared to other models.

Chapter 6 reviews techniques like augmented/virtual reality in healthcare through IoT perspective. Today's consumer-augmented reality (C-AR) technologies are developed for a wide range of possible industries of use. Augmented Reality (AR) and Virtual Reality (VR) technologies are used to improve the integrated IoT healthcare system. There is a high need for such products that can enhance present clinical practice in IoT-enabled healthcare monitoring applications. With the development of technology, mobile devices have evolved into sensor-based wearable ones, and AR/VR has found increasing applications. AR/VR is used in medical disciplines such as telemedicine, neurological rehabilitation, surgical simulation, and education and training in medicine. This chapter involves related studies which present that AR/VR lessens the drawbacks of conventional medical care, cuts down on medical malpractice brought on by inexperienced operations, and minimizes the price of medical education and training. Additionally, the application has improved patient-doctor interaction, elevated the standard of diagnosis and treatment, and increased the effectiveness of medical education and training. This chapter provides a case study for the detection, treatment, and guidance for Alzheimer's patients based on their VR-based IoT-enabled environments. This chapter introduces VR applications in medical practice, IoT-enabled device monitoring with the goal of educating health professionals about these applications and piquing their interest in using technology to enhance medical care quality.

Chapter 7 analyzes different shooting methods to solve two-point boundary value problems in ODEs numerically and its related applications in medical science. Boundary value problems (BVPs) in ODEs arise in modeling many physical situations from microscale to mega scale. Such two-point BVPs are complex and often possess no analytical closed form solutions. So, one has to rely on approximating the actual solution numerically to a desired accuracy. To approximate the solution numerically, several numerical methods are available in the literature. In this chapter, numerical solutions are discussed for two-point BVPs that arise in higher-order ODEs using the shooting technique. To solve linear BVPs, the shooting technique is derived as an application of linear algebra. In one-dimensional case, Newton-Raphson iterates have rapid convergence. This is not the case in higher dimensions. Nevertheless, it is discussed as a class of BVPs for which the rate of convergence of the underlying Newton iterates is rapid. Explicit examples are highlighted to demonstrate implementation of the numerical scheme. Such BVPs arise in nonlinear dynamics of blood flow through arteries, where blood is a typical Casson fluid and the inner wall of the artery acts as a stretching sheet, which is important in view of hemodynamics in medical and health sciences.

Chapter 8 reviews the role of key management in healthcare using Internet of Medical Things (IoMT). The revolution of the healthcare sector through adoption of the IoMT provides significant benefits, including providing efficient and timely medical support by accurate continuous monitoring data. This chapter introduces an essential framework of IoMT monitoring system comprising a platform key management layer that establishes ad-hoc, point-to-point secure channels between devices within the IoMT system and a knowledge key management layer that provides keys for end-to-end encryption of patient data. In Health Insurance Portability and Accountability (HIPAA) Act, privacy and security regulations are crucial in protecting healthcare privacy. A versatile cryptographic key management solution must facilitate interoperation among the applied cryptographic mechanisms to follow regulations. IoMT, via wireless networks, watches patients' conditions and recovery progress anytime and anywhere, maintaining the security, privacy, honesty, and genuineness of patients' health records. Effective key management and circulation are obligatory to ensure IoMT in a wireless environment. An enhanced vital management scheme to spot the safety and privacy problems with patients' information through solid encryption management is essential for IoMT applications. This colossal joint effort supported by other technologies will exponentially improve the standard of medical research, leading to radical change within the healthcare model and offering key management in healthcare.

Chapter 9 deals with security issues related to COVID data using AI. AI application during the pandemic (COVID-19) is being explored in this chapter due to its beneficial aspects. AI is going to stay in the field of patient care and research. The legal and ethical issues include privacy and surveillance, bias, and discrimination. Currently, there are no well-defined regulations to address the legal and ethical issues that may arise due to the use of AI in healthcare. This chapter further focuses on the potential that AI has in augmenting provider performance and playing a key role, but like other disruptive technologies in the past, causing a significant impact should not be underestimated.

Chapter 10 presents a review on security issues and defense mechanism using IoMT. IoMT is an expeditiously expanding technology that holds the capacity to transform the healthcare sector by furnishing patients with more individualized and streamlined healthcare services through the implementation of connected devices, sensors, and other medical equipment. This chapter reviews the use of IoMT, as it brings significant security risks that must be addressed to protect patient privacy and safety. One of the major security concerns with IoMT is the vast amount of sensitive patient information generated and transmitted, which can be attractive targets for cybercriminals. In addition, the use of diverse devices, including personal technology integration, poses an additional challenge to implementing uniform security protocols across all systems. Defense mechanisms such as encryption techniques, access control measures, and network security protocols have been discussed to mitigate these risks. However, the effectiveness of these security measures depends on the security awareness of healthcare users, vendors, and novice IoMT adopters.

Chapter 11 discusses the threat modeling mechanism in healthcare. Healthcare sector in terms of data generation is way ahead of any other data generation systems. The data involved in this case belong to patient records, medical history of patients in the form of various test reports and the different parametric values contained by these records. Heavy storage is one of the requirements of this bulky data. After the storage part the remote communication among different end users regarding the exchange of this information is also a kind of challenge, as this data can be at risk while exchanging information by means of some unauthorized attack. To maintain and use this huge amount of data smoothly the risk analysis has to be performed. For the secure communication and storage a proactive approach of threat modeling is the requirement. In this chapter, the threat modeling issue related to healthcare data system has been addressed. The threat analysis technique SRTIDE is discussed in detail in this chapter. Different aspects of risk involved have been discussed along with the possible solution to each risk category.

Chapter 12 presents the use of blockchain technology for privacy and threat detection. Blockchain technology has emerged as a potential solution for privacy protection and threat detection in the digital world. This chapter outlines the use of blockchain technology for privacy and threat detection. It first discusses the blockchain-based privacy solutions, including their advantages, use cases, and limitations. This chapter moves forward by presenting the hybrid solutions that combine blockchain technology with other privacy and threat detection techniques. It also highlights the benefits and challenges of combining blockchain with other techniques. The inference abridges are the key points of the chapter and highlights the implications for the future of privacy and threat detection.

Chapter 13 outlines blockchain-based decentralized biometric authentication system for vulnerability analysis. In today's world, security is an essential factor in nearly all types of applications due to the increasing frequency of cyberattacks. While biometric authentication is considered one of the safest and most advanced authentication methods, traditional centralized systems still have security flaws that need to be addressed. However, the use of blockchain technology has shown potential for improving security and reducing vulnerabilities, thereby minimizing the risk of data breaches. This chapter proposes a decentralized biometric authentication method that uses blockchain technology to address security concerns. The system authenticates users using their biometric data, and this data is stored on a decentralized blockchain, which enhances security by preventing unauthorized access. Additionally, the system utilizes vulnerability analysis capabilities to detect and prevent attacks. By leveraging the power of blockchain technology, the proposed system ensures the confidentiality, integrity, and authentication (CIA Triad) of biometric data while offering improved security, privacy, and attack resistance. Overall, the proposed approach in this chapter enhances the security of biometric authentication, reduces the likelihood of data breaches, and provides a more robust solution for applications that require high-level security.

Chapter 14 highlights the bibliometric analysis for security issues related to cervical cancer research. The treatment and prevention of cervical cancer depend heavily on early detection, which is a severe public health concern. In this chapter, a bibliometric study is carried out to determine trends in cervical cancer research. The findings indicate an increase in publications, with the US and China leading in terms of scientific output and citation influence. However, data privacy and confidentiality are significant issues in cervical cancer research due to the collecting and analysis of sensitive health information about specific individuals. The privacy and confidentiality of study participants could be jeopardized by data breaches or unauthorized access to such information. The quality and accessibility of research data and infrastructure are at risk from cyberattacks like ransomware and phishing scams, which can also pose a serious threat to cervical cancer research. The data from this chapter can help researchers, decision-makers, and other stakeholders develop cervical cancer screening, diagnosis, and treatment. Future studies seek to use AI and biomarker identification for early detection and prevention.

About the Editors

Dr Neha Sharma is working as Assistant Professor in the Department of Computer Science and Engineering at Chitkara University Institute of Engineering & Technology, Chitkara University, Rajpura, Punjab, India. She has received the MTech (CSE) and PhD (Computer Science) degrees in the area of Computer Science with vast teaching experience of more than 12 years in a reputed organization. She has more than 25 international publications in the reputed peer-reviewed journals including IEEE Xplore, SCOPUS, and SCI indexed. Her main area of research is the image processing, machine learning, deep learning, and cyber security. She has also published several National & International Patents under the Intellectual Property Rights of Government of India & Abroad. She is actively associated with NAAC preparations at Universities interface. She is associated with many high impact society memberships like IEEE (Senior Member), ACM, ISTE (Life-time Member).

Dr. Durgesh Srivastava is an associate professor in the Department of Computer Science and Engineering at Chitkara University Institute of Engineering & Technology, Chitkara University, Rajpura, Punjab, India. He received his PhD degree in Computer Science & Engineering from IKG Punjab Technical University, Jalandhar, Punjab, India, in 2020. He received a B Tech degree in Information & Technology (IT) from MIET, Meerut, UP, in 2006 and an ME in Software Engineering from Birla Institute of Technology (BIT), Mesra, Ranchi, Jharkhand, India, in 2008. He has 14 years of teaching experience. His research interests include machine learning, soft computing, pattern recognition, software engineering, modeling, and design. He has authored several research papers/book in reputed international/national journals and conference/seminar.

Dr. Deepak Sinwar is an Associate Professor at the Department of IoT & Intelligent Systems, School of Computing and Intelligent Systems, Manipal University Jaipur, Jaipur, Rajasthan, India. He received his Ph.D and M.Tech degrees in Computer Science and Engineering in 2016 and 2010, respectively; and his B.Tech (with honors) in Information Technology in 2008. He is an enthusiastic and motivating academician with more than 13 years of teaching experience. His research interests include Meta-heuristics, Ad-hoc Networks, Data Mining, Reliability Engineering, Machine Learning, and Computer Vision. On his credit, he has published more than 50 articles in peer-reviewed journals, conference proceedings, and book chapters. He has been involved in many editorial activities like editing books/ special issues with publishers of repute like Taylor & Francis, SpringerNature, Wiley, IGI Global, etc. He has organized and attended various Conferences and Workshops during his teaching career. He is a life member of Indian Society for Technical Education (ISTE), senior member of IEEE and member of ACM professional society.

Contributors

M Bhagampriyal, Thiagarajar College of Engineering, Madurai, Tamil Nadu, India

Anupam Bonkra, Department of Computer Science and Engineering, Maharishi Markandeshwar (Deemed to be University), Mullana-Ambala, Haryana, India

Sunil Kumar Chawla, Chitkara University Institute of Engineering and Technology, Chitkara University, Rajpura, Punjab, India

Pummy Dhiman, Chitkara University Institute of Engineering and Technology, Chitkara University, Rajpura, Punjab, India

Rajan Kumar Dudeja, Chitkara University Institute of Engineering and Technology, Chitkara University, Rajpura, Punjab, India

Shubham Gargrish, Chitkara University Institute of Engineering and Technology, Chitkara University, Rajpura, Punjab, India

Rupali Gill, Chitkara University Institute of Engineering and Technology, Chitkara University, Rajpura, Punjab, India

D K Girija, Department of Computer Science, Government First Grade College, Madhugiri, Karnataka, India

Kirti Kangra, Department of Computer Science and Engineering

Guru Jambheshwar University of Science and Technology, Hisar, Haryana, India

Amandeep Kaur, Chitkara University Institute of Engineering and Technology, Chitkara University, Rajpura, Punjab, India

Rajwinder Kaur, Chitkara University Institute of Engineering and Technology, Chitkara University, Rajpura, Punjab, India

A Malini, Thiagarajar College of Engineering, Madurai, Tamil Nadu, India

Mamta, Chitkara University Institute of Engineering and Technology, Chitkara University, Rajpura, Punjab, India

Ramkrishna Mondal, Department of Hospital Administration, AIIMS Patna, India

Monika, Department of Fashion Communication, National Institute of Fashion Technology, Patna, India

Umamaheswari Rajasekaran, Thiagarajar College of Engineering, Madurai, Tamil Nadu, India

Manisha Rajput, Chitkara University Institute of Engineering and Technology, Chitkara University, Rajpura, Punjab, India

P Ramyavarshini, Thiagarajar College of Engineering, Madurai, Tamil Nadu, India

Divyanshu Ranjan, Chitkara University Institute of Engineering and Technology, Chitkara University, Rajpura, Punjab, India

Lekha Rani, Chitkara University Institute of Engineering and Technology, Chitkara University, Rajpura, Punjab, India

M Rashmi, Department of Computer Science, GFGC, Vijayanagar, Bengaluru, Karnataka, India

Pradeepta Kumar Sarangi, Chitkara University Institute of Engineering and Technology, Chitkara University, Himachal Pradesh, Punjab, India

Mohd Asif Shah, Dean of Faculty, Department of Economics, Kardan University, Parwane Du, Kabul, Afghanistan

Kriti Sharma, Chandigarh University, Gharuan, Punjab, India

Neha Sharma, Chitkara University Institute of Engineering and Technology, Chitkara University, Rajpura, Punjab, India

H K Shilpa, Faculty in Computer Science, Mandya University, Mandya, Karnataka, India

S Shrinivas, Thiagarajar College of Engineering, Madurai, Tamil Nadu, India

Gurpreet Singh, Chitkara University Institute of Engineering and Technology, Chitkara University, Rajpura, Punjab, India

Jaswinder Singh, Department of Computer Science and Engineering, Guru Jambheshwar University of Science and Technology, Hisar, Haryana, India

Jitender Singh, Department of Mathematics, Guru Nanak Dev University Amritsar, Punjab, India

Sakshi Sinha, Department of CPG Unit, TCS Hinjewadi, Pune, India

G K Sriram, Thiagarajar College of Engineering, Madurai, Tamil Nadu, India

P Sai Swetha, Thiagarajar College of Engineering, Madurai, Tamil Nadu, India

N Yogeesh, Department of Mathematics, Government First Grade College, Tumkur-572102, Karnataka, India

1 Artificial Intelligence in Healthcare
A Paradigm Shift

Kirti Kangra and Jaswinder Singh

1 INTRODUCTION

Artificial Intelligence (AI) is a branch of science and engineering concerned with computational understanding that is generally referred to as intelligent behavior, as well as the development of objects that exhibit this behavior. It is now a well-known field in computer science, as it has improved human life in a variety of ways. In several areas, it has recently outperformed humans, and this is the reason to believe that this trend will continue in healthcare too. It was meant to enhance the human capacity to provide healthcare and to mimic the diagnostic capabilities of doctors [1].

AI in healthcare can be increasingly rising availability of data, associate with the rapid growth of analytical methods in big data. It is incapable of "learning" aspects from very large volumes of healthcare data that are being used to gain information to be applied in clinical practice. It is incapable of enhancing its quality by using the input to understand and self-correct. It will harness the recent medical knowledge from the literature that will help to provide optimum patient treatment by assisting physicists. It will substantially help to minimize human detection and therapeutic errors. More precisely, a significant portion of the literature on AI examines data from electrodiagnosis, genetic testing, and diagnostic imaging at the diagnostic level. Earlier, Radiologists were encouraged to use AI technologies in the analysis of diagnostic images with extensive data knowledge [2].

The advancement of AI in the medical world will add clear and continuous monitoring of the patient's well-being to innovations linking the trained physician to the medical system. The processing of recorded biosignals, imaging, and diagnostic information can be consistent with AI expertise from millions of related observational cases that include indicative preventive actions, warnings about health status changes, and care predictions. This direct monitoring increases the risk detection of emergency incidents by monitoring the patient's health condition [3].

DOI: 10.1201/9781003377818-1

Testing should be performed regularly to lessen errors in AI, and to perform AI algorithms significantly from the actions of humans. The algorithms are simple if you set a target. They cannot modify themselves and can only understand exactly what has been instructed. It is hard to think about the healthcare future without understanding it entirely. Working on AI started in 1956, making important contributions to medical practice [4].

The key objective of this chapter is to provide an overview of how AI can help in the healthcare sector without the intervention of humans.

This chapter is subdivided into various sections. The beginning section is a precise introduction to AI and in the second section, different types of AI are discussed; the next section discusses some important works by researchers (see Table 1.1) in the domain of healthcare using AI algorithms. In the later sections, applications, benefits, and problems of AI in the healthcare sector have been discussed. In the last section, Healthcare 4.0 has been discussed.

1.1 EVOLUTION OF AI

To solve complex mathematical problems and build "thinking machines", the concept of AI was initiated in the 1950s. Later "John McCarthy, Alan Newell, Arthur Samuel, Herbert Simon, and Marvin Minsky" conceptualized the theory of AI. Although AI research has grown gradually over the past 60 years, early AI promoter assurances have proved overly optimistic. The "AI winter ended in the 1990s, as computational power and data storage" progressed to the point where complex tasks became feasible. AI made an important step in 1995 with the advancement of the "Artificial Linguistic Internet Computer Entity" by Richard Wallace which was able to hold basic conversations. IBM also created a machine called Deep Blue in the 1990s which used a brute force approach to play against Gary Kasparov, the world chess champion. In 2011, Apple gave a smart language-based assistant to their iPhone 4s i.e. Siri. The program understands and processes the language of nature and can thus serve as a personal assistant. Siri provides answers and executes commands that are spoken by the user, rather than entering via the keyboard. The user clicks the Home button or says "Hi, Siri" to wake it up. Siri operates according to previous "experiences". In 2014, another smart language-based assistant with Amazon's Alexa is welcomed into several people's kitchens, living rooms, and bedrooms. Contrary to a smartphone's language-based assistants, Alexa needs to be plugged into a socket and only responds when "Alexa" addresses. In 2017 the software "AlphaGO" created by Google, defeated the world's best "Go" player Ke Jie after winning the previous year against Lee Sedol. Since the "GO" game was far more complex than the chess game, it was considered impossible for a computer to master. Apart from the Deep Blue chess machine, which analyzes all movements to find the optimum, "AlphaGo" learns like a human being, the program was presented with the data of millions of movements by human players and played millions of games against themselves.

In the last decade, AI's influence has continued to grow rapidly. Eventually, Deep Learning is one of the most popular strategies to be explored today. Some of the most challenging issues in the fields of Machine Learning (ML), data science, and AI are generated by the ability to identify correlations and complex patterns far better than other approaches. There are several techniques developed to reduce human effort and increase efficiency.

1.2 Evolution of AI in Healthcare

In 1970, a physician interested in using computer science in medicine, William B Schwartz, issued a significant article in the New England Journal of Medicine titled "Medicine and the Computer: The promise and problems of change". In the article he argued, "Computing science will probably exert its major effects by augmenting and, in some cases, largely replacing the intellectual functions of the physician". Early attempts to implement AI in healthcare comprised developing "rules-based systems" that would support healthcare reasoning [5]. However, severe medical problems are much more challenging to deal with, with straightforward "rules-based" techniques to solve the problem. In 1976, the "Scottish surgeon Gunn" used statistical methods to medicate severe stomach disease [6]. This was obtained via computer-based clinical audits of structured case records, whereby diagnosis done this way was asserted to have about 10% more accuracy than the conventional route. By the 1980s, AI researchers were well recognized, particularly in US learning centers [7]. This innovation has helped to expand the use of the latest technological medical diagnostic techniques to AI. At this point, several AI medical applications are grounded on expert systems [8]. In the late 1990s, medicine AI studies began using new technologies such as ML and ANNs to support clinical decision-making. The next segment discusses the emerging use of AI in different sectors of healthcare. In India, the number of doctors is less compared with other countries because of its huge population. By using AI in healthcare, this problem will be overcome up to a certain limit. With the help of this technology, doctors work as consultants. It also reduces the cost of healthcare up to a point.

2 TYPES OF AI

There are two subfields of AI: ML and DL. AI, ML, and DL allow the organization of healthcare to evaluate an enormous quantity and data variety. They are slowly developing perspectives that contribute to constructive treatment, raising potential risks, and streamlining work processes. AI, ML, and DL allude to distinct intelligence aspects. An understanding of the interaction among these technologies is necessary [4].

2.1 Machine Learning

ML is the study of computing techniques that enhance outcomes by automatically acquiring information from the past [9]. Expert performance needs domain significant information and has formed several AI expert systems that are now used continuously in organizations. ML goals are to deliver growing stages of computerization in the software engineering process, switching much time-consuming human operation with automated strategies that enhance quality or productivity by finding and utilizing phenomena in training data [10]. The most important ML metric is how frequently they produce systems that are employed in a variety of fields, including business, education, and others. There are two types of ML techniques: "Inductive, and Deductive".

"Deductive learning" relies on current knowledge and evidence and discovers new information from the past one. Techniques of inductive ML construct computer programs by drawing principles and correlations from large data sets. Inductive learning considers cases and generalizes the idea of learning rather than beginning with specific knowledge, which is one major subset of inductive learning.

ML also coincides with statistics. Besides, several ML strategies have been discovered to construct computer programs by retrieving principles and correlations from large data sets to have exact counterparts with statistics ML methods. Some ML techniques are – NN, CART, Case-based reasoning, etc.

2.1.1 ML Algorithms

In this section, different algorithms used by researchers in their work will be discussed.

2.1.1.1 SVM

SVM is a supervised ML algorithm that categorizes data points by building a hyper-plane that can distinguish them. To identify the best hyper-plane, it is necessary to maximize margins. SVM has the advantage of being able to separate data points in both linear and nonlinear ways using different kernels. It works well with data with a lot of dimensions. SVM classifier's potential can be utilized using different kernels namely "linear, RBF, and polynomial" [11].

2.1.1.2 ANN

The acronym "ANN" refers to a parallel architecture that is modeled after biological neural processing. MLP is the most popular ANN architecture [12], even though there are many others. There are three layers in the ANN architecture: "Input layer, Hidden layer, and Output layer". The output of one layer is passed to the next layer, i.e., the input layer passes its outcome to the hidden layer, which then passes it to the output layer. After that, the user will get the result.

2.1.1.3 NB

It is based on the Bayes theorem, which uses the "probability of occurrence, class prior probability, and predictor prior probability to calculate the posterior probability" [13]. It uses a similar method to predict the likelihood of several classes based on a variety of factors. Text classification and multi-class classification problems are solved using this algorithm.

2.1.1.4 DT

As it resembles the human decision-making process, DT is simple to comprehend. It can solve issues using both discrete and continuous data input. It consists of root nodes, branches, and leaf nodes. Every internal node performs an attribute test, the result of which is displayed on the branch, and the class label is displayed on the leaf node as a result [14].

2.1.1.5 RF

RF is a cluster of unpruned classification or regression trees that result from a random sampling of training data. Random features are picked during the induction phase. To make predictions, the ensemble's predictions are compiled by majority voting for classification or average for regression [15]. By cross-validation accuracy can be increased. It can handle missing values very efficiently and maintain accuracy for the data used.

2.1.1.6 LR

LR, one of the most important statistical and ML approaches, is used by "statisticians and researchers to analyze, classify binary and proportional response data sets". LR has several key recompenses, including the ability to provide probabilities naturally and the ability to handle multi-class classification issues [16].

2.1.1.7 K-NN

K-NN algorithm compares unknown instances with training instances in the feature space. It classifies the dataset based on the value of K, unlike other methods, developing a model does not require a learning process. The main concern is deciding on the K value. If K is minimal then outliers can dominate, it is computationally expensive if K is high [17].

2.2 DEEP LEARNING

DL approaches have generated a lot of exuberance in the research community in fixing numerous complicated tasks by observing the unprocessed sensor data. It started using back in 1971 [18]. DL is a subclass of the modern approach to ML that has been of immense global significance over the past few years. To evaluate input without interruption, automated engineering uses representation learning techniques for different levels of the procession, thus identifying the complex structures in high-dimensional data by projection onto a lower-dimensional manifold. Compared to classical techniques, DL has been shown to achieve substantially higher error margins in many areas, including NLP, computer vision, and voice recognition [19]. DL was primarily practical for healthcare imaging studies in drugs and healthcare. DL systems displayed excellent diagnostic efficiency in the detection of various medical diseases, including T.B., chest X-rays, skin images of malignant melanoma, and secondary lymph node metastases from portions of breast cancer tissue. Similarly, DL especially fundus images and OCT were applied to ocular imaging. DL approaches have been used for severe ophthalmic diseases, such as DR, glaucoma, AMD, and ROP. DL has also been used to assess cardiovascular refractive error and health conditions.

3 LITERATURE REVIEW

Table 1.1 specifically discusses recent research in AI in the healthcare sector:

AI is generally used in many fields; healthcare is one of them. By studying some research paper that provides important information regarding how AI is helping in healthcare. Inference concluded from the above literature survey that a lot more work can be done in the field of AI related to healthcare. AI provides much help in the healthcare sector, and a number of techniques are thereby used which can diagnose the disease early. There are several techniques in AI and each technique can be used to diagnose the disease.

4 BENEFITS OF AI IN HEALTHCARE SECTOR

Healthcare is one important field where AI adoption is accelerating and the effects are profound. AI is a self-sustaining growth engine for the healthcare industry.

a. Prognosis & Diagnosis

AI techniques will operate in the most effective way to diagnose and treatment of the disease. AI plays a vital role in the timely and accurate diagnosis of serious diseases that are primarily dependent on the timely identification of symptoms for their diagnosis and treatment. Human beings usually make mistakes when examining images and samples and trying to make appropriate decisions but AI techniques can study and examine hundreds of thousands of samples in rapid succession and disclose valuable trends rapidly [41].

b. Error-prone

AI has the power to cut down on medical errors dramatically. Without hesitation, AI is the best way for hospitals and medical facilities to reduce medical mistakes and make healthcare safer and effective. With the introduction of AI assistants, a substantial part of the clinical and ambulatory facilities of the specialist can be handled by and assigned to these AI assistants, thereby offering the doctors more time to deal more effectively with severe patients and thus lowering the possibility of medical failures. AI assistants are often less likely to make errors than human doctors [42].

c. Health Care using gadgets

All users now have access to gadgets with sensors capable of gathering valuable health information. An increasing proportion of health-related data is collected on the go from smartphones with activity trackers in smart devices that can detect a pulse all around the clock. Accumulating and examining this data, and combining it with the information given by

TABLE 1.1

Recent Contribution of Researchers

Author Name [Ref.no], Year	Title of Paper	Findings	Results
Chang et al., [20] 2022	"An artificial intelligence model for heart disease detection using machine learning algorithms"	• Focuses on applying ML techniques to design to detect cardiac problem. • LR and RF classifiers were used	Accuracy – 83%.
Manimurugan et al., [21] 2022	"Two-Stage Classification Model for the Prediction of Heart Disease Using IoMT and Artificial Intelligence"	• Focuses on predicting cardiac disease. • Hybrid Faster R-CNN with SE-ResNet-101 model was used to classify • Hybrid linear discriminant analysis with modified ant lion optimization was used for classification of echocardiogram images	Precision – 98.06%, Recall – 98.95%, Specificity – 96.32%, F-score – 99.02%, Accuracy – 99.15%.
Kishor & Chakraborty [22] 2022	"Artificial Intelligence and Internet of Things Based Healthcare 4.0 Monitoring System"	• Suggest ML based healthcare model for early prediction of diseases. • Nine fatal diseases were selected. • DT, SVM, adaptive boosting, NB, RF, ANN, and K-NN • RF classifier works better	Accuracy – 97.62%, Sensitivity – 99.67%, specificity – 97.81%, AUC – 99.32%.
Arroyo & Delima, [23] 2022	"An Optimized Neural Network Using Genetic Algorithm for Cardiovascular Disease Prediction"	• Proposed an optimization system to predict heart disease • ANN and Genetic Algorithm were used	Accuracy – 73.43%
Lu et al., [24] 2022	"A patient network-based machine learning model for disease prediction: The case of type 2 diabetes mellitus"	• Discussed Type 2 Diabetes disease • Eigen vector centrality and Closeness centrality of the network, and patient age, were the most crucial parameters for the model	AUC values ranged from 0.79 to 0.91 for the suggested framework using ML classifiers

(Continued)

TABLE 1.1
(Continued)

Author Name [Ref.no], Year	Title of Paper	Findings	Results
Neha Sharma et al., [25] et al 2022	"Optimized multimedia data through computationally intelligent algorithms"	• Proposes a method for image steganography • Firefly optimization algorithm and ant colony optimization algorithm with Huffman encoding were used	Achieves the PSNR of 68.06 dB and the embedding capacity of 985,682 bits.
Nagaraj M. Lutimath, Neha Sharma, Byregowda B K [26] 2021	"Prediction of Heart Disease using Biomedical Data through Machine Learning Techniques"	• Proposed technique for diagnosing heart disease • RF classifier was selected • Performance measured by MAE, RMSE and MSE	Random forest regression model provides better accuracy than decision tree regression model
PARLAR, [27] 2021	"A heuristic approach with artificial neural network for Parkinson's disease"	• Proposed an optimization technique for diagnosing Parkinson's disease • Wolf Search Algorithm with the ANN model • Feature selection methods Information Gain (IG), ReliefF, and WSA were used. • ANN classifier presented the most accurate classification results	F-1 score – 92.5%
Pramanik et al., [28] 2021	"Machine learning methods with decision forests for parkinson's detection"	• Discussed Parkinson's detection method that consists of incremental decision trees and training instances • Systematically Developed Forest, Decision Forest and RF were used	Decision Trees detect highest accuracy of 94.12% to 95.00%.

(Continued)

TABLE 1.1
(Continued)

Author Name [Ref.no], Year	Title of Paper	Findings	Results
Prasath et al., [29] 2021	"A comparative and comprehensive study of prediction of Parkinson's disease"	• Discussed various ML techniques for the prediction of Parkinson's disease	
U. J. Khan et al., [30] 2021	"Hybrid Classfication for Heart Disease Prediction using Artificial Intelligence"	• Focuses on predicting cardiac disease. • RF and DT-based hybrid system	Accuracy – 94.4%.
Akgül et al., [31] (2020)	"Diagnosis of heart disease using an intelligent method: A hybrid ANN – GA approach"	• Focuses on predicting cardiac disease. • Hybrid ANN-GA, ANN with default parameters, C4.5, KNN, and NB.	Accuracy – 95.82%
J. Rahman et al.,[32] (2020)	"Classification and prediction of diabetes disease using machine learning paradigm"	• Focuses on predicting diabetic disease • LR used for feature selection and RF for classification	Accuracy – 94.25%
Tripathi & Kumar, [33] 2020	"Early Prediction of Diabetes Mellitus Using Machine Learning"	• Focuses on predicting diabetic disease • linear discriminant analysis (LDA), KNN, SVM, and RF were used for classification • RF exceeds other classification algorithms	Accuracy – 87.66%.
Revathy et al., [34] 2020	"Chronic Kidney Disease Prediction using Machine Learning Models"	• Suggested prediction system for the early identification of CKD • ML models such as DT, RF, and SVM were used to diagnose CKD • RF Classifier works better	Accuracy – 99.16%

(Continued)

**TABLE 1.1
(Continued)**

Author Name [Ref.no], Year	Title of Paper	Findings	Results
B. Khan et al., [35] 2020	"Improving Heart Disease Prediction Using Feature Selection Approaches"	• Focuses on cardiac disease. • NB, LR, MLP, J48, SVM, NBTree, and Composite Hypercube on Iterated Random Projection were used for classification • CHIRP attained the highest accuracy level	Accuracy – 99.75%
Rodríguez-ruiz et al., [36] 2019	"Detection of Breast Cancer with Mammography : Effect of an Artificial Intelligence Support System"	• Used an AI support program to detect breast cancer • NN was used for classification	
Al-mufti et al., [37] 2019	"Artificial Intelligence in Neurocritical Care"	• Used AI to neurocritical treatment • Model-based method and Data driven method	
Dankwa-mullan & Rivo, [38] 2019	"Transforming Diabetes Care Through Artificial Intelligence"	• Focuses on predicting diabetic disease	
Nasser & Abu-naser, [39] 2019	"Lung Cancer Detection Using Artificial Neural Network"	• Focuses on predicting Lung Cancer • ANN was used for classification	
Watanabe et al., [40] 2019	"Improved Cancer Detection Using Artificial Intelligence : a Retrospective Evaluation of Missed Cancers on Mammography"	• Focuses on predicting breast cancer	7.2% escalation in the AUC curve shown by the suggested approach

patients through applications and other home monitoring tools, may provide different views on person and community health. Wearable fitness trackers such as those from "FitBit, Apple, Garmin" and others – track heart rate and fitness level. They can send user warnings to get an extra workout and can share this information with doctors (and with AI systems) for further analysis of patients' requirements and routines.

5 APPLICATIONS OF AI IN HEALTHCARE

This section of the chapter explains the applications of AI in the healthcare sector.

a. Health virtual assistant helps in observing and monitoring patients and healthcare providers.

b. Customer facility and medicine apps are the emerging sectors in AI that will be adopted as part of what medical professionals are offering soon. AI application with the help of which patients can communicate via a dialog window on a website or over the phone to get help with their issues.

c. The much-admired technique of AI is a medical Decision Support System (DSS). This expert system primarily focuses on detecting the state of a patient by providing demographic data and its symptoms. It suggests antibiotics to treat patients who are infected. This method (DSS) uses the Bayesian network to diagnose different types of cancer and unpredicted cardiac diseases.

d. Fuzzy Logic is a procedure that is used for data processing purposes that lets ambiguity, especially in the healthcare sector. This method is used in many sectors of medicine such as "multiple logistic regression analysis and also used for the diagnosis of many diseases like lung cancer, acute leukemia, breast, and pancreatic cancer". It could also determine the survival of breast cancer sufferers.

e. AI enables to analyze anomalies in "X-rays and MRIs, in genomics" to conduct difficult analyses and in precise medication to treat specific patients and build highly personalized treatments.

6 PROBLEMS USING AI IN HEALTHCARE

The main problems using AI in healthcare are [43]:

a. Lack of specific architecture at enterprises: The dilemma is for companies to use various compute motors to obtain multiple storage choices. Big companies prefer to store commonly used data such as "consumer, financial, supply chain, product", and the like in high-performance, high-speed I/O environments, whereas less commonly used big data sets including "sensor readings, web, and rich media" are stored in inexpensive cloud object storage.

b. Privacy and information safety: By using AI there is an issue of information protection in healthcare. Data from history is used to train the AI system, and steps should be taken to prevent such data from reaching third persons. There should also be effective security against cyber-attacks, as it is a significant problem in any sector, but it's becoming critical in healthcare because the sector is directly linked to people's lives, and cyber-attacks can directly lead to death [44].

c. Training is required not just for the systems which are based on AI but also for physicians to improve precise, safe, and reliable AI solutions as information experts. By using AI, doctors become confident and not be confronted with the confusion of the risks involved with medical technology advances. Doctors should know, design, implement, and optimize AI for better clinical care [3].

d. Gender Biasedness: Both the internet users and mobile internet customers in India are projected to rise – to 420 million and 300 million respectively in 2017 "(IAMAI and Kantar IMRB 2017)". Mobiles are the primary Internet access point, especially in rural India, where mobile phones account for 60% of internet access. Females in South Asia are 38% less likely than men to own a cell phone; combined with masculine and misogynistic social expectations means that the actual rate of access may be much lower. A second concern is that gender ratios are being seriously distorted at all rates in India's tech industry. Therefore a real risk that the AI in which whole humanity will experience strong male bias.

7   HEALTHCARE 4.0

The healthcare sector is dealing with a number of issues, such as growing expenses for healthcare services, healthcare experts, a lack of qualified healthcare workers, growing requirement for high-quality healthcare services, the necessity of cooperation between healthcare providers and related businesses and organizations, and a fierce competition between healthcare providers [45]. Due to these difficulties, healthcare professionals are being compelled to think about adopting and using novel healthcare models that make use of cutting-edge "Information and communication technology (ICT)". The industry sector, which is already attempting to benefit from ICT advancements, is kicking off the Industry 4.0 era with the help of innovations like the Internet of Things (IoT), cyber-physical systems (CPS), and analytics [46]. The continuous development of the industrial revolutions is the foundation for the 4.0. "Industry 1.0 (manual machining), Industry 2.0 (powered machining), Industry 3.0 (computerized machining), and now Industry 4.0", which ushers in the age of autonomous and intelligent industrial activities, have all come before. Industry 4.0 uses optimization, industrial automation, and the utilization of digital applications to optimize operations, save charges, and boost productivity.

Healthcare is a significant industry that stands to gain from adopting Industry 4.0 principles. "Healthcare Industry 4.0, Healthcare 4.0, or Health 4.0" terms used were formed by applying Industry 4.0 principles to the healthcare sector [47]. The 4.0 in Health 4.0 was carried over from Industry 4.0, and does not denote the presence of Health 3.0, 2.0, or 1.0 because healthcare systems developed independently of industrial systems. Implementing interconnected healthcare infrastructures with real-time, distributed, and virtualized healthcare services for patients, specialists, and both formal and informal healthcare facility providers is known as "health 4.0". As one alternative for improvement, it focuses on fostering, facilitating, and optimizing coordination, consistency, and integration to shift healthcare services from being founded on "empirical data" to "precision medicine". This is consistent with the worldwide transition from a professional-oriented, hospital-based model to a dispersed, patient-centered model. Alternative direction includes expediting convergence, coordination, and optimal use of healthcare service assets, and specialists, for smoother operations and at lesser expenses. Health 4.0 can be expanded significantly to improve every component of the healthcare system and its value chain. Healthcare expenditure is expected to exceed $18.28 trillion globally in 2040 [48], necessitating the use of Industry 4.0 principles and technology [49] to increase effectiveness and efficiency everywhere.

7.1 HEALTH 4.0 AND ITS TECHNOLOGIES

The establishment of public health and disease management information websites, on the Internet, signified the initiation of the growth of ICT use in healthcare. This was preceded by the occurrence of electronic health records (EHR) and cloud-based and mobile-based internet applications. The rise of Health 4.0, which combines all these techniques with real-time information gathering, growing usage of AI, and advanced statistical solutions made possible by engaging digital interfaces, is something we are currently witnessing. The basic concept of Health 4.0 is that healthcare providers are building an intelligent health network along the overall healthcare value chain by integrating patients, private medical equipment, hospitals, clinics, pharmaceutical and medical suppliers, and other healthcare-related elements. This digital health network transforms the ways that healthcare services are delivered and makes it possible for improved and highly efficient communication throughout the whole healthcare value chain. Medical CPS, the Internet of Health Things, health clouds, health fogs, big data analytics, ML, blockchain, and intelligent algorithms are all combined to make healthcare sector more effective.

7.2 HEALTH 4.0 SIX DESIGN PRINCIPLES

The six principles of Health 4.0 are discussed below [50]:

a. Interoperability: potential to integrate various healthcare systems and gadgets.
b. Virtualization: potential to duplicate various healthcare systems, tools, and procedures digitally or virtually;
c. Decentralization: competence of health systems to make intelligent judgments and maintain self-control.
d. Real-time ability: potential to proactively collect and examine health data to conduct the appropriate action.
e. Service Oriented: the capability to design software services that communicate with healthcare systems and equipment.

f. Modularity: potential to modify components to satisfy new specifications and reuse existing components to create brand-new healthcare systems.

7.3 HEALTH 4.0 OBJECTIVES

Two key goals will be accomplished with the support of Health 4.0 capabilities: (1) high-quality healthcare offerings; and (2) enhanced productivity and performance, by keeping an eye on expenses and equipment consumption. These goals are established and organized based on the requirement of the healthcare sector. Health 4.0 offers a range of expertise, including fine-grained information acquisition and management, better connections and cooperation opportunities throughout diverse healthcare services, equipment, client records, and medical practitioners, better data analysis, enhanced automation deployment, and increased healthcare system quality. If all these tools are used wisely, they can help with both goals [51].

1. Offering high-quality medical care to patients requires boosting the overall system efficiency and quality, prioritizing the consumption of resources, and utilizing the equipment to strengthen the perspectives of both the healthcare providers and the patients. To accomplish this goal, some examples of potential change areas are as follows:

    a. Enhancing patient services such as setting up meetings, treatment regimens, continuous monitoring, and communications with medical staff. This will enhance patient happiness and lead to a positive experience.

    b. With a more thorough examination of present and past operations and requirements, better distribution of resources and schedules for the healthcare industry. This will permit more efficient use of resources and staff resulting in increased personnel contentment and improved patients' interactions.

    c. Using automated technology, intelligent monitoring, and decision-making services to improve the effectiveness and precision of patient care. As a result, it will be feasible to expedite many of the services offered, minimize the dependence on humans for menial or repetitive work, and lessen the likelihood of errors having a detrimental impact on the patients.

    d. Care providers can develop more individualized treatments and healthcare plans for each patient by using thorough and accurate patient health information and maintaining additional aspects that may be impacting their health.

    e. Analyzing past and current information accumulated from tools and resources to set "proactive maintenance schedules, perform preventive maintenance", and have improved estimates of future requirements. Thus, minimizing service problems and being ready to modify speedily according to patients' requirements.

2. Increasing the efficacy and efficiency of operations and resource use for healthcare services is another goal of Health 4.0. To attain this goal, some examples are as follows:

   a. Applying continuous tracking and measurements to enable predictive maintenance, which lowers the cost of maintenance, increases equipment operational efficiency, and lowers the number of malfunctions leading to unplanned repairs.

   b. Giving patients the chance to review their whole medical history over an extended duration of time to enhance diagnoses, lessen the need for unnecessary testing and laboratory work, and boost medication usage.

   c. Developing the capability to compile data on infectious diseases from huge patient database. This will make it possible to properly anticipate the resources that will be required to address the issue and determine infection trends and hotspots. This will facilitate directing the required resources as quickly as possible to the most damaged regions. Also, it might point to more effective methods for reducing the transmission of infections and lower infection rates, which would ease the burden on medical resources.

   d. To provide a base for analytics using patient information gathered, allowing for a better knowledge of common diseases. This will enhance diagnosis and offer additional information about the connections between diseases and a patient's past health history, lifestyle, and culture. As a result, procedures for disorders will be improved, resources will be allocated more effectively, and projections of the medications required will be made.

   e. Enabling the use of CPS-supported medical equipment and intelligent decision-making software would help automate numerous operations and lower the demand for staff. The end outcome will be lower overall expenses and more effective operations with decreased error probabilities.

7.4   HEALTH 4.0 APPLICATIONS

Several healthcare applications have successfully leveraged cutting-edge ICT to accomplish particular objectives. There are also numerous initiatives to apply Health 4.0 ideas to enhance some of these applications. Understanding the abilities and resources provided by Health 4.0 is essential for designing and deploying apps within the larger context.

   a. Patient Management: Patients can use a number of applications to discover qualified healthcare providers, book consultations, check-ins, complete medical paperwork, claim for insurance coverage, order drugs, and access data on self-care and welfare. These programs, as well as many more with related features, can be merged into a single system under Health 4.0. Patients will enter the system, specify their requirements, and the system will automatically guide them through every stage and smoothly transfer the pertinent data from their patient history among the many parties involved, such as doctors, nurses, laboratories, and pharmacies. This can be developed further by incorporating more elements and systems that can enable these abilities [52].

b. Personalized Healthcare: Healthcare practitioners may make more accurate evaluations and offer extremely precise solutions for each instance by merging data gathered in all areas by using cutting-edge analysis and visualization tools. For instance, two people with cardiac disease who also have various other medical illnesses lead different lifestyles and possibly have various genetic predispositions to certain diseases. Although each person with cardiovascular disease may require the same medication, they most likely need a distinct overall treatment strategy to account for their variances. This accumulated knowledge may also lessen the potentially bad effects of various medicines and enable dynamic therapy adjustments depending on wider changes. It may also lead to greater insights into which drugs will work best for each patient.

c. Management: Using state-of-the-art data integration, analysis, and visualization tools, healthcare professionals may provide more precise assessments and solutions for each situation. Consider two individuals with cardiovascular disease who also have a number of other illnesses or disorders, maintain diverse lifestyles, and maybe have a variety of genetic predispositions to particular diseases. Even though every patient with cardiovascular disease may require the same treatment, they almost certainly require a different overall treatment plan to take into account their differences.

d. Scheduling: Scheduling the professional healthcare staff, such as doctors, surgeons, nurses, and therapists, involves many aspects that make it extremely hard to arrive at an ideal timetable, with the possible exception of routine workers like clerks, custodians, and administration. Applications for Health 4.0 can be created that can gather information about the staff, equipment, requirement levels, and even data. They can then employ sophisticated scheduling algorithms to generate efficient schedules, make backup plans, and take emergency situations into account. This strategy will assist in providing better timetables, more consistent demands, better work for the professionals, and an improved work environment.

e. Remote Access: Numerous healthcare facilities are tiny in size and lack several pieces of pricey or sophisticated devices. Also, certain instruments and skills are specialized for certain facilities. The applicant will benefit greatly and get greater usage out of the device if there is a simple and safe way to access and use it. Clinics, for instance, might have high-tech, pricey tools for evaluating MRI results. It is also possible to design a business model to specify usage terms, charges, rules, and management practices. Health 4.0 integration can support such remote connection, tracking, and costing tools. Using cutting-edge techniques like blockchain can also be helpful because it offers means to log all transactions, encrypt the data, and negotiate usage agreements remotely.

f. Telemedicine in Real-Time: Real-time telehealth, also referred to as "synchronous telehealth", involves two-way, live video interactions between a physician and a client. It can partially substitute for face-to-face physician-client encounters.

8 COMPARING TRADITION HEALTHCARE WITH AI IN HEALTHCARE

In traditional healthcare system, there are lots of problems regarding analysis, detection, maintenance, and cost but by shifting on to automated healthcare system these problems are tackled in an efficient manner. Manual processing of records makes errors, but by using an AI analysis system, these errors can be reduced. Detection of disease using AI becomes easy and more accurate, but by using traditional detection methods, the chances of errors increase which results in cost increase; moreover, it is time-consuming and requires more efforts. Keeping records related to patients requires more efforts in traditional methods when compared to AI systems.

9 CONCLUSION

AI is a rapidly growing science that has applications in different sectors, as well as the basis for medicinal services. Studies show that AI is a dynamically evolving healthcare sector. Different AI techniques are used for making effective choices that will increase the achievement of healthcare institutes and the health of the patients. This study covers different aspects of AI. It has two subfields, namely ML and DL. In this chapter, different ML techniques like SVM, NB, ANN, DT, RF, K-NN, and LR are covered. The literature covered in this chapter has discussed research related to AI, ML, and DL. It also emphasizes the applications, advantages, and difficulties associated with implementation. All these covered aspects are centered around healthcare. But healthcare still faces lots of problems i.e. maintenance of data, Data analysis, and storage of data. Data collected from different technologies i.e. IoT, different healthcare applications, hospitals, clinics, etc. To analyze such huge data there is a need for more strong technology i.e. Healthcare 4.0. Healthcare 4.0 works on the principles of industry 4.0. Industry 4.0 uses optimization, industrial automation, and the utilization of digital applications to optimize operations, save charges, and boost productivity. This gives the origin of Healthcare 4.0. Healthcare 4.0 improves the patient experience and successfully raises the standard of treatment while also increasing efficiency, consistency, and cost-effectiveness. Medical CPS, the Internet of Health Things, health clouds, health fogs, big data analytics, ML, blockchain, and intelligent algorithms are all combined and utilized. This chapter will help the researcher to understand Healthcare 4.0, its principles, objectives, and applications.

REFERENCES

[1] A. Meiliana, "Artificial Intelligent in Healthcare," no. September 2019, doi:10.18585/inabj.v11i2.844.

[2] E. Trivizakis and A. Kouroubali, "The Vision of Integrating Artificial Intelligence in Health-Care The Vision of Integrating Artificial Intelligence in Health-Care," no. February 2020, pp. 11–12, 2019, doi:10.13140/RG.2.2.15304.67848.

[3] S. Kalyanakrishnan, R. A. Panicker, S. Natarajan, and S. Rao, "Opportunities and Challenges for Artificial Intelligence in India," In *Proceedings of the 2018 AAAI/ACM conference on AI, Ethics, and Society*, 2018 pp. 164–170,.

[4] Z. Sharma, P. Vepanattu, and A. Chauhan, "The Impact of Artificial Intelligence on Healthcare," *Indian J Public Health Res Dev.*, vol. 10, no. 8, 2019.

[5] O. Access, "We are IntechOpen, the World ' s Leading Publisher of Open Access Books Built by Scientists, for Scientists TOP 1%."

[6] A. N. Ramesh, C. Kambhampati, J. R. T. Monson, and P. J. Drew, "Artificial Intelligence in Medicine," *Ann. R. Coll. Surg. Engl.*, vol. 86, no. 5, pp. 334–338, 2004, doi:10.1308/147870804290.

[7] J. N. Kok, E. J. W. Boers, W. A. Kosters, P. Van Der Putten, and M. Poel, "Knowledge for Sustainable Development: An Insight into the Encyclopedia of Life Support Systems: Artificial Intelligence: Definition, Trends, Techniques and Cases," *Encycl. Life Support Syst.*, pp. 1096–1097, 2010, [Online]. Available: https://www.eolss.net/Sample-Chapters/C15/E6-44.pdf.

[8] J. Scott and R. Scott, "Artificial Intelligence: Its Use in Medical Diagnosis," *J. Nucl. Med.*, vol. 34, no. 3, pp. 510–514, 1993.

[9] D. Shu *et al.*, "Artificial Intelligence and Deep Learning in Ophthalmology," pp. 167–175, 2019, doi:10.1136/bjophthalmol-2018–313173.

[10] Y. Singh, P. K. Bhatia, and O. Sangwan, "A Review of Studies on Machine Learning Techniques," *IJCSS*, vol. 1, no. 1, pp. 70–84.

[11] J. Goyal, P. Khandnor, and T. C. Aseri, "A Comparative Analysis of Machine Learning Classifiers for Dysphonia-based Classification of Parkinson's Disease," *Int. J. Data Sci. Anal.*, vol. 11, no. 1, pp. 69–83, 2021, doi:10.1007/s41060-020-00234-0.

[12] S. Bashir, Z. S. Khan, F. H. Khan, A. Anjum, and K. Bashir, "Improving Heart Disease Prediction Using Feature Selection Approaches," *2019 16th Int. Bhurban Conf. Appl. Sci. Technol.*, pp. 619–623, 2019, doi:10.1109/IBCAST.2019.8667106.

[13] A. H. Gonsalves, "Prediction of Coronary Heart Disease using Machine Learning : An Experimental Analysis," in *ACM International Conference Proceeding Series (2019)*, 2019, pp. 51–56.

[14] H. H. Patel and P. Prajapati, "Study and Analysis of Decision Tree Based Classification Algorithms," *Int. J. Comput. Sci. Eng.*, vol. 6, no. 10, pp. 74–78, 2018, doi:10.26438/ijcse/v6i10.7478.

[15] J. Ali, R. Khan, N. Ahmad, and I. Maqsood, "Random Forests and Decision Trees," *Int. J. Comput. Sci.*, vol. 9, no. December 2013, pp. 272–278, 2012.

[16] M. Maalouf, "Logistic Regression in Data Analysis: An Overview Logistic Regression in Data Analysis : An Overview Maher Maalouf*," *Int. J. Data Anal. Tech. Strateg.*, no. July 2011, 2015, doi:10.1504/IJDATS.2011.041335.

[17] S. Meesri, S. Phimoltares, and A. Mahaweerawat, "Diagnosis of Heart Disease Using a Mixed Classifier," *ICSEC 2017–21st Int. Comput. Sci. Eng. Conf. 2017, Proceeding*, vol. 6, pp. 118–123, 2018, doi:10.1109/ICSEC.2017.8443940.

[18] G. V. K. S. Abhinav, "Artificial Intelligence in Healthcare," no. October, pp. 7–10, 2019, doi:10.22270/jddt.v9i5-s.3634.

[19] A. Carrio, C. Sampedro, A. Rodriguez-ramos, and P. Campoy, "A Review of Deep Learning Methods and Applications for Unmanned Aerial Vehicles," *J. Sens.*, vol. 2017, 2017.

[20] V. Chang, V. R. Bhavani, A. Q. Xu, and M. Hossain, "An Artificial Intelligence Model for Heart Disease Detection Using Machine Learning Algorithms," *Healthc. Anal.*, vol. 2, no. January, p. 100016, 2022, doi:10.1016/j.health.2022.100016.

[21] S. Manimurugan *et al.*, "Two-stage Classification Model for the Prediction of Heart Disease Using IoMT and Artificial Intelligence," *Sensors*, vol. 22, no. 2, 2022, doi:10.3390/s22020476.

[22] A. Kishor and C. Chakraborty, "Artificial Intelligence and Internet of Things Based Healthcare 4.0 Monitoring System," *Wirel. Pers. Commun.*, vol. 127, no. 2, pp. 1615–1631, 2022, doi:10.1007/s11277-021-08708-5.

[23] J. C. T. Arroyo and A. J. P. Delima, "An Optimized Neural Network Using Genetic Algorithm for Cardiovascular Disease Prediction," *J. Adv. Inf. Technol.*, vol. 13, no. 1, pp. 95–99, 2022, doi:10.12720/jait.13.1.95–99.

[24] H. Lu, S. Uddin, F. Hajati, M. A. Moni, and M. Khushi, "A Patient Network-based Machine Learning Model for Disease Prediction: The Case of Type 2 Diabetes Mellitus," *Appl. Intell.*, vol. 52, no. 3, pp. 2411–2422, 2022, doi:10.1007/s10489-021-02533-w.

[25] N. M. Lutimath, N. Sharma, and B. K. Byregowda, "Prediction of Heart Disease using Biomedical Data through Machine Learning Techniques," *EAI Endorsed Trans. Pervasive Heal. Technol.*, vol. 7, no. 29, pp. 1–6, 2021, doi:10.4108/eai.30–8-2021.170881.

[26] N. Sharma, C. Chakraborty, and R. Kumar, "Optimized Multimedia Data through Computationally Intelligent Algorithms," *Multimed. Syst.*, no. 0123456789, 2022, doi:10.1007/s00530-022-00918-6.

[27] T. Parlar, "A Heuristic Approach with Artificial Neural Network for Parkinson's Disease," *Int. J. Appl. Math. Electron. Comput.*, vol. 9, no. 1, pp. 1–6, 2021, doi:10.18100/ijamec.802599.

[28] M. Pramanik, R. Pradhan, P. Nandy, A. K. Bhoi, and P. Barsocchi, "Machine Learning Methods with Decision Forests for Parkinson's Detection," *Appl. Sci.*, vol. 11, no. 2, pp. 1–25, 2021, doi:10.3390/app11020581.

[29] N. Prasath, V. Pandi, S. Manickavasagam, and P. Ramadoss, "A Comparative and Comprehensive Study of Prediction of Parkinson's Disease," *Indones. J. Electr. Eng. Comput. Sci.*, vol. 23, no. 3, pp. 1748–1760, 2021, doi:10.11591/ijeecs.v23.i3.pp1748–1760.

[30] U. J. Khan, A. Oberoi, and J. Gill, "Hybrid Classfication for Heart Disease Prediction Using Artificial Intelligence," *Proc. -5th Int. Conf. Comput. Methodol. Commun. ICCMC 2021*, no. April, pp. 1779–1785, 2021, doi:10.1109/ICCMC51019.2021.9418345.

[31] M. Akgül, Ö. E. Sönmez, and T. Özcan, "Diagnosis of Heart Disease Using an Intelligent Method: A Hybrid ANN – GA Approach," *Adv. Intell. Syst. Comput.*, vol. 1029, pp. 1250–1257, 2020, doi:10.1007/978-3-030-23756-1_147.

[32] J. Rahman, B. Ahammed, and M. Abedin, "Classification and Prediction of Diabetes Disease Using Machine Learning Paradigm," *Heal. Inf. Sci. Syst.*, pp. 1–14, 2020, doi:10.1007/s13755-019-0095-z.

[33] G. Tripathi and R. Kumar, "Early Prediction of Diabetes Mellitus Using Machine Learning," in *ICRITO 2020- IEEE 8th International Conference on Reliability, Infocom Technologies and Optimization (Trends and Future Directions) (2020) 1009–1014*, 2020, pp. 1009–1014, doi:10.1109/ICRITO48877.2020.9197832.

[34] S. Revathy, B. Bharathi, P. Jeyanthi, and M. Ramesh, "Chronic Kidney Disease Prediction Using Machine Learning Models," no. May, 2020, doi:10.35940/ijeat. A2213.109119.

[35] R. M. Barber *et al.*, "Healthcare Access and Quality Index Based on Mortality from Causes Amenable to Personal Health Care in 195 Countries and Territories, 1990– 2015: A Novel Analysis from the Global Burden of Disease Study 2015," *Lancet*, vol. 390, no. 10091, pp. 231–266, Jul. 2017, doi:10.1016/S0140–6736(17)30818-8.

[36] A. Rodríguez-ruiz, E. Krupinski, J. Mordang, and K. Schilling, "Detection of Breast Cancer with Mammography : Effect of an Artificial Intelligence Support System," *Radiology*, vol. 290, no. 2, 305–314, 2019.

[37] F. Al-mufti *et al.*, "Artificial Intelligence in Neurocritical Care," *J. Neurol. Sci.*, 2019. doi:10.1016/j.jns.2019.06.024.

[38] I. Dankwa-mullan and M. Rivo, "Transforming Diabetes Care through Artificial Intelligence," vol. 22, no. 3, 2019, doi:10.1089/pop.2018.0129.

[39] I. M. Nasser and S. S. Abu-naser, "Lung Cancer Detection Using Artificial Neural Network," *IJEAIS*, vol. 3, no. 3, pp. 17–23, 2019.

[40] A. T. Watanabe *et al.*, "Improved Cancer Detection Using Artificial Intelligence: A Retrospective Evaluation of Missed Cancers on Mammography," *J. Digit. Imaging*, vol. 32, pp. 625–637, 2019.

[41] Y. Pan *et al.*, "Brain Tumor Grading Based on Neural Networks and Convolutional Neural Networks," *Proc. Annu. Int. Conf. IEEE Eng. Med. Biol. Soc. EMBS*, vol. 2015-Novem, no. August 2015, pp. 699–702, 2015, doi:10.1109/EMBC.2015.7318458.

[42. T. Davenport and R. Kalakota, "The Potential for Artificial Intelligence in Healthcare," *Futur. Healthc. J.*, vol. 6, no. 2, pp. 94–98, 2019, doi:10.7861/futurehosp. 6-2-94.

[43] O. Iliashenko, Z. Bikkulova, A. Dubgorn, G. St, P. Polytechnic, and S. Petersburg, "Opportunities and Challenges Intelligence in Healthcare." In *E3S Web of Conferences*, vol. 110, p. 02028. EDP Sciences, 2019.

[44] N. Sharma, C. Chakraborty, and R. Kumar, "Optimized Multimedia Data through Computationally Intelligent Algorithms," *Multimed. Syst.*, vol. 29, no. 5, pp. 2961–2977, 2023.

[45] T. J. Douglas and J. A. Ryman, "Understanding Competitive Advantage in the General Hospital Industry: Evaluating Strategic Competencies," *Strateg. Manag. J.*, vol. 24, no. 4, pp. 333–347, 2003, doi:10.1002/smj.301.

[46] H. Lasi, P. Fettke, H. G. Kemper, T. Feld, and M. Hoffmann, "Industry 4.0," *Bus. Inf. Syst. Eng.*, vol. 6, no. 4, pp. 239–242, 2014, doi:10.1007/s12599-014-0334-4.

[47] A. Carolina, B. Monteiro, R. P. França, B. Monteiro1, R. Padilha, and V. V Estrela, "Health 4.0: Applications, Management, Technologies and Review Type of article: Review," *Med. Technol. J.*, vol. 2, no. March 2018, pp. 262–276, 2019, [Online]. Available: https://www.researchgate.net/publication/330412784.

[48] J. L. Dieleman *et al.*, "National Spending on Health by Source for 184 Countries between 2013 and 2040," *Lancet*, vol. 387, no. 10037, pp. 2521–2535, 2016, doi:10.1016/S0140–6736(16)30167-2.

[49] M. Hermann, T. Pentek, and B. Otto, "Design Principles for Industrie 4.0 Scenarios: A Literature Review," *Tech. Univ. Dortmund*, vol. 1, no. 1, pp. 4–16, 2015, doi:10.13140/RG.2.2.29269.22248.

[50] C. Chute and T. French, "Introducing Care 4.0: An Integrated Care Paradigm Built on Industry 4.0 Capabilities," *Int. J. Environ. Res. Public Health*, vol. 16, no. 12, 2019, doi:10.3390/ijerph16122247.

[51] J. Al-Jaroodi, N. Mohamed, and E. Abukhousa, "Health 4.0: On the Way to Realizing the Healthcare of the Future," *IEEE Access*, vol. 8, pp. 211189–211210, 2020, doi:10.1109/ACCESS.2020.3038858.

[52] M. Beri, B. Kumar, S. Tiwari, N. Sharma, H. Vashishtya, and P. Chaudhary, "IoT Based Health Monitoring System Built on ESP32." In *2022 2nd International Conference on Advance Computing and Innovative Technologies in Engineering (ICACITE)* (pp. 454–458). IEEE, 2022, April.

2 AI's Implications in Healthcare and Medical Systems

*P Ramyavarshini, P Sai Swetha,
A Malini, and Mohd Asif Shah*

1 INTRODUCTION

The term "Artificial Intelligence" (AI) was formed by John McCarthy in 1995 which he said as "Science and Engineering of making intelligent machines, especially intelligent computer programs". The optimal attribute of AI is its ability to account for a problem and take necessary steps to arrive at a solution to the problem. AI is divided into weak AI and strong AI. Weak AI depends on a single work to solve it more efficiently rather than multi-tasking, whereas strong AI focuses on more complex and manually solvable problems. Researchers and developers are making good progress in representing various human activities like problem-solving skills and interpersonal skills. The application of AI is more prevalent in sectors like business and education, and it is beginning to be applied in the healthcare sector also. AI, which is based on minimization of human input, has the capacity to change healthcare and address several problems and tackle them quickly. It has the capacity to improve patients' health as well as improve the healthcare given to them. The recent improvements in AI have made people wonder what if AI could replace humans. In practical terms, it may not be a substitute, but it can assist physicians to achieve better results and accuracy. AI comprises technologies like machine learning (ML), deep learning, and natural language processing (NLP). ML used here helps to better treat patients and better understand medical images [11]. Deep learning has many aspects of healthcare that are helpful in healthcare like its superior performance, end-to-end learning system, with various features [12]. NLP helps to sort the unstructured data to improve patient care and disease diagnosis. Medical education, clinical practice, and healthcare delivery have benefited from these technologies [14]. The Covid-19 pandemic brought a positive effect on AI and its improvement in the healthcare industry. It has made the healthcare sector more effective by analyzing large datasets computationally to improve care given to patients. In most of the hospitals, AI technology is implemented. Moreover, this technology bridges the gap between the developing countries and the developed countries in terms

DOI: 10.1201/9781003377818-2

of healthcare. It has various benefits like: minimizing the needs of nurses to take care of patients, new tools that help for effective operations. It is essential for healthcare providers to be well versed in the potential applications of different aspects of healthcare [9]. While the hospitals store huge sets of information in their database in the form of images and clinical trials, AI technology helps to analyze those data. AI algorithms are trained to identify the pattern of data and it can detect the patterns that are not identifiable by humans [14]. In deep learning, the data is being analyzed by the computer [13]. The usage of AI helps improve the work of doctors, helps the staff in hospitals, and develops innovative treatments to cure diseases faster. The differentiation of AI from human beings is done as follows. According to the program designed, the algorithm analyzes the input data and functions accordingly. The black box algorithm gives the accurate function but the logic behind the function is not known [9]. The AI field is a growing field all over the world, and a study shows that the United States has invested nearly 600 million dollars. As AI in healthcare is widespread, research is going on the applications in various medical fields. Apart from diagnosing the patients this technology also provides the best experience for the patient. The timeline of AI, the role of AI in healthcare and its advancement, and the implementation of AI in clinical practice are discussed below (refer Figure 2.1).

2 TIMELINE OF AI IN HEALTHCARE

- In the year 1995, the term "Artificial Intelligence" was coined by John McCarthy which he defined as "science and engineering of making intelligent machines".
- The first problem-solving program called "Dendral" was produced in the year 1960–1970, which identified bacteria and recommended antibodies. The main goal of this program was to study the assumptions made. It is the first system found to solve the problem.
- The microcomputer development took place in the year 1970–1980s. This was the period when researchers identified the problem that took place in the absence of doctors and data and initiated the AI system that must be built to solve these problems. Later AI system design was made to accommodate the problems.
- The genomic sequencing database was developed in the year 2010–2019 There was a tremendous growth of AI in the electronic medical record system, in which, based on the illness of patients, their treatment, etc. the algorithms are being trained and used [19]. There was an advancement of NLP in the healthcare industry that took place at this time, through which the unstructured data was analyzed very easily. Robot-assisted surgery was initially started in 1960s and there was a huge progress in the field. It helps patients engage in a conversation and helps them to take medicines on time. Moreover it performs a basic checkup and analyzes their health conditions.
- From the year 2019 onwards, the discovery and development of drugs took place. AI played a major role in drug discovery to find medicines

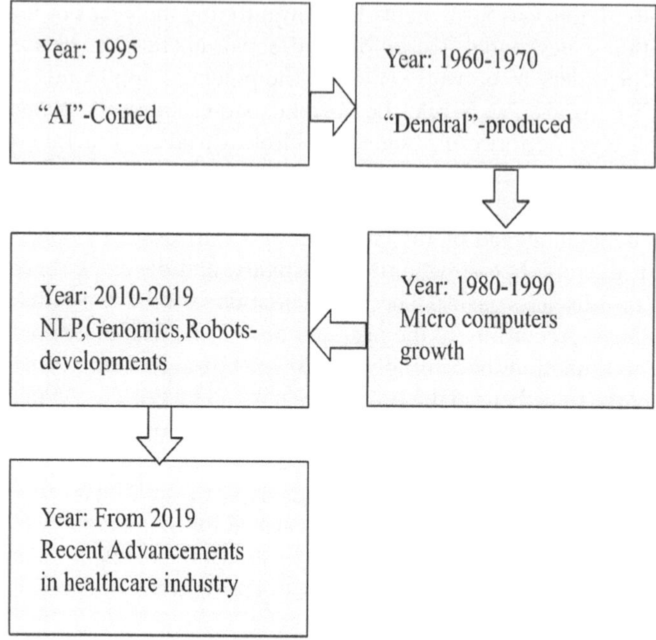

FIGURE 2.1   Timeline of AI in Medical Field

that can help to treat diseases and its prevention. Pre-clinical research started, which identifies suitable cohorts for clinical trials by analyzing medical records and social media consent. Personalized healthcare was given to patients, in order to improve their health conditions. Virtual health medical assessment was done which helped the patients to recover in a short span of time]. Report says that these Virtual Health assessments show good results in patients' health conditions.

3   ROLE OF AI IN HEALTHCARE

3.1   AI in Telemonitoring

Telemonitoring means with the help of technology monitoring the patients from their home and checking their health conditions regularly. This technology has helped mainly in treating all the patients over distant, difficult topography and communication. Moreover it is cost-effective and easier to access. AI monitors the patients and checks their blood pressure, level of oxygen, pulse rate, sugar level, and provides advice to them based on their symptoms and their past health records [1]. For example, the patients would be asked to upload their Computed Tomography (CT) scan and X-rays to a server that is safer and the AI system takes a deep look into the images and provides the required suggestions to the doctors. It can be used to provide personalized treatment based on their needs and health conditions, and the most effective treatment that must be given to patients are identified through the algorithms in ML [1]. The algorithms in ML are handed down for predicting the patients' denouement. AI manages chronic disease by telemedicine applications.

3.2 AI IN HEALTHCARE ROBOTS

AI and robots bridge the gap between the medical and healthcare industry. Some of the existing examples of implementation of AI along with the integration of robotics in healthcare sectors will be discussed. Supplementary robots provide continuous supply of medicines and equipment throughout the hospital floors while the staff are busy assisting the patients. The Exo-Skeleton robots help the disabled patients to walk and become more independent on themselves [2]. Robots assist patients engage in a conversation and help them to take medicines on time. Moreover it performs a basic checkup and analyzes their health conditions. They help with rehabilitation and surgery [2]. The HAL exoskeleton places the sensors on the skin and the electrical signals are found in patients' body and movements in their body and using observations made it helps them to recover from spinal cord injuries and heart strokes.

3.3 AI IN DRUG DISCOVERY

The main purpose of AI in the field of drug discovery is to find medicines which in turn help in the treatment of diseases and its prevention. The pharmaceutical companies have started to speed up their process in drug discovery using the AI technology [4]. Here are four methods using which the AI can do the process of drug discovery and they are listed as follows: the growth of biology is measured, improvement in chemistry, the increase in rate of success, and the fastest drug discovery method [3]. It creates cutting-edge algorithms by utilizing the most recent and sophisticated biology and chemistry techniques. At present, many pharmaceutical companies face challenges in discovery of drugs due to hike in price and less effectiveness [4]. AI methods have made it more cost efficient and time efficient. An example of this is use of AI in drug screening.

3.4 AI IN GENOMICS

Generally, genomics contains large and complex genomics dataset and the understanding of the dataset is quite difficult and the AI technology is used here. Several estimations have predicted that the enormous amount of data will be produced within the next decade. Hence, the sequencing of DNA and other biological data has increased the complexity of datasets. This is the reason why AI has to elucidate the hidden information within the big data [5]. Some of the existing examples of AI in genomics are as follows: the people's faces are examined to identify the genetic disorder with the assistance of facial analysis of AI program; liquid biopsy is done to identify the variety of cancer using the algorithms in ML; also with the assistance of ML algorithm in identifying the disease causing genetic variance, the deep learning algorithm is used to improve the various gene editing tools. The Covid-19 has a positive impact on AI in genomics. Integrating AI into genomics has several advantages like identifying the origin of virus, structure of the virus, and its behavior, and using all these observations the new vaccines for curing the disease was developed [6]. Based on the application, functionality, and end user perspective, the offerings available in the genomics market are divided on the global level in AI technology.

4   ADVANCEMENT OF AI IN HEALTH

There is a huge demand for healthcare globally and many countries are in need of medical professionals, especially doctors. Increase in advancement of wireless technology and smartphones have pathed the need for healthcare and have given various chances using the applications to monitor healthcare and search platforms. Due to the advancements and several improvements in medical field, the use of AI has started to become crucial. It is known that AI technology can reduce the cost more efficiently and according to a study it is found that AI is expected to reduce the US healthcare industry cost by USD 150 billion by 2026 [7]. By monitoring the patients regularly and by early diagnosis in treating their disease the AI has helped people to stay healthy. The advancement of AI is increasing rapidly in the medical field.

Some of the advancements are:

4.1   MEDICAL IMAGING AND HOMECARE TECHNOLOGY DEVELOPMENT

By using AI in medical imaging the doctors can identify patients' condition in a quick manner, promoting early intervention. For example, it helps in identifying cardiovascular abnormalities. The AI technology is used in the identification of enlargement of left atrial from the analysis of chest X-ray which solves the cardiovascular problems [18].

4.2   SURGICAL TECHNOLOGY AND HEALTH AUTOMATION IMPLEMENTATION USING AI

It is more beneficial for doctors and patients for assisting AI in surgery [7]. For example, by using CT, ultrasound, and Magnetic Resonance Imaging (MRI), the surgical plans have improved consistently, which when combined with robotic assistant, will improve the patients recovery [7].

4.3   ROBOTIC PROCESS AUTOMATION IN PATIENTS HEALTHCARE

Robots are used in hospitals for assisting doctors and nurses. They are used to assist the healthcare professionals and improve patients' health [21]. The hospitals arranged robots to monitor the reduction of pathogens that were found during the Covid-19 [2].

4.4 Intelligence Inhalers

Smart inhalers are one of the biggest advantages that were found in clinical pharmacy. The patients and healthcare professionals face several issues related to respiratory problem and it is all managed by the smart inhaler. This inhaler has several features like noting the time, location, and dosage given in a particular day, and it sends reminders regarding the dosage.

4.5 Internet of Things -Based Sensors

The wearable IoT is a smart device which keeps track of all the patients' activities. It has sensors, software connected to the cloud which helps monitor the healthcare of patients [8]. Some of applications of this wearable sensors and trackers are health condition monitoring, patient therapy delivery, rehabilitation of patients, activity tracking, and early disease diagnosis.

4.6 Healthcare Data Analytics

The predictive analysis comprises a large amount of data from Electronic Healthcare Records and medical images and finds the search pattern to analyze it. Some of the applications of the analysis are preventing the admissions of patients again, management of huge patients, improving cyber security, and speeding up insurance claims submission [20]. FitBits and smartwatches are the software where AI is used to monitor the patients' health and analyze the data and report their health conditions from time to time.

4.7 AI Analyzes the Unstructured Data

Four steps to manage unstructured data are: making content accessible, organized, and searchable; improving the quality of unstructured data; analyzing the unstructured data; and visualizing the data [21]. AI analyzes the unstructured data using the deep learning techniques and NLP techniques. For example, from unstructured data the NLP finds the medical conditions and treatment to be given.

4.8 AI in Drug Discovery

In recent times, there is an enormous growth in drug discovery due to AI [3]. It creates cutting-edge algorithms by utilizing the most recent and sophisticated biology and chemistry techniques. Several pharmaceutical companies have built their own drug discovery.

4.9 Forecasting Kidney Disease

Most widely applied deep learning model is Convolutional Neural Network (CNN) for image processing, which has helped in diagnosing kidney disease [16].

The forecasting of kidney disease is done based on the neural network pattern that has been pre-trained which identifies the glomerular and nonglomerular regions.

4.10　AI CONTRIBUTES TO RADIATION THERAPY

AI in radiotherapy has improved the quality, standards of treatment, and several time consuming steps with automation assistance. With respect to a study, it stated that automatic segmentation is the most supported application.

The progress of deep learning has a positive effect on AI tools. Deep learning helps to find correlations that are complex to solve using the ML algorithms. AI integrated with advanced technologies like block chain provides innovative solutions for the healthcare industry. AI is being used in maternal care, and it helps to predict whether mothers who are nearing delivery time are at risk during delivery. Unlike the traditional stethoscope, AI powered stethoscope takes readings in any place even if it's noisy, which makes a more accurate diagnosis. The advancements of AI in healthcare have made people realize that AI can perform equal to humans and better than humans.

5　RESEARCH SURVEY

5.1　ML IN HEALTHCARE

The subcategory of AI is called ML, and its ultimate goal is to optimize productivity and consistency of the doctors in the medical field. There are several changes observed in the field of healthcare due to the improvisations in AI. ML yields better results here [11]. The doctors are able to make better decisions in order to take care of the ill patients with the help of AI technology. This automated ML offers a fresh perspective and useful programming interfaces to make use and analyze the healthcare records, which helps for the medical practitioner and other staffs in this field. The ML algorithms are being implemented in Data Science, which helps to solve many practical problems and makes the healthcare industry to work faster [12]. There have been several reports of the ML concept's adaptable qualities helping the health domain. Some of the applications of ML in medical fields are shown below in Figure 2.2 [2]:

5.1.1　Robot-Assisted Surgery

The health information to treat the patients is added to the surgeon's monitor during robotic surgeries, and ML is really useful in this. To connect to several patient databases and evaluate a complex diversity of data types, which supports robotics procedures, strong and fast AI assisted services are necessary.

5.1.2　Disease Prediction

According to the symptoms shown by the patients, the disease by which they are affected is being evaluated and found using the disease prediction ML system. The system will analyze a patient's health condition and predict the probability

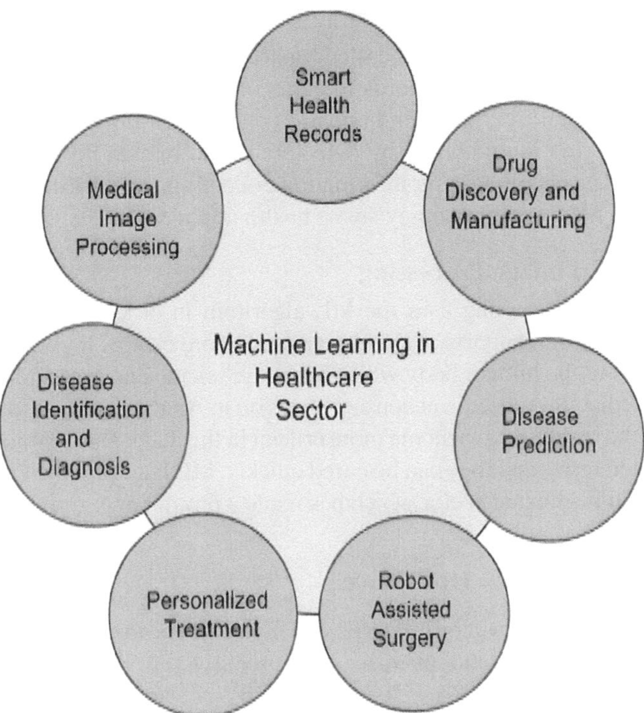

FIGURE 2.2   Applications of ML in Medical Field

level of the disease. In order to predict the disease for patients, the naive bayes classifier is being used. The probability of disease is calculated using naive bayes algorithm. Diseases like jaundice, malaria, and dengue are predicted using linear regression and decision tree.

5.1.3   Personalized Treatment

Personalized medicines and treatment would reduce trial and error-based treatment decisions. It brings down the burdens associated with a condition both in terms of health and conditions. It provides patient centric medication through integration of multiple data. There's a reduction in time and cost in clinical trials. It is suitable for disease identification and diagnosis. The disease detection system identifies different diseases like liver disorders, heart disease, and diabetes. The support vector system (SVS) is used in various disciplines like facial expression, protein fold, and speech recognition. The k-nearest neighbor classification is used for disease diagnosis and it is suitable for classification as well as regression analysis.

5.1.4   Drug Discovery and Management

The various fields in drug discovery in ML are materials finding and consumables, chemical synthesis, data mining, and research in biology. AI offers a variety of methods for training and assessing in the pharmaceutical research process.

5.1.5 Smart Health Records

The emerging field in e-health is called Smart Health Records (SHR) which uses the already available health records to better study and understand healthcare to provide better facilities. The fundamental concept behind this technology is to utilize all information gathered by detectors in the human body. The system is characterized as encompassing information collecting, networking, and information security. ML is used in many smart health applications.

5.1.6 Medical Image Processing

Medical Image Processing uses the ML algorithm in order to analyze the inner structures and different parts of the human body more clearly. It gives clear images of the organs in the human body which helps the scientist and researchers to study on it and predict the subsequent consequences on it. Analyzing the information and predicting the results have become more crucial in this field. Due to this the patients can be treated faster and they can be cured quickly. ML have provided path for various studies in healthcare sector which has made a promising future.

5.2 DEEP LEARNING IN HEALTHCARE

Deep learning has the capability to solve many health problems, but many studies have not shown the benefits of utilizing it properly yet. The versatility to learn intricate and multisensory data, its outstanding performance, its complete training system, and its combined feature learning are only a few of the elements of healthcare that are beneficial in the field. Deep learning is being differentiated from the neural layers of AI by the amount of underlying layers and potential to understand significant generalization of inputs. Some of the deep learning algorithms and their systems which are listed along with their applications mentioned in some of the papers are as follows [13]:

5.2.1 Stacked Sparse AE

- Using the MRI of the human brain the Alzheimer's disease can be predicted earlier and it can be cured
- Diagnosing the cancer
- Analyzing the proteins' structure

5.2.2 RBM (Restricted Boltzmann Machine)

- The variant modes of Alzheimer's disease are found using multiple MRI scan
- Multiple Schizophrenia tumors in simultaneous 3D MRIs are divided
- Imposing treatments to patients immediately relying on their medical conditions
- Identification of photoplethysmography signals for health monitoring

5.2.3 CNN

- Self-division of knee cartilage MRI to find the risk of osteoarthritis
- Finding out the blood vessels in the eyes

- Differentiating the stages of skin cancer
- Finding out the stage when the heart doesn't pump blood
- Estimate the unique properties of proteins that bind DNA and RNA

5.2.4 LSTM RNN (Long Short Term Memory History Recurrent Neural Network)

- Based on patient data, a temporal storage system for forecast medicine
- Estimating the disease
- Re-estimating the patient's health issues

An unsupervised training system called stacked sparse AE – AE makes use of the loaded value as the goal value. It consists of a processor which translates the feed into a subliminal version and subsequently decodes the processor from its representation [13]. The reconstruction errors are reduced at most. Finding pertinent patterns in information is possible.

RBM – RBM gains knowledge of the likelihood pattern across the given domain. RBM has restrictions that neurons in the human body must be of the bipartite graph. There can be symmetric connection between pairs of nodes from each of two groups and not from same group that makes use of the most efficient learning algorithms. It can do dimensionality reduction and collaborative filtering [13] CNN – The basic CNN design consists of a completely linked network for trained forecasting and a sharing layer [13]. Conducive to train them efficiently they are in need of huge data collection of label documents. They focus on neighborhood relationships and links between the component weights, followed by a highlighted consolidation. LSTM RNN (Long Short Term Memory Recurrent Neural Network) – They are useful in filtering relevant information. Each output is dependent on the preceding calculation and they are built up of homogeneous webwork that completes similar chores for each component in a series [13]. LSTM and GRU addressed the problem by modeling the hidden states. These led to excellent performance in NLP. Generative Adversarial Networks (GANs) contain neural networks which replace the needed information with synthetic data. Synthetic medical images would potentially allow researchers to create large datasets with high-quality images and a more balanced distribution of pathological findings. GAN helps to protect patient privacy by decreasing the need to use real medical images for research [13]. The deep learning algorithm works better than the ML algorithms and it has the capability to deliver solutions to the data in the healthcare sector and its assessment.

5.3 NLP in Healthcare

NLP is the capacity of computer systems to apprehend human phrases and textual content. NLP inside the healthcare zone can appropriately give voice to the unstructured information, giving remarkable perception into know-how high-quality, improving techniques and better outcomes for sufferers. The NLP in healthcare makes use of specialized engines which might be able to scrub a big set of unstructured information to locate the improperly coded affected person situations [14]. NLP clinical statistics and the usage of gadget-studying algorithms can discover the disorder that might not have been formerly coded. NLP software can quickly analyze clinical material and generate the information that is needed. Some of the NLP assets are listed below:

- Massive expansion of unrelated vocabulary in the medical fields
- Handling of medical items
- Terms and acronyms for formal insight markers

6 ETHICS OF AI IN HEALTHCARE

Although AI has numerous applications and benefits in the medical field, researchers must also take a look at the ethics and its effects. There's a benefit of integrating AI into healthcare, as it helps for improving healthcare delivery. However, it's important to reduce ethical hazards such as those that pose a threat to patient autonomy and confidentiality [10]. The stakeholders must be encouraged to be adaptable in implementing AI as a supplementary tool rather than seeing it as a replacement for doctors. Using AI in precision medicine raises additional pressing issues. For instance, when one-sidedness is present in the dataset, AI technology can learn them which may lead to inaccurate predictions. Moreover steered and misconception of data can be done. The usage of the black box algorithm raises legal difficulties including medical misfunctionality and feasibility of products because the logic behind the working is not known, which was suggested by Hanna R Sullivan and Scott J Schweikart [9]. There's also a talk on how AI may be useful in medical education, both in terms of training aspiring doctors for building their careers in AI and also using this technology in teaching. The ethical and clinical issues that emerge between patients and machines should also be taken into consideration during the reframe. To ensure the health conditions and comfort of patients AI used in healthcare must constantly adapt to the changing surroundings by upholding the ethical values. Depending upon the capacity to check out the software, the protection of software can be assessed and the failure of the software can be found. For instance, the mechanism by which the organ system works in the drugs can be used in software applications [10]. There's a social gap due to the development of AI, where the gap between the developing and developed countries has increased as a result of computerization and advancement in economies. There is also unemployment occurring continuously due to the development of robots. The development of robotic nurses and robots used in surgery in the health sector rather than nurses as caretakers threatens their future job opportunities [2]. Robotic doctors are unable to provide the understanding and tenderness needed for clinical evaluation. The use of robots in psychiatric hospitals may affect the patients' health condition more [2]. There's not much data privacy as the data collected through AI technology may be hacked. The upgrading of AI in the healthcare industry is more beneficial. However, the drawbacks can shadow the positives. The resource person must take into account the morality to overcome this.

7   IMPLEMENTATION OF AI INTO CLINICAL PROCESS

AI can be incorporated into clinical processes in different ways. For instance, the screening tool that analyzes the images initially and then with the help of the chances for disease to occur is used as a criteria for using which the radiologists decipher the images. Drug development in clinics has been unchanged due to the systematic needs and avoidance of risks [3]. In clinical processes which include image processing, segmentation of medical images, and creation and classification of clinical datasets, ML has improved many elements of the human ability to perceive the surroundings [3]. Biotechnology Corporation, research labs, and technological companies are using AI in the following fields:

- Predicting the pharmaceutical qualities of chemical components with the help of algorithms in ML and drug discovery [3]
- Segmenting the medical images for faster diagnosis and tracking of disease progression [4]
- Developing deep learning techniques on genomics and data in clinics for the detection of new models to predict them [11]

Pharma companies are engaged in the following in order to realize the full capacity of AI in the development of clinics:

- Data Interpretation
    In order to incorporate the ML algorithm into clinical practice, the customer field must include specialists in the field.
- Availability of large healthcare datasets
    Implementing the ML algorithm into the clinical process will be successful only when the data can be accessed [15]. Multiple international healthcare databases will be accessible through the most efficient platform.
- Depth understanding of pharmaceuticals
    For intelligence analysis, the experts must possess a thorough understanding of healthcare datasets, physician and patient knowledge, and therapeutic knowledge [2].
- Ability to integrate different datasets
    The healthcare datasets are usually unstructured making them difficult to analyze. An expert must be present to remove errors in the data so that the algorithms can analyze and understand the solution and change them into actions (refer Figure 2.3).

    - The AI search tool is used by doctors to find a clinical trial using the patients' clinical datasets.
    - The patients are then screened to see if they are eligible for clinical trials. AI algorithm finds a match with the recruiting phase by mining various datasets and patients can enroll.

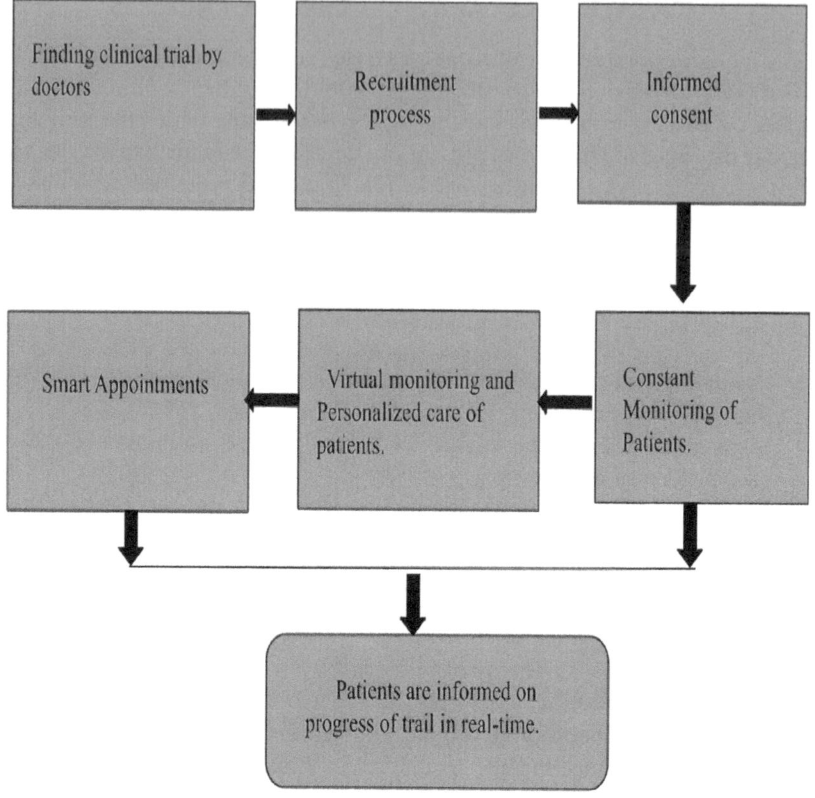

FIGURE 2.3   Patient's Journey through AI-clinical Trial

- The study is explained in detail and the patients can also inquire about the study. The patients receive mobile support with detailed information. Later, the patients are given a choice if they want to enter the trial.
- Patients are assigned to treatment groups randomly in order to receive new drugs or standard of patient care.
- The smartphones and watches provide constant monitoring and support and the progress of each trial is informed to the patients.
- Virtual monitoring and telemedicines reduce site visits and moreover personalized care of patients is also done.
- Smart Appointments are created using local information and patients' own calendars if site visits are required. Patients can make hospital visits for follow-ups, based on the smart appointments given.
- The information collected during each trial will be analyzed to decide on the next step. The patients are informed on the progress of each trial up-to-date.

The ability to foresee how AI will affect medicine practice, patient care, and quality of life is being overtaken by advancements in technology. In the near future, AI will support clinical decisions in a decision loop alongside human decisions [15]. Hence, AI technology puts the power in the hands of life sciences and healthcare organizations that provide patients faster access to safer medicines and save their lives.

8   FUTURE OF HEALTHCARE WITH FEDERATED LEARNING

Generally, the data sets are stored in a computer system, the federated learning trains these using its algorithm without interchanging them, as this is also a technique of ML [16]. It allows for the creation of a single model which is trained using multiple datasets without any of those datasets being shared. Compared to distributed learning, federated learning algorithms are fundamentally different and are mainly for addressing data privacy. Although AI, ML/DL algorithms have a lot of benefits in the medical field as they have improved the healthcare delivery and have better disease diagnosis system, they are not used much due to some of their problems like security and privacy. The recent development in this field has paved the way to train the models under ML which is complex [17]. For analyzing medical data at network's nodes in a federated manner to safeguard privacy and security contents which has become an active study area. FL is a promising solution to improve ML-based systems. Recent study suggested that federated learning can be used in various IoT applications like e-healthcare [16]. Federated learning has helped the healthcare industry by making availability of e-health in spite of lack of data in healthcare industry. The federated learning has brought an efficient healthcare system due to its advantages. For example, Mellody project was implemented in which the project's ultimate goal was to provide a learning model in federated learning that is used in pharmacies [17]. Its goal is to make a federated learning model which is predictable which in turn infers the way by which proteins are binded to chemical compounds which optimizes drug discovery processes. This federated learning would enhance and improve the medical judgment and so it can be implemented on large scale [16]. This system provides help to people living in remote areas. The federated learning can also help for early diagnosis and arrival of diseases and has the capability to prevent them.

9   AI IN COVID-19

December 2019 witnessed the rise of Corona Virus (Covid-19) which triggered the syndrome virus called SARS-CoV-2 and was propagated to almost all the countries rapidly. There was a rapid spread of the virus among people with face to face contact. The disease gets transmitted through respiratory droplets and causes severe infections in respiratory tracts. At the initial stage, there were more patients affected by this disease, and after few months the count decreased. There was a fluctuation in the number of cases of affected patients. Initially, there was a shortage of medicines to provide treatment to the patients. This shortage of medicines was also one of the reasons for increase in the cases all over the world. SARS-CoV-2 got spread rapidly to more than 150 nations all over the world by the middle of March 2021 in which a report says that more than 2 million deaths were confirmed. This exerted more pressure on limited healthcare resources. Rapid increase in cases caused a pressure to doctors since only limited health-care resources were available, and that was the time when AI was brought into the healthcare sector. There were several advantages when the AI technology was brought into healthcare sector. Some of the applications are listed below:

9.1 Prediction and Tracking of Diseases

By pulling data from news sources and social media, AI can be used to esti-mate the transmission of viruses and then provide crucial data about danger-ous regions. For instance, using the ML algorithm, Bluedot found the places where the Covid-19 got spread and cases over there. Using AI technology, smart watches, mobiles phones, and more items used by people are made to diag-nose the Covid-19 disease. While the structure of the proteins must be known to study about the arrival of Covid-19 and its impact, AI has a pivotal role in structuring proteins. The results pave the way for development of antibiotics. The SARS-CoV-2 structure is very complex and difficult to understand and hence a program was developed to thoroughly study about the complex nature of proteins.

9.1.1 Monitoring of Covid-19 Cases

AI provides vital information for allocating resources and making decisions based on data gathered from demographics and disease manifestations [13]. AI technol-ogy keeps continuous track of patients in healthcare and suggests the course of treatment for them. It predicts patient's chances of recovery by monitoring the patients and provides daily updates, storage, and course of treatment.

9.1.2 Diagnosis of Disease

A deep learning model for testing and comparing Covid-19 with other diseases was developed which was called as CovNet. This model was developed for sep-arating Covid-19 with other community disorders [30]. Later on a better deep learning model was developed which is known as Covid-ResNet which per-formed better than CovNet in diagnosing Covid-19. AI found Covid-19 from the scanned images of patients.

9.1.3 Development of Antibiotics

AI was used in the development of drugs by the industries in the medical field to provide a more efficient solution to Covid-19. Some of the examples for successful implementation of AI into clinical processes are the development of Pfizer and Moderna. It used AI in development of mRNA sequences.

9.2 Development of Therapeutics

Deep learning is used in antibodies development. A study was conducted to find the most viable drugs suitable for fighting against Covid-19 which used several

AI technologies. Many ML, deep learning algorithms were implemented to find more medicines.

There was a reduction in the proportion of people who were admitted in the hospital due to Covid-19 after the middle of 2021. The use of AI along with other technologies was also a reason for curing the disease. AI technology was on par with human experts. It was even more accurate than human experts.

10   MEDICAL IMAGE PROCESSING

The term "Image processing" refers to the operations that are performed on an image which could help in either enhancing the image otherwise it can be said as taking out the needed data from the image. The images are being imported and scrutinized to know about their features. Medical image processing is the process of visualizing the inner structures of a body to diagnose and treat medical conditions. It helps for disease identification and management. It comprises microscopic and macroscopic modalities. It has a database of structure and functions of organs to observe the abnormality. Digital image processing is done using a computer in combination with computer simulation algorithms to perform digital image analysis. It includes techniques such as image gaining, storage, presentation, and communication. Medical image processing plays a crucial role in the health industry for diagnosis of the disease. Deep Learning focuses on medical image analysis like bioimaging, neuroimaging, and DNA sequencing. The deep learning technique used in image processing is the Super Resolution Convolutional Neural Network (SRCNN), which improves the quality of images from low quality to high quality. The SRCNN consists of following activities: Preprocessing, feature extraction, non-linear mapping, and reconstruction. CNN and Generative Adversarial Network (GNN) are deep learning algorithms used for image restoration. CNN is one of the finest models available for the majority of everlasting problems, even with very little training data. CNN is regarded as the foundation method of deep learning. The development in deep learning paved the way for the rise of medical image processing.

The Faster Region Convolutional Neural Network (R-CNN) helps in object detection by finding objects in an image. The autoencoders are a neural network that comprises encoders and decoders. The encoder creates fingerprints of input image and decoder reconstructs it from the original image. The autoencoder deep learning technique helps to decrease the file dimensions of the picture by keeping the same standard of the picture. Generative Adversarial Network (GNN) deep learning technique generates synthetic images that are artificially generating images that have a desired content.

CLASSIFICATION: Image classification means it intakes a picture and gives output of the classification label of the image with some probability like loss, accuracy, and probability. The three types of image classification are unsupervised image classification, supervised image classification, and object based image classification. The unsupervised bunches the pixels into groups based on their characteristics. The supervised classification lets the user to choose the sample pixels in an image.

OBJECT DETECTION: Object detection is a type of image classification technique and object localization. It is useful for identifying objects in image or video. It uses boundary boxes to indicate each object in an image or video. There are various algorithms for detecting the objects like Single Shot Detector (SSD), YOLO (You Look Only Once), Spatial Pyramid Pooling (SPP), Haar Cascade, etc. Example: HAAR CASCADE: Haar cascade algorithm detects the object in an image irrespective of their scale in image and location. For example, the face mask detection algorithm to find whether a person is wearing mask or not is as follows. The data set is collected to partition the person with mask and without mask and then the data preprocessing (resizing the image and converting image into array) is done. Next the information obtained is divided into training (80%) and testing (20%). The training of the structure is done with the train dataset and testing is done with the test dataset. A consecutive convolutional network is built with multiple layers after splitting the dataset. The CNN model is pre-trained after the model is built. Training the required model is the next step after the process. The model is being trained with faces of people with mask and without mask. After training and creating the model there are two possible results: zero for person without mask (indicated by red color) and one for person with mask (indicated by green color). Next step is cascading face detection model. The haar cascade algorithm is used for finding out the facial features. The openCv makes use of this algorithm to capture the front faces of people. Then with the help of this algorithm the person with mask and without mask can be identified.

IMAGE SEGMENTATION: The term Image Segmentation refers to breaking the images into small cells and each cell represents the part of image and it makes the image analysis procedure more clear. Medical image segmentation, also known as natural image segmentation, is the process of manually or automatically taking out the necessary object, such as an organ, from a medical image which is either two dimensional or three dimensional.

FEATURE MAP: Feature map also called an activation map refers to the stimulation of various regions of image through mapping and also specific features are mapped. A certain attribute was discovered if there was a considerable engagement.

FEATURE EXTRACTION: The necessary area is extracted during the feature solvent extraction in order to examine the image. The image quality is improved from low quality to higher quality. The feature extraction is divided into two broad categories: low level and high level feature extraction.

KERNEL: Kernel or convolutional matrix is a matrix which contains numbers and it is used all over images to activate it. It is used for blurring, sharpening, edge detection, and feature extraction (a technique for determining the important portions of an image). The main objective of kernels is to retrieve valuable information from the convolution with fewer dimensions.

CONVOLUTION: Convolution is an integer-based mathematical procedure that involves fitting a matrix on an image. A tweaked filtered image is generated by multiplying the red green blue (RGB) image of a pixel and its relevant information by a matrix.

CORRELATION: Correlation is more closely related to convolution. It computes the response of the mask on an image. The results of the pixel got in output in the correlation are also determined as a weighted sum of nearby pixels. Deep learning terms are used in medical image processing:

EPOCH: Epoch denotes a single neural network pass across the full dataset. A forward and backward pass together is counted as one pass.

OPTIMIZER: Optimizer makes changes in the model based on the results from the loss function. It helps to minimize the loss function.

LOSS FUNCTION: A loss function or cost function quantifies the error between output of the algorithm and given target value. It measures how efficiently the neural network models the training data.

CALLBACK: Callback is an object that can perform certain actions at various stages of training. For example, the action can go ahead and stop the training since the validation accuracy is reached.

FULLY CONNECTED LAYER: Each node in a fully connected layer is linked to both the nodes, one before it and another after it. In CNNs the hidden layers are called fully connected layers.

WEIGHTS AND BIASES: Artificial neural network is made up of multiple processing units called nodes which are organized into layers that are connected to each other by weights. Each weight in the network will have corresponding values which is the strength of the connection between two nodes that it connects. Bias value allows the neural network to better fit the data. It is added to the sum of the weighted input.

IMAGE FILTERING: Image filtering is a technique for improving the technique of the images. Image filtering has different operations like sharpening, smoothing, and edge detection. In order to overcome the noise in image they are passed through filters. Some of the general filters are:

SOBEL FILTER: The Sobel filter is a gradient-based edge recognition technique. The images are divided into pixels and image intensity for each pixel is being calculated. From light to dark the direction of increase and the rate of change is found, which shows the change of image at each pixel, and also shows the way the pixel is represented. It uses 3*3 kernels, one for change in horizontal and one for change in vertical direction. The two kernels are mixed up with the actual image to know the results.

PREWITT FILTER: A relative approach of feature extraction and recognition of edges is the Prewitt filter. The Sobel filter, which is used to find vertical and horizontal edges, is comparable to it. In Prewitt filter the edges are calculated by using the difference between corresponding pixel intensities of an image.

GAUSSIAN FILTER: The distortion in an image is removed using a Gaussian filter. In this the weight of the central pixel is greater than surrounding pixels. The two dimensional Gaussian function is used while working with images. It is more effective at smoothing images.

NON-LOCAL MEANS FILTER: It removes the noise from the image and protects the sharpness of strong edges. In this method the average of all pixels is calculated and this value is weighted depending on the similarity of all pixels and hence less details are lost unlike the details lost in other methods of filter are used.

11 CONCLUSION

AI has a pivotal part in the medical field. AI can not only aid in the development of pharmaceuticals but also improve the efficiency of the current ones. We have reviewed various applications of AI in healthcare like telemonitoring, drug discovery, genomics and we have seen about healthcare robotics. All the applications are discussed in detail. The recent advancements of AI in the medical field is discussed which include some of the advancements like medical image processing, smart inhalers, software like Fitbits, etc. We then discussed in detail the three major categories of AI: ML, deep learning and NLP. AI has a lot of positive impact on healthcare. The ethics of AI in healthcare is also mentioned in detail. The growing expense of healthcare will remain controversial among healthcare stakeholders. However, there's still more improvement in AI which in turn will improve the patients' conditions better. The implementation of AI in the clinical process and patient clinical trial journey is discussed in detail. Research papers and reports state that federated learning has a future scope in the healthcare sector than ML and deep learning. The potential for healthcare cost reduction and service quality improvement is enormous, and it is quite likely that AI will advance quickly in the medical industry with help from the government.

REFERENCES

[1] Beri, M., Kumar, B., Tiwari, S., Sharma, N., Vashishtya, H., & Chaudhary, P. (2022 Apr). IoT Based Health Monitoring System Built on ESP32. In *2022 2nd International Conference on Advance Computing and Innovative Technologies in Engineering (ICACITE)* (pp. 454–458). IEEE.

[2] Srivastava, D., Sharma, N., Sinwar, D., Yousif, J. H., & Gupta, H. P. (Eds.). (2023). *Intelligent Internet of Things for Smart Healthcare Systems*. CRC Press, Boca Raton. https://www.taylorfrancis.com/books/edit/10.1201/9781003326182

[3] Shaheen, M. Y. *Applications of Artificial Intelligence (AI) in Healthcare: A Review.* ScienceOpen Preprints. doi:10.14293/S2199-1006.1.SOR-.PPVRY8K.v1.

[4] Chan, H. S., Shan, H., Dahoun, T., Vogel, H., & Yuan, S. (2019). Advancing Drug Discovery via Artificial Intelligence. *Trends in Pharmacological Sciences*, 40(8), 592–604.

[5] Lutimath, N. M., Ramachandra, H. V., Raghav, S., & Sharma, N. (2022). Prediction of Heart Disease Using Genetic Algorithm. In *Proceedings of Second Doctoral Symposium on Computational Intelligence: DoSCI 2021* (pp. 49–58). Springer Singapore.

[6] Sharma, N., Soni, M., Kumar, S., Kumar, R., Deb, N., & Shrivastava, A. (2023). Supervised Machine Learning Method for Ontology-based Financial Decisions in the Stock Market. *ACM Transactions on Asian and Low-Resource Language Information Processing*, 22(5), 1–24.

[7] Rigby, M. J. (2019). Ethical Dimensions of Using Artificial Intelligence in Health Care. *AMA Journal of Ethics*, 21(2), 121–124.

[8] Farhud, D. D., & Zokaei, S. (2021 Nov). Ethical Issues of Artificial Intelligence in Medicine and Healthcare. *Iran J Public Health*, 50(11), i–v. doi:10.18502/ijph. v50i11.7600. PMID: 35223619; PMCID: PMC8826344.

[9] Javaid, M., Haleem, A., Singh, R. P., Suman, R., & Rab, S. (2022). Significance of Machine Learning in Healthcare: Features, Pillars and Applications. *International Journal of Intelligent Networks*, 3 (2022), 58–73.

[10] Jabbar, M. A., Samreen, S., & Aluvalu, R. (2018). The Future of Health Care: Machine Learning. *International Journal of Engineering & Technology*, 7(4, 6), 23–25.

[11] Miotto, R., Wang, F., Wang, S., Jiang, X., & Dudley, J. T. (2018). Deep Learning for Healthcare: Review, Opportunities and Challenges. *Briefings in Bioinformatics*, 19(6), 1236–1246.

[12] Panchbhai, B. S., & Pathak, V. M. (2022). A Systematic Review of Natural Language Processing in Healthcare. *Journal of Algebraic Statistics*, 13(1), 682–707.

[13] Magrabi, F., Ammenwerth, E., McNair, J. B., De Keizer, N. F., Hyppönen, H., Nykänen, P., & Georgiou, A. (2019). Artificial Intelligence in Clinical Decision Support: Challenges for Evaluating AI and Practical Implications. *Yearbook of Medical Informatics*, 28(1), 128–134.

[16] Antunes, R. S., André da Costa, C., Küderle, A., Yari, I. A., & Eskofier, B. (2022). Federated Learning for Healthcare: Systematic Review and Architecture Proposal. *ACM Transactions on Intelligent Systems and Technology (TIST)*, 13(4), 1–23.

[17] Harger, C., Chen, G., Farmer, A., Huang, W., Inman, J., Kiphart, D., Schilkey, F., Skupski, M. P., & Weller, J. (2000 Jan 1). The Genome Sequence DataBase. *Nucleic Acids Research*, 28(1), 31–32. doi:10.1093/nar/28.1.31. PMID: 10592174; PMCID: PMC102463.

[18] Yao, L., Zhang, H., Zhang, M., Chen, X., Zhang, J., Huang, J., & Zhang, L. (2021). Application of Artificial Intelligence in Renal Disease. *Clinical eHealth*, 4, 54–61.

[19] Kaul, V., Enslin, S., & Seth A. (2020). Gross, History of Artificial Intelligence in Medicine. *Gastrointestinal Endoscopy*, 92(4), 807–812, ISSN 0016–5107, doi:10.1016/j.gie.2020.06.040.

[20] Sharma, A., Virmani, T., Pathak, V., Sharma, A., Pathak, K., Kumar, G., & Pathak, D. (2022 July 6). Artificial Intelligence-based Data-driven Strategy to Accelerate Research, Development, and Clinical Trials of COVID Vaccine. *BioMed research international*, 2022, 7205241. doi:10.1155/2022/7205241. PMID: 35845955; PMCID: PMC9279074.

[21] Bharodiya, A. K. (2022). Feature Extraction Methods for CT-Scan Images Using Image Processing. In (Ed.), *Computed-Tomography (CT) Scan*. IntechOpen. doi:10.5772/intechopen.102573.

3 Advancements of Artificial Intelligence in Healthcare

G K Sriram, S Shrinivas, A Malini, and Mohd Asif Shah

1 INTRODUCTI.ON

In this modern technological globe, one of the booming sectors is Artificial Intelligence (AI) or artificial intelligence. AI is essentially a machine that has been programmed by computers to tackle human issues more effectively than humans. AI can have a huge potential impact on all aspects of society. It makes life simpler and more effective than we may imagine. One component of living a happy life is being healthy, but we are not doing that. AI in healthcare may offer a way to lead a healthy lifestyle. As an example, AI can analyze a patient's medical history to make a cancer diagnosis as early as feasible. The risk of a premature child is analyzed by AI, which provides the doctors with a clear report. The identification of brain disorders and tumors is then increasingly used [1]. Even radiological scans, which can provide an accurate picture of a patient's present health, incorporate AI. They increase the accuracy and efficiency of magnetic resonance imaging (MRI) scanning [34]. AI is utilized to track the health of the liver and lungs as well as in medication discovery. We often encounter delays in receiving reports, but owing to these technologies, we can do it immediately. As an illustration, consider radiology scans like MRI, CT, X-rays, and PT scans. Although the results of all these scans are not provided immediately, we can obtain the results fast and receive a diagnosis as soon as possible by using these techniques. Simple terms, they assist us to lead healthy lives by providing us with red flags before we fall. The processes and roles employed in order to offer these services and conveniences are pretty intriguing, such as image analysis, classification, segmentation, and visualization. Other examples include integrated analytics, medical imaging, big data computing, ML, and deep learning (DL). These techniques and features can advance healthcare to the next generation. The functions employed here depend on one another. For instance, image segmentation and visualization processing can be aided by machine learning (ML) [5].

Numerical data analysis is performed through big analytics. Similar to that, each function used here is combined to the others and as a whole, they improve

DOI: 10.1201/9781003377818-3

the outcomes. As an illustration, PACS is one of the techniques used to safely store and digitally transfer electronic images and reports with therapeutic relevance. They can be used to check for preterm birth risk and aid in the detection of breast cancer. DL is identical to ML in that it examines the patient's current condition and provides a clear image of how to diagnose it. AI can aid in the diagnosis of disorders affecting the heart and nervous system as well as stroke issues. Natural language processing and cutting edge DL techniques are employed to assess the patient's current condition. The implementation of AI, which is a dynamically growing technology, in healthcare is motivated by the need for more accurate diagnosis and outcomes. Numerous tools are used in the radiology tests and to interpret the data, but the process is labor-intensive and time-consuming. There are situations where patients may require quick assistance, but the analyzing procedure delays it, which can lead to diagnosis failure. Therefore, when AI enters the picture, it decreases this process delay and can suggest very effective diagnosing approaches, which can also build trust and produce better outcomes in the healthcare sector. AI tools are already employed in healthcare facilities to diagnose patients ethically and they are observing excellent outcomes. Despite their interconnections, they share several traits and characteristics that are evocative. Each function has unique advantages and capabilities. These are the hot new technologies that will emerge in the upcoming years. The world is going to witness a huge evolution with AI in healthcare. Therefore, using these technologies will undoubtedly aid in better patient care and medical diagnosis.

2 ADVANCEMENT OF AI IN HEALTHCARE

While AI is a popular topic in tech right now, the technology was first discovered during World War II. AI was developed to automate human and animal activities. When people required immediate solutions for their medical issues, AI in healthcare began to boom. People needed to simplify their lives as they evolved on the planet. Instead of simplifying their lives, they began to introduce new issues within themselves. One of the things that leads to difficult diseases in humans is poor eating habits. This demand for quick fixes was brought on by the urge to replace the conventional good practices. AI in healthcare is used to diagnose and treat patients with high-quality treatment using the techniques mentioned in Figure 3.1. The transition to AI in healthcare is already halfway complete. AI in healthcare uses many ML algorithms [4]. AI technology will be used to improve every aspect of the healthcare system. The majority of healthcare fields use AI to assess the patient and make the appropriate diagnosis, as expected. Domains are using AI effectively and witnessing immense good response.

2.1 AI in Treating Tumors

One of the dangerous diseases that kills people is tumors. According to reports from 2020, brain tumors impact between 85% and 90% of those who suffer

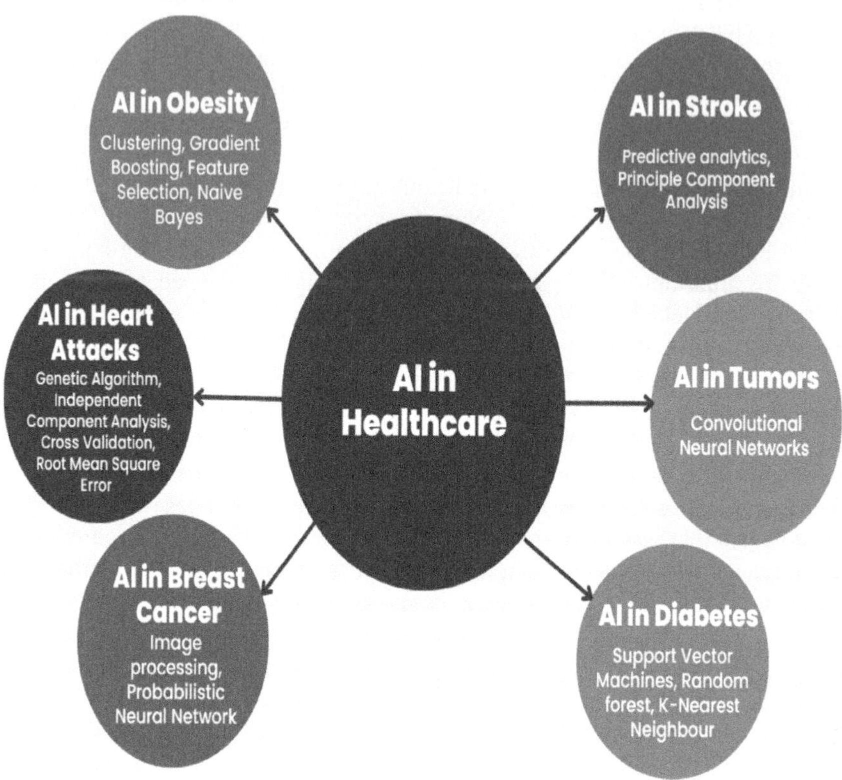

FIGURE 3.1   AI in Healthcare

tumors. Three groups comprise the classification of tumors: (1) Cancerous tumors, which are extremely likely to spread to other body organs and have a high rate of mortality. (2) Non-cancerous tumors, which differ with cancerous tumors in that they only damage the organ or gland that the tumor has already afflicted and do not build out to other parts of the body. Rarely does this result in fatalities. (3) Pre-cancerous tumors are tumors that develop before becoming malignant. Therefore, AI may be utilized to solve this, and diagnosis can be completed as rapidly as is known. The tumors and their risk level can be identified using a variety of methods. Binary particle swarm optimization is one such approach that mostly functions on continuous datasets [2]. Due to its usefulness in graphical depiction, this technique can accurately capture the structure of tumors. Each swarm contains an internal route called a velocity vector that is accustomed to predict the next motion of the particle. Each particle updates its current vector and the vector is restated to a fixed number of times or until it reaches the minimal error. PSO is used in identifying the various types of tumors with accurate condition and stage of it. Another algorithm that works well in diagnosing tumors is the CNN [3].

2.1.1   CNN

1. The Convolutional Layer: It extricates diverse features from the input. This carries out a few mathematical operations between the provided input and the term known as filter of specific size MxM. Following a dot operation on the input and filter, various features from the input image are extracted. Additionally, it detects the input image's outer and inner layers as well as its borders.
2. The Pooling Layer: The data acquired in the convolutional layer is generalizable in this way. It reduces and makes independent the connections between the layers. There are numerous approaches to pooling. The largest element picked from the independent set is identified using max pooling. Between the convolutional layer and the fully constructed layer, this literally serves as a bridging layer.
3. Fully Connected Layer: The FC layers receive the flattened stage image from the pooling layer. The categorization procedure begins in the extra layers, where various mathematical operations are typically performed. This CNN layer decreases the amount of human oversight.
4. Dropout: The training dataset is overfitted after the FC layer, and the more the overfitting in the training dataset, the worse the model will perform when seeking new data. A layer is used to ignore this process, whereby during training, neurons are eliminated from the neural network and its size is minimized.
5. Activation Functions: It is regarded as an essential component of CNN. Using mathematical processes, it determines whether the neuron may be triggered or deactivated and whether it is relevant or not.

2.2   AI IN STROKE

A stroke is an illness that can have catastrophic effects on a person's health. Stroke symptoms commonly include difficulties speaking and hearing, as well as sudden weakness in the face, legs, and particularly one side of the body. Brain stroke is another name for stroke. Hemorrhagic stroke, transient ischemic attack, ischemic stroke, and brain stem stroke are the four different forms of stroke. A multiple number of AI algorithms are utilized to the effects of stroke in advance. AI-based stroke impact identification can aid in a speedy diagnosis [6], [7]. Principle component analysis and decision trees are the two most common algorithms used to analyze the stroke. Decision trees fall in the category of supervised ML which can make predictions like humans. Regression and classification are both handled by decision trees. They are used to illustrate decisions and the decision-making process. Decision trees are frequently used in data mining to derive a plan and achieve a specific goal. The primary steps in the decision tree are data splitting into several split points and cost function testing. Cost function displays the analysis error between the value that was predicted and the actual value. The splitting process is broken down into three parts, starting with the precision that can be acquired from each split. The highest or lowest split choice is next. This procedure is recursive and is considered as a greedy algorithm overall. After splitting, one of the most important stages is pruning, when irrelevant nodes are eliminated to increase the model's accuracy [9].

Principle component analysis (PCA) plays a vital role for both 2D and 3D data visualization [10]. It is a useful tool for illustrating the scope of brain problems. Dimension reduction is its main objective. Its goal is to decrease the data dimension without sacrificing any information. It entirely gets rid of duplicates and irrelevant data. By knocking off a few criteria, such as identifying the covariance matrix of any dataset used, PCA can be conducted on a dataset. Covariance between the selected pair of variables refers to what is meant by a covariance matrix. The dataset must be normalized before the covariance matrix is computed. In order to determine the principle components that can lower the dimensions, the Eigen vectors are sorted after being identified with the covariance matrix of the data.

By detecting the health-related insights of the patient, the technique of predictive analysis makes diagnosing patients easier [8]. This method aids in forecasting the kind of diseases that the patient may encounter in the future and the appropriate treatments. It will provide a detailed image of all the specifics of your health. In four layers of predictive analysis, there are 4 types of analytics: descriptive, diagnostic, predictive, and prescriptive. The first and most important step in diagnosing a patient is descriptive analytics, which is the basic observation of the patient's current state of health. The finest part of diagnostic analytics is that the patient will also clearly understand the cause of their illness. Here, the diagnosers will examine the reason for the illness and inconvenience. How these three phases may function well is the main emphasis of predictive analytics. It seeks to make predictions that, when it comes to healthcare, can have a greater success rate. Although predictive analytics makes treatment considerably more effective, many diagnosers currently focus on descriptive and diagnostic analytics. Predictions are used in prescriptive analysis to determine the best course of action. The most advanced approaches in healthcare today are thought to be predictive and prescriptive analytics.

2.3 AI IN DIABETES

In this world, diabetes is viewed as a global disease. Diabetes affects people of all ages, including newborns and nonagenarians. People with diabetes must alter every aspect of their lifestyle, including their eating habits, place of employment, and many other aspects of their daily lives. Whether they like it or not, they must adhere to it in order to live comfortably. Some major indicators of diabetes are constant fatigue, frequent urination, dry skin, and an excessive thirst at all time. Type-1, Type-2, and gestational diabetes are the three predominant types of the disease. Children and teenagers are the most common type-1 diabetes victims.

Their immune system is harmed, and the pancreatic cells that produce insulin are also affected. The most pervasive kind of diabetes is type-2, which is inherited. During pregnancy, gestational diabetes affects the sufferer and might result in high blood pressure. With automated retinal scans, diabetic treatment, self-management tools, and clinical support, AI can benefit diabetes patients. To diagnose diabetes, a variety of powerful AI algorithms can be applied.

The most popular ML formula is called support vector machine. It is an ML category of supervised ML. Labeling the data points is a requirement of supervised ML. Diabetes patients can be identified by their type of diabetes when they enter a hospital, for example. Analysis of the non-linearity between the data points is done using support vector machines [11]. A regression model is an SVM. The continuous outcome will be predicted using a regression model, which will assess the interaction of the independent variables. Its goal is to use hyperplanes to classify the data points into different groups. For example, first category data points are arranged on one side of the boundary line, while second category data points are placed on the other side of the boundary line, using hyperplanes to separate the data points. The extreme data points are called support vectors. SVM can be categorized into two varieties: linear SVM in which the data is separable into two different classes using a single straight line and non-linear SVM, which is vice versa of linear SVM. In SVM, the points that are most near the hyperplane are termed as support vectors and the space separating them from the hyperplane are described as margins. A hyperplane with most support vectors is called an optimal hyperplane.

Another algorithm that can be used to study diabetes is random forest. A form of supervised ML is random forest [12]. A collection of decision trees where the average is determined and subsets are created can be described as a random forest. An algorithm for ensemble learning is random forest. A multitasking approach that uses classifiers, regression, function approximation, and predictions can be described within a few terms as ensemble learning. The model's performance may be enhanced by it. Its goal is to resolve challenging computational and intellectual challenges. Compared to other ML algorithms, random trees will train faster. Because it almost consistently accurately predicts the future, random forest is a high accuracy ML model. K data points from the training dataset are selected, and after being grouped into decision trees, a total of N decision trees are selected to form the random forest.

K-Nearest Neighbor is a supervised ML [13]. By analyzing their similarities, it seeks to fit new data points into existing data points. When new data sets are discovered, they are quickly categorized into categories based on their characteristics. Due to the non-parametric nature of K-NN, it will not focus on the underlying data. K-NN is also referred to as the "lazy learner algorithm" since it gains knowledge while classifying data. In contradiction to many other ML algorithms, K-NN learns while performing categorization. It has classification and regression capabilities. Data points in the space region and recently joined data points in the vector region are used for the comparison. In K-NN, target function in ML analyzes the training data set to find solutions to any problems that are presented. In

K-NN, the target function may have discrete or continuous values. Many datasets can be implemented quickly and easily.

Popular supervised ML algorithm that involves prediction is logistic regression [14]. The dependent variables will be predicted using logistic regression using the independent set of variables. It determines if the dependent variables have a probability between 0 and 1. The values could be discrete or categorical. Similar to linear regression, logistic regression predicts data through classification rather than regression; both techniques are used to predict data. It is effective to find the predominant variables among the data points. Sigmoid functions are used in logistic regression. A curve with a "S" shape can be termed as a sigmoid function or logistic function. The predicted values are plotted in the curve. Threshold values are probabilities of 0 to 1. The maximum threshold value is 1 and minimum threshold value is 0. Binomial, Multinomial, and Ordinal are the three different forms of logit regression.

2.4 AI IN BREAST CANCER

People are affected by breast cancer when there is an irregular growth in breast cells, which can result in dangerous symptoms like skin blisters, heat in the breast skin, and irritation. While there are several kinds of breast cancer, invasive ductal carcinoma and invasive lobular carcinoma are the most prominent among them. Image is compressed in terms of resolution and size. It focuses on compressing the image without any information loss. Before it reaches a critical level, AI uses a variety of ways to recognize and forecast the impact and stage of breast cancer. Probabilistic neural networks are necessary for making breast cancer predictions. It is a pattern recognizer and helpful in determining how data points should be classified. Input layer, pattern layer, summation layer, and output layer are the four primary layers that are utilized in probabilistic neural networks [17]. The input layer will use the data to uncover any hidden layers, and this data is then delivered to the pattern layer, which will train the cells. The geometric separation between the anticipated outputs will be calculated by the concealed geometric cells. Each cell will be assigned to a PNN category in the summation layer, and each layer's weight will be specified. Weighted categories will be compared in the output layer [15]. Image processing with AI can be a superpower when it comes to analyzing breast cancer. Image processing is processing the input image into machine readable form and used to analyze it. It converts the image into matrix form and calculates the intensity. Intensity can be termed as x and y coordinates of an image. Image processing is done with several steps that are discussed in [16] and the same has been summarized with Figure 3.2.

2.5 AI IN DETECTION OF HEART ATTACKS

One of the most unpredictable catastrophes that can affect a person's heart is a heart attack. It will instantly strike humans speechless and leave them stunned for a while. It can easily end a life in a matter of minutes. People experience heart

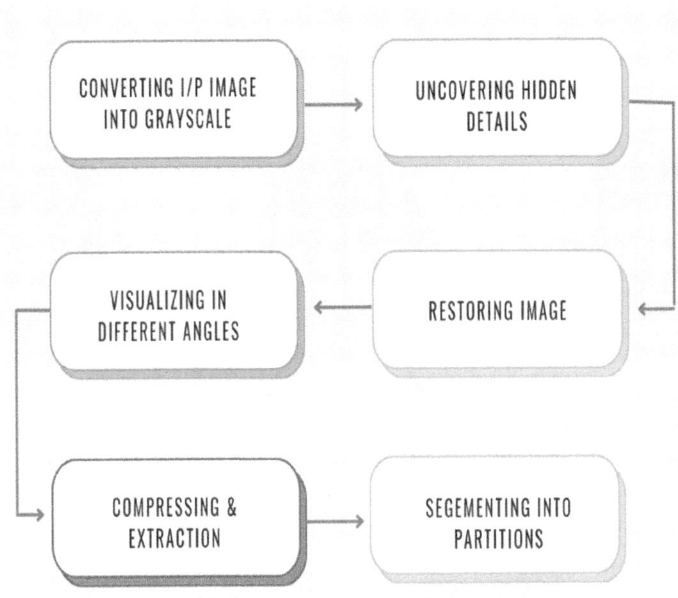

FIGURE 3.2 Image Processing

attacks when the heart muscle is not getting enough blood flow. Many times, heart attacks lead to strokes. Unstable pressure, generalized weakness, pain in other areas of the body, uncomfortable breathing, and excessive sweating are some basic signs of a heart attack. There are numerous effective ways for heart attack detection using AI. Of the algorithms, the genetic algorithm is one that can be used to detect heart attacks early. It helps to solve difficult problems that are complex and cannot be solved easily. Its goal is to simplify complex problems through optimization. In evolutionary processes, the complicated problem is simplified through a number of stages to arrive at the best potential solution as depicted in Figure 3.3.

Electrocardiogram (ECA) testing can be effectively employed with Independent Component Analysis (ICA), a ML algorithm. The required signal will be extracted from the ECG's mixed signals using independent component analysis (ICA). This division will provide a clear image for the patient's diagnosis. Although this approach resembles PCA in aspect, there are few differences.

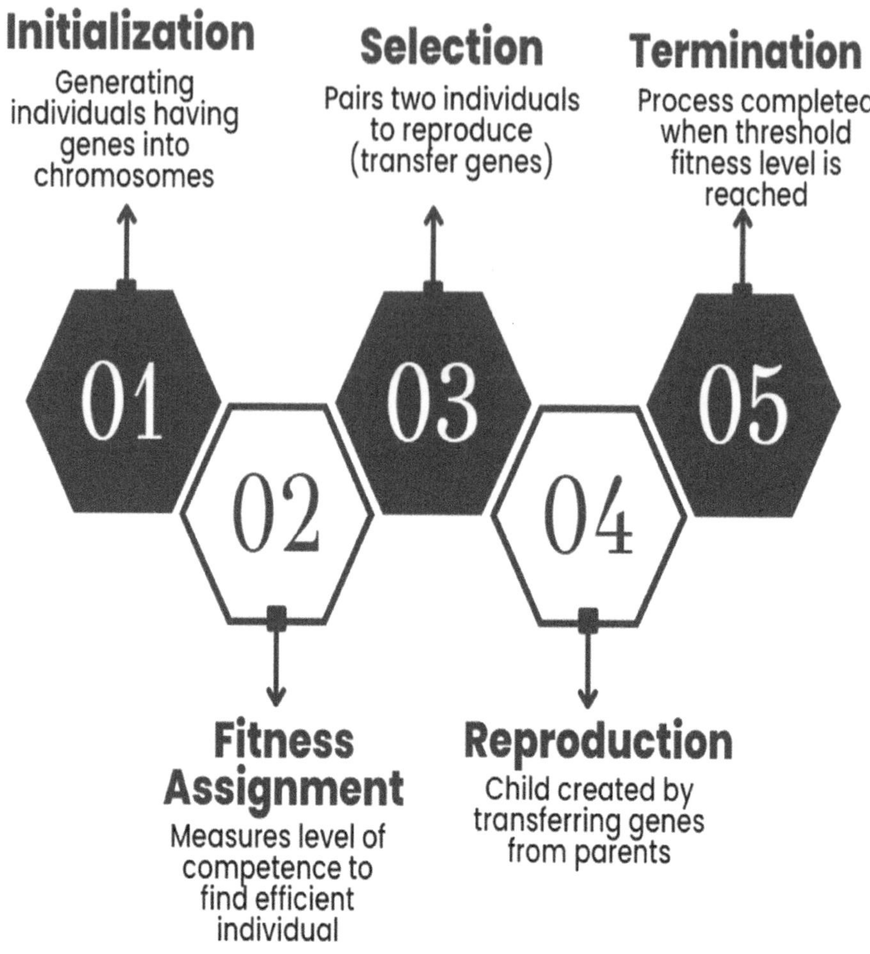

FIGURE 3.3 Genetics Algorithm

While ICA seeks to identify the separate signals, PCA seeks to compress the signals. PCA will not prioritize mutual independence between the mixed signals, whereas ICA will prioritize it highly [19].

The Root Mean Square Error technique is used to assess the model's correctness. The value difference between the projected results and the expected value is often referred to as the RMSE. It is helpful for determining the model's accuracy and precision. The regression model's error rate is determined here. It is the distance between expected value and obtained value [18].

The cross validation method is a very significant tool for evaluating the stability of the trained model. A subset of the provided dataset will be used in cross validation to predict the necessary data points. In most ML algorithms, at least 75% of the data points are trained, and the trained data points are tested for 25% of the time. However, in cross validation, we'll use one half data points for training and the other half for examining. Cross validation can be categorized into several categories as follows: (1) Leave One Out Cross Validation (LOOCV):. every data point from the dataset is used for the validation's training portion and just one is used for testing. It uses almost all of the dataset's data points; however, it takes a long time. (2) K – Fold Cross Validation: the data points in the dataset is splitted into k numbers of subsets called folds. Each subset is put under training and (k-1) subset is reserved for testing the data. (3) Stratified Cross Validation: with a few modifications, this procedure is comparable to K-Fold cross validation. The subsets are examined for representation in each subset during stratified cross validation. It examines the dataset's information to determine whether everything is categorized properly. (4) Hold Out Cross Validation: the data points are trained as usual, and some of them enter the testing phase, however in this case, only the training set is used to make the prediction. A dataset's training subset is used for the prediction [20].

2.6 AI IN OBESITY

Obesity is something that quickly lowers a person's self-esteem. It prevents individuals from performing tasks easily. Teenagers and adults alike are being affected by obesity. Early obesity can prevent many experiences throughout life. An individual's confidence level is significantly influenced by their physical appearance. Even a skilled individual can lose confidence in speaking their mind. The complex disease of obesity is thought to cause excessive body fat. They have a significant role in the enlargement of heart disease, stroke, diabetes, excessive blood pressure, and occasionally even cancer [21]. The Body Mass Index value, which is determined using the person's height and weight, is used to categorize obesity. With the help of the BMI, obesity can be split into three main categories: Class 1 people have a BMI of 30 to 34.9. BMI values in the 35 to 39.9 category are in Class 2. Class 3 ranges more than 40. Class 1 can be insignificant, Class 2 should be closely watched, and Class 3 is extremely risky [22]. Obesity's primary symptoms are fatigue, depression, joint discomfort, and drowsiness. The first stage in every ML method is data preprocessing. The raw data will be transformed into formatted data through data preparation. The data will benefit from its use in cleaning. An effective ML approach for predicting obesity is gradient boosting [23]. Boosting algorithms can be thought of as a catalyst that enhances the model's efficacy. ML algorithms are created to significantly raise the precision of predictions, and this boosting approach will strengthen the model even more. A boosting method known as gradient boosting aims to eliminate the errors of its predecessor. The Adaboost algorithm is fundamentally different from gradient boosting (adaptive boosting). All of the weak subsets will be combined into a strong one in the name of adaptive boosting methods [26].

Clustering is a useful tool for data analysis in ML. An unsupervised ML algorithm is clustering. Unlabeled data points or datasets are a definition of unsupervised ML. The process of clustering is the classification or grouping of the data points into clusters or groupings. A collection of related data points is referred to as a cluster. Clustering will provide a clear image for assessing the necessary individual data points [24]. The dataset's similarities and dissimilarities will be divided using clustering. Clustering is classified into:

1) Hierarchical-based clustering: It will divide the data into clusters based on two methods, namely (a) Agglomerative hierarchical clustering: It takes a bottom-up strategy. The data points are clustered from bottom to top in the dataset. (b) Divisive hierarchical clustering: It follows a top-to-bottom strategy. The data points are clustered from top to bottom in the dataset. 2) Centroid-based clustering: It will cluster the data points with closeness between the data points. It is an iterative process. It will measure the disparity between the information. Based on distance measures data points will be added to one cluster and the rest of the data points will be added to the other cluster. 3) Density-based clustering: The density in the region will be determined by density clustering. In less dense areas, it will identify differences and similarities between the data points. 4) Distribution-based clustering: Data points are grouped together based on proportions according to their probability to belong into a given distribution. In clustering based on distribution, Gaussian distributions are dominant. 5) Fuzzy clustering: Here the same data point can be grouped into other clusters as well. It is termed as Fuzzy C-means clustering. 6) K-means clustering: It will group the data points which are unlabeled. It is an iterative process which will divide the clusters into k sets.

The Naive Bayes classifier is a classification of supervised ML techniques that applies the Bayes theorem from probability. It is applied to categorization problems. It is regarded as the most accurate classification algorithm. It can make an efficient model in a quick time. Because it is a probabilistic classifier, the classification of the data points is built upon likelihood of the data. It is frequently applied to text classification as well [25].

Another approach used to minimize the dataset's dimensions without sacrificing any information is dimensionality reduction [28]. It is quite effective in cluster analysis and biometrics. All redundant data points in the dataset will be eliminated when dimensionality reduction is implemented. It will take less time to decrease the dataset. When the data points are incorrect, there could be information loss. Feature selection is accomplished after this step. The module methods for feature selection include ANOVA, PCA, and others [27].

3 CHALLENGES OF AI IN HEALTHCARE

AI has been assisting the medical industry in clinical decisions for over a decade. The major challenge faced during this advancement was the problem with misrepresentative, inadequate, and biased data that are potential enough to lead to fatal outcomes and lack of generalization in the model outcomes. Although many have come up with solutions that can provide research with large datasets there still exists a problem of bias, irregularity, lack of labeled data, etc. Due to decreased promptness in uploading clinical data, the data preprocessing steps have become tedious. When taking the medical domain under consideration, regular data preprocessing for filling the missing values such as imputation and reinforcement learning cannot be completely relied upon and hence there is a constant need for domain experts to provide suggestions with respect to the condition for which the data is obtained.

The model or framework being implemented is another hurdle in the medical field. Although there are a number of techniques such as clustering, heatmaps, word count, and other scores to test and prove the accuracy of the model, DL models are still considered black boxes. Having a deterministic model with interpretability is of utmost importance in this field as here the situation is not a controlled one for which the model has been trained and hence there are a number of possibilities for the model to classify certain patients with certain diseases based on probability [29].

The development of the DL algorithms is a must in cases where chronic and acute cases need to be addressed. This requirement can be satisfied only when the model and data are shared across research areas for further insights and efficiency improvements but that comes with the cost of sharing the datasets containing patient-sensitive information. As mentioned above the lack of parametrics in the data can lead to poor models and hence the point of "what extent to share the data" is still unknown. Scalability and availability of the model is another important thing to be taken into consideration as cloud computing has made it possible to bring the models close to the data origin point. This is required as the datasets and conditions of different regions may differ based on the medical and lifestyle practices of that region.

4   RECENT DEVELOPMENTS IN HEALTHCARE

Numerous implementations and practices of AI are used in the healthcare sector. Healthcare AI solutions have fast become essential for processing and managing the sea of data and information effectively. AI in healthcare has led to modified versions of currently used methods and treatments as that mentioned in Figure 3.4. The trickiest challenges are quickly solved for hospitals and doctors because of it. Additionally, it provides better quality. AI can rapidly tackle medical errors. Numerous thousands of individuals all across the world may suffer harm or perhaps eventually die due to medical mistakes. These mistakes are frequently the result of inadequate medical histories and analyses. AI is proficient in that. Data can be predicted more accurately by AI. Faster than medical professionals, it can forecast and diagnose patients. With AI in healthcare, diagnosing has become faster. Robotic surgery with AI assistance is a revolutionary advancement in medical technology. It has given rise to a brand-new premium version that can be used in surgical situations. By giving the exact measurements needed for micro surgeries, AI-assisted robotic surgery can assist surgeons in performing their work with a higher level of accuracy, precision, and control. It can operate patients with less pain and more reliability. Utilizing a health tracking system, people's lives have already seen a radical transformation. Smart watches now come with built-in health tracking software that provides transparent statistics on oxygen saturation, heart rate, blood pressure, and the reminder time for sleeping and being active. Applications that make use of healthcare Informatics improve accessibility for people. Using AI, vocal biomarkers are causing yet another revolution in the healthcare sector. For patient remote monitoring, vocal biomarkers are utilized. It can be easy for patients to plan ahead for future health issues and medications with the information provided in a short 30-second voice sample. It operates by using electronic devices to gather and store health and medical information in one area, then having diagnosticians review that information in a different location. Aging patients, people with chronic illnesses, and others can better manage their health remotely by Remote Patients Monitoring (RPM). This worked well during the COVID-19 pandemic. Remote patient tracking from one location to another allowed diagnosers to follow patients. Although it is currently a wearable device, it has already begun to become more straightforward and persistent. No more straps and bands. Everything will be integrated directly into the everyday devices that we use. Patient convenience is increased through at-home lab tests. Pregnancy screenings and blood sugar checks for diabetics were among the laboratory tests available at home. Acquiring knowledge can help people make better decisions about their future treatment and health maintenance. It is accessible for less money and produces precise results. Frequent trips to diagnosticians have decreased as a result. Increasingly, people may perform DNA tests in their homes using saliva swabs, which can provide a good understanding of diseases. It is accessible for testing for food sensitivity tests, infertility tests, HIV, and other illnesses like hepatitis C and COVID-19. Compared to hospital lab testing, it only requires less equipment. They can be carried anywhere conveniently and are disposable when using portable equipment. Using chatbots in traditional medicine and healthcare: Patients and the healthcare system can connect continuously and diligently using chatbots. Patients might express their personal opinions and any difficulties they had with the treatment. It gives the hospital patients a reason to feel confident. It can assist with routine data collection, appointment scheduling, reminders, tracking improvements, checking for medical facilities, and caring for the patients' mental health during tough situations. Patients can ask chatbots questions about almost everything. It can keep monitoring each patient, individually. It can manage all of the patient data from numerous hospitals. Patients will feel free to express themselves when these chatbots are used in hospitals, giving them hope for a quick recovery from illness. As a multidimensional idea, digital health insurance provides a framework from the points where technology and healthcare converge. The internet of things (IoT) and augmented reality can make digital health insurance feasible. It can provide improvised, affordable medical care. A cultural revolution is beginning with digital health insurance. Through applications that are insurance-oriented, it may provide individuals with easy explanations and clear thoughts. The digitalization of insurance is offered at extremely cheap cost and minimal risk, and it links individuals with ease. Data is kept in a highly secure way.

With the use of past records on health conditions and current health information, preventative medicine serves as a precaution to ward off diseases. It emphasizes the protection of humans against diseases. We have long practiced preventative medicine. One such approach we have used for children is vaccination. Children of all ages will receive immunizations until they reach a particular age. AI-based preventative medicine has improved the medical sector. It is helpful in forecasting the disease's potential effects in the future. Medical errors are being eliminated by preventative medicine. The data is visualized using diagnostic and visual data. Data visualization can aid diagnosticians in making diagnoses that take into account the patient's potential future effects. AI is frequently used to identify diseases that are spreading in a community and is helpful in studying the causes of the illness spread. It can also determine which group of people will be afflicted and how long it will take them to recover. AI is used to foresee the chemical and pharmacological properties of drug discovery and design. Delivering the appropriate care to the appropriate patients with great efficiency and accuracy is the goal of a developed healthcare system. AI plays a significant impact on the mental health of people. Patients with mental illnesses typically have a lot to say, but they avoid doing so due to their own assumptions and judgments about other people. Here, AI will assist these individuals in speaking up, expressing their viewpoints, and expressing their emotions. By analyzing their current mental state, AI can provide these individuals with counseling and therapeutic interventions. Depending on their emotional condition and the results of the report analysis, each patient receives a unique treatment. Digital nurses represent yet another AI revolution. In hospitals, nurses typically care for patients more effectively than doctors do. When this is digitalized using AI, it will have some exciting striking similarities to those of doctors as can be seen in Figure 3.4. It can handle routine patient monitoring, check for medical availability, and assure individualized care for each patient.

5 WEARABLE TECHNOLOGY IN HEALTHCARE

Wearable technologies with AI have made huge changes in the life of people making life more convenient and even providing great assistance for a number of daily activities. Providing care for the aged population is a challenging task, as with advancements in aging, the body conditions such as disabilities, risk of falling down, and chronic conditions have increased. A fraction of these issues can be addressed with the help of wearable devices [30]. Fall indication algorithms for wearable devices have been developed in recent years that take motion information from the movement of individuals through two tri-axle accelerometer bracelet devices in order to analyze the data based on which intimation to the concerned will be sent when there is a risk of the patient showing uncoordinated movements.

Physical activity monitoring is another such area where wearable devices have been shown to be useful. One study where a student's posture can be changed

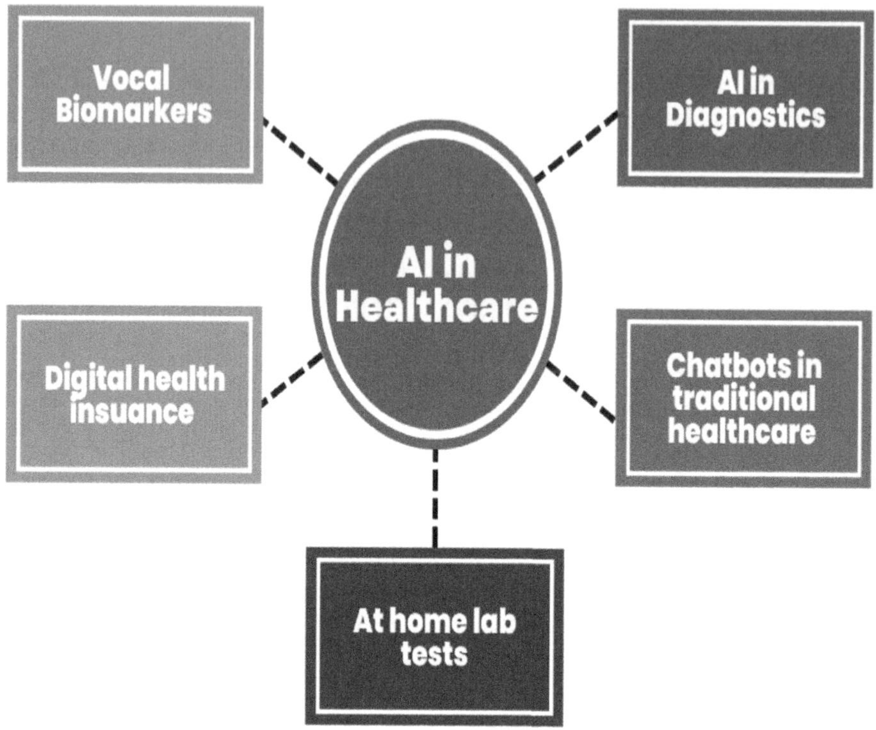

FIGURE 3.4　Recent AI Developments in Healthcare

based on frequent reminders was conducted with the help of a wearable device that produced vibrations for a fixed period of time in regular intervals thereby making it an effective strategy for habitual changes. Human physiological status detection has been a widely incorporated feature in wearable devices these days and the same is also found to be used for collecting information about mental status if modified slightly. The sensors of heart rate monitoring and audio sensor in the wearable device are combined with an ML algorithm and are used for stress detection in small children. Similarly, a slightly elegant way of using of electro-dermal activity sensor for stress detection has been used as skin conductance has been shown to have a greater correlation with the stress level of an individual.

In the field of sports, wearable technologies are being incorporated in order to record the status of the player during training and during the game. Similarly, the field of fitness is also greatly assisted by these devices as they track the physical activity that is being done. Although these devices assist, it has been observed that when compared to the gold standard dedicated sensors that are made specifically for tracking a particular exercise these perform at a much lower level thereby proving a minimal stimulus mechanism. Recently, point-of-care diagnostic devices and garments that are integrated with portable sensors are being tested for incorporation in the intensive care units, emergency medical services, or emergency room environments for continuous detection of parameters such as patient's blood oxygen saturation, breathing rate, the temperature of the body, heart rate and even external environmental variables such as temperature and pressure of the unit. Wearable digital watches have been studied for monitoring the vital signs of the patient remotely. Results of the studies showed that the device provided a reliable heart rate recording throughout all the activities performed by the individual. This provided an out-of-the-laboratory assessment feature therefore not interfering with the everyday activity of that individual.

6 ARTIFICIAL INTELLIGENCE-BASED PRODUCTS IN HEALTHCARE DOMAIN

There are medical devices that are effectively being used by people all around nowadays. Most of these medical gadgets are cooperating with AI to produce high-quality results with improved latency. Automated medical care devices are something that will focus on treating the patients with high accuracy, notifying the redundant healthcare tasks, patient chat bots, managing health records, virtual assistants, contacting the doctors in the emergency periods, etc. Having the AI trained to monitor and diagnosing devices it can separately become a personal doctor in many situations. The lifestyle where patients need to meet and contact for every single issue they face after any surgery or treatment is changing as patients just need a device to clarify all kinds of doubts and questions they have.

6.1 KARDIA

As a forerunner in mobile health technologies, AliveCor created the iPhone ECG recorder Kardia. A medical device called Kardia is used to track heartbeats and identify disorders like atrial fibrillation. It is the first portable, medical-grade ECG monitor that has received FDA clearance. The tool uses an app to record and analyze your ECG and is Bluetooth-connected to your smartphone. The app has features that let you share your results with your healthcare practitioner and provides feedback on heart rate, rhythm, and arrhythmia detection. AFib, bradycardia, tachycardia, and other arrhythmia can all be found using the instrument. For those who wish to monitor their heart health without the burden of seeing a doctor, the device is the best option because it is simple to use and understand. Kardia's tiny size and portability make it simple for users to carry and use anywhere, making it simple for people to frequently monitor their heart health.

- Simple electrocardiogram reading with Kardia simply takes a little touch to the chest, making it simple for users to use independently.
- Results are available instantly, enabling users to see their heart health status in real-time, following an ECG reading performed with Kardia.
- Mobile device integration: Kardia works with tablets and smartphones, making it simple for users to monitor their heart health and communicate the data with their doctors.

6.2   EMBRACE 2

A wearable device called Embrace 2 is intended to detect potential seizures and notify the user of them. It is a smart bracelet featuring sensors that can track the wearer's temperature, skin conductance, and activity. The wearer and any designated carers will receive a vibrating alert if the device notices a seizure-like pattern. Embrace 2 is designed to assist epilepsy sufferers and their carers to feel more secure and informed about their disease. The wearer's seizures can also be tracked by the device, and insights into their causes, frequency, and length can be provided. This data can help medical experts manage the wearer's condition. It is essential to remember that Embrace 2 is not a medical gadget and shouldn't be used in place of expert medical guidance and care. The gadget is not meant to be used to diagnose or treat epilepsy; rather, it is meant to offer additional information and assistance to those who have it.

- Comprehensive health tracking: Embrace2 tracks various aspects of health, including sleep, stress, physical activity, and seizures, providing individuals with a comprehensive view of their health.
- Advanced sensing technology: Embrace2 uses advanced sensors to accurately and continuously monitor health, providing real-time data on various aspects of health.
- Seizure detection: Embrace2 is capable of detecting and alerting caregivers in the event of a seizure, allowing for prompt intervention and care.
- Long battery life: Embrace2 has a long battery life, allowing individuals to wear the device for extended periods without needing to recharge.
- Customizable notifications: Embrace2 allows individuals to customize notifications, so they can receive only the information that is relevant to them.

6.3   CLOUDMINDS

A technological startup called CloudMinds focuses on building cloud robotics platforms and intelligent robots. The company's goal is to develop intelligent robots that can help people live better lives in a variety of industries, including healthcare, logistics, and customer service. The company is known for its focus on AI and cloud computing. It is a company that promotes patients' health by reducing readmissions.

6.4   VIZ LVO

This is AI-based technology which is treating stroke using a CT scan. The stroke can be classified whether it is hemorrhagic or ischemic. It detects the stroke using Large Vessel Occlusion and provides faster real-time notifications on track. This acts to be one of the best technologies used by doctors to treat LVOs in quick time. The highlighting point of this product is, they are providing accurate results 52 minutes faster than usual time and more importantly, it can do that for multiple patients in a single toss. Across 139 hospitals in the US, they make real use of this device. With 96% of sensitivity and 94% specificity the LVOs are identified.

6.5 AIDOC

Aidoc is a healthcare technology business with its headquarters in Israel that offers AI solutions for the radiology sector. By assisting with the interpretation of medical pictures, offering decision support, and enhancing workflow effectiveness, its AI technology supports radiologists in their daily tasks. Radiologists can immediately priorities patient care by using Aidoc's AI algorithms, which are trained to spot severe conditions including strokes, traumatic injuries, and other medical crises in real time. By utilizing AI in medical imaging, the company hopes to enhance patient outcomes and save healthcare expenses.

6.6 SENSELY

Virtual healthcare solutions are offered by the healthcare technology firm Sensely to both individuals and businesses. Its main offering is Molly, a virtual nurse who combines NLP and AI to assist patients in managing their health. The virtual nurse from Sensely may assist customers to manage chronic diseases, giving health information, and, if necessary, connecting them with a live healthcare expert. By making healthcare services easily accessible to people, Sensely hopes to ease the strain on existing healthcare systems and aid in improved health management. The company's virtual healthcare platform may be adapted to match the unique requirements of various organizations and populations, and it can be incorporated into current healthcare systems.

- An intuitive and user-friendly interface is provided for patients by Sensely's virtual nurse, Molly, using conversational AI and natural language processing.
- Personalized care: Sensely's platform may be altered to cater to the unique requirements of various patients and demographics, offering individualized support.
- Integration with current healthcare systems: The Sensely platform may be easily incorporated into current healthcare systems, facilitating seamless integration and enhancing provider workflow.
- Accessible and practical: Sensely's virtual healthcare platform offers people practical healthcare services that are also accessible, relieving pressure on traditional healthcare systems.
- Evidence-based care: Sensely's virtual nurse helps people make educated decisions about their health by providing evidence-based health information and assistance.

7   PRIVACY-PRESERVING DISTRIBUTED LEARNING

Distributed learning is a methodology in which data safety is ensured by avoidance of sharing the original data across research areas and thus sharing the mathematical parameters or metadata of the entire data or its instance. This methodology thus reduces or completely annihilates the concept of tracking back the original data from the one that was provided for analysis resulting in the privacy of patient-oriented data such as name, date of birth, ID, and others varying from one source to another [31]. AI and Big data for healthcare have been potential solutions for typical problems in the healthcare domain. However, with this rapid growth and application, privacy of data and regulatory concerns are raising in an alarming manner. Thus, the distributed learning technique is found to produce a solution as if the data were centralized even by working with different instances. The data here is also fully anonymized with the help of cryptographic algorithms such as hashing algorithm therefore the model learns the data without any personal data leaving the medical centers.

8   EXAMPLES OF MACHINE LEARNING ALGORITHMS

There are three main categories of ML algorithms: Supervised algorithms which have a function that maps the input values to the output values based on the variable studied; unsupervised learning in which the algorithm is not aware of the output variable and hence creates a mapping function for the structure of the data; and lastly, reinforcement learning algorithms which are trained on limited scenario-based dataset and then provides learned outcome from the experience of the previously learned data when a new scenario is provided as input. These categories of algorithms along with the availability of distributed algorithm are tabulated in Table 3.1.

9   CASE STUDY

In the modern medical industry, AI is widely applied. The healthcare industry makes some kind of advancement every day. The goal of AI is to diagnose humans more accurately and effectively. The medical industry currently uses a wide range of new technologies. The ability to treat a patient's specific issue precisely actually helps doctors. In general, hospitals typically manage a lot of data. In order for the AI model to predict the future of the specific patient, handling each patient's radiological data is absolutely necessary. In the United States, Bronx is a community where it is termed as the poorest in the urban countryside. People there cannot afford to pay as much as those in other urban nations. When compared to the previous 10 to 20 years, there is a concurrent rise in the number of ill patients. There, Acute respiratory distress syndrome (ARDS) affects more than 40% of the population. ARDS is a respiratory condition that can be devastating and is brought on by lungs that are unable to supply enough oxygen to other vital organs. Sepsis, a disorder that develops in the bloodstream, is often what leads to ARDS. After the

TABLE 3.1
Availability of Distributed Algorithm for Machine Learning Algorithms

Type of Algorithm	Algorithm	Description	Availability of Distributed Algorithm
Supervised learning	Logistic regression	It is used for discrete value estimation of a set of independent variables by conditional probability of the occurrence of a particular event	Available
	SVM	It does classification by constructing hyperplanes in the multidimensional space separating different class labels	Available
	Decision tree	It is a non-parametric method for classification and regression problems based on conditional control statements	Available
	Random forest	This algorithm is a composition of two techniques, a decision tree and a forest algorithm that randomly selects features to put into various decision trees	Not available
	KNN	It can be used for both classification and regression but it's mostly used for classification problems. In this the algorithm works on the assumption that data items that are similar are close to each other and then it chooses K closest data and tests the data	Available

(Continued)

**TABLE 3.1
(Continued)**

Type of Algorithm	Algorithm	Description	Availability of Distributed Algorithm
Unsupervised learning	Apriori algorithm	It is one of the most popular Data mining algorithm that is used for finding frequent item-set for Boolean association rule in given database	Available
	K-means	It is a clustering algorithm. In this the data is partitioned into K clusters based on the nearest cluster mean	Available
Reinforcement learning	Q-learning	It is a type of learning algorithm in which the agent is provided with the actions and a function action-value for the action taken at a particular situation	Available
	MDP	This algorithm is similar to of other algorithms until the point to which the agent is supposed to decide the best action out of the set for the provided scenario and the repetition of this optimized step. This makes the output of the algorithm to depend on the current state and not the previous state thus following Markov's Property	Not Available

COVID-19 outbreak, ARDS cases increased. Smoking and drinking alcohol both promote ARDS throughout the body. Regular ventilation was required for these individuals, which was difficult at first. They had to decide which of the numerous patients with comparable illnesses were to be treated first because they were checking each patient one at a time, which was the traditional procedure. As a result, they were unable to identify the high-risk patient. In the community, this led to a high death toll. They applied AI to find a solution for this issue. The institution's core part is the Patient Centered Analytic Learning Machine. The patient's BP level, oxygen saturation, heart rate, and changes in their physiologic vital signs are just a few of the different types of data that PALM will gather from them. Calculating each patient's risk and informing them of it is its mission. Using this, medical professionals may quickly identify high-risk individuals.

The use of AI has already begun to replace key tasks currently carried out by human diagnosticians. Doctors perform surgeries, which are crucial portions that require a lot of patience and precision. Doctors will perform procedures with the utmost care, but it's like a knife with two sharp edges. Doctors performing surgeries won't have a clear view of the body portion or organ they're operating on. They will need to exercise greater caution in those conditions. Despite the addition of some technology to the surgical chapter of healthcare, it fell short of expectations. They lacked 3D visualization and only had 2D, as well as wrist access to the equipment. The Da Vinci System was introduced to overcome all of these issues [32]. This technology can meet the demand for improving surgical outcomes. A camera and surgical equipment will be included in the system. The display of 3D pictures of the functioning process will aid in the diagnosis. The organs will be operated by the system more precisely like what doctors do. It may produce a visual system with great performance. With few difficulties and a speedy recovery, this technology is capable of performing head, neck, heart, and gynecological procedures. It can operate on organs by itself with minor incisions, which will be a less frightening time. The controller, which will be inspected by the surgeon and controlled by hand and foot motions with a 3D high definition image, is one of the three primary modules employed in this system. All of the surgical tools and equipment, as well as the camera, will be stored on the patient cart. All surgeons will be able to see what is happening during surgery on the Vision Cart [33]. Only a few countries have access to this mechanism. The length of this procedure is up to an hour. In hospitals around the world, more than 6700 da Vinci machines are in place. The procedures differ depending on the surgery. Special training will be provided to the surgeons before they use this treatment. Open surgery and this are extremely similar. This system has created a mind-blowing system by extensively utilizing AI capabilities. This system has significantly altered the medical industry. Patients are able to resume their daily activities because of this method. Surgery is performed painlessly and without difficulties. Therefore, this has been one of the most innovative and amazing solutions that AI has delivered to the healthcare industry.

10 CONCLUSION

AI has made significant progress toward improving healthcare compared to traditional approaches. Existing AI-based methods have exponentially minimized the difficulties in diagnosis and treatment. Also AI-based tools and devices have been incorporated for a wide variety of use including personal healthcare monitoring that provides results that are near accurate to those that are produced in a dedicated lab. It also makes it possible for patients to be kept under surveillance even outside the premises of healthcare center. Noticeably, in the last few years AI haws come up with a huge number of solutions for improved treatment accuracy and decreased medical errors. Many hospitals have begun implementing AI technologies in medical suits and in intensive care unit in order to provide patient with timely support and real-time monitoring. With this enormous adaption, we also face the problem of privacy and security of the data that is being used and to mitigate this problem several approaches have been proposed out of which distributed learning algorithms have proved to be the best option. Thus adoption of AI in healthcare is crucial and with this constant improvement and research it would one time be a major part of healthcare domain.

REFERENCES

[1] Davenport, T., & Kalakota, R. (2019). The potential for artificial intelligence in healthcare. *Future Healthcare Journal*, 6(2), 94.

[2] Khanesar, M. A., Teshnehlab, M., & Shoorehdeli, M. A. (2007, June). A novel binary particle swarm optimization. In *2007 Mediterranean Conference on Control & Automation* (pp. 1–6). IEEE.

[3] Khalifa, N. E. M., Taha, M. H. N., Ali, D. E., Slowik, A., & Hassanien, A. E. (2020). Artificial intelligence technique for gene expression by tumor RNA-Seq data: a novel optimized deep learning approach. *IEEE Access*, 8, 22874–22883.

[4] Hailemariam, Y., Yazdinejad, A., Parizi, R. M., Srivastava, G., & Dehghantanha, A. (2020, December). An empirical evaluation of AI deep explainable tools. In *2020 IEEE Globecom Workshops (GC Wkshps* (pp. 1–6). IEEE

[5] Panesar, A. (2019). *Machine Learning and AI for Healthcare* (pp. 1–73). Coventry: Apress.

[6] Singh, M. S., & Choudhary, P. (2017, August). Stroke prediction using artificial intelligence. In *2017 8th Annual Industrial Automation and Electromechanical Engineering Conference (IEMECON)* (pp. 158–161). IEEE.

[7] Biswas, M., Saba, L., Omerzu, T., Johri, A. M., Khanna, N. N., Viskovic, K., ... & Suri, J. S. (2021). A review on joint carotid intima-media thickness and plaque area measurement in ultrasound for cardiovascular/stroke risk monitoring: artificial intelligence framework. *Journal of Digital Imaging*, 34(3), 581–604.

[8] Pawar, U., O'Shea, D., Rea, S., & O'Reilly, R. (2020, June). Explainable ai in healthcare. In *2020 International Conference on Cyber Situational Awareness, Data Analytics and Assessment (CyberSA)* (pp. 1–2). IEEE.

[9] Mastoli, M. M. M., Pol, U. R., & Patil, R. D. (2019). Machine learning classification algorithms for predictive analysis in healthcare. *Machine Learning*, 6(12), 1225–1229.

[10] Kherif, F., & Latypova, A. (2020). Principal component analysis. In (Eds.) Andrea Mechelli & Sandra Vieira, *Machine Learning* (pp. 209–225). Academic Press.

[11] Ellahham, S. (2020). Artificial intelligence: the future for diabetes care. *The American Journal of Medicine, 133*(8), 895–900.

[12] Kaur, P., Kumar, R., & Kumar, M. (2019). A healthcare monitoring system using random forest and internet of things (IoT). *Multimedia Tools and Applications, 78*(14), 19905–19916.

[13] Oza, A., & Bokhare, A. (2022). Diabetes prediction using logistic regression and K-nearest neighbor. In (Eds.) Mukesh Saraswat, Harish Sharma, K. Balachandran, Joong Hoon Kim, Jagdish Chand Bansal, *Congress on Intelligent Systems* (pp. 407–418). Singapore: Springer.

[14] Daghistani, T., & Alshammari, R. (2020). Comparison of statistical logistic regression and random forest machine learning techniques in predicting diabetes. *Journal of Advances in Information Technology, 11*(2), 78–83.

[15] Osareh, A., & Shadgar, B. (2010, April). Machine learning techniques to diagnose breast cancer. In *2010 5th International Symposium on Health Informatics and Bioinformatics* (pp. 114–120). IEEE.

[16] Cahoon, T. C., Sutton, M. A., & Bezdek, J. C. (2000, May). Breast cancer detection using image processing techniques. In *Ninth IEEE International Conference on Fuzzy Systems. FUZZ-IEEE 2000 (Cat. No. 00CH37063)* (Vol. 2, pp. 973–976) IEEE.

[17] Sadhukhan, S., Upadhyay, N., & Chakraborty, P. (2020). Breast cancer diagnosis using image processing and machine learning. In (Eds.) Jyotsna Kumar Mandal & Debika Bhattacharya, *Emerging Technology in Modelling and Graphics* (pp. 113–127). Singapore: Springer.

[18] Aghamohammadi, M., Madan, M., Hong, J. K., & Watson, I. (2019, June). Predicting heart attack through explainable artificial intelligence. In *International Conference on Computational Science* (pp. 633–645). Springer, Cham.

[19] Mercuri, M., Liu, Y. H., Lorato, I., Torfs, T., Wieringa, F., Bourdoux, A., & Van Hoof, C. (2018). A direct phase-tracking Doppler radar using wavelet independent component analysis for non-contact respiratory and heart rate monitoring. *IEEE Transactions on Biomedical Circuits and Systems, 12*(3), 632–643.

[20] Krishnani, D., Kumari, A., Dewangan, A., Singh, A., & Naik, N. S. (2019, October). Prediction of coronary heart disease using supervised machine learning algorithms. In *TENCON 2019–2019 IEEE Region 10 Conference (TENCON)* (pp. 367–372). IEEE.

[21] Singh, B., & Tawfik, H. (2019, June). A machine learning approach for predicting weight gain risks in young adults. In *2019 10th International Conference on Dependable Systems, Services and Technologies (DESSERT)* (pp. 231–234). IEEE.

[22] Singh, B., & Tawfik, H. (2020, June). Machine learning approach for the early prediction of the risk of overweight and obesity in young people. In *International Conference on Computational Science* (pp. 523–535). Springer, Cham.

[23] Montañez, C. A. C., Fergus, P., Hussain, A., Al-Jumeily, D., Abdulaimma, B., Hind, J., & Radi, N. (2017, May). Machine learning approaches for the prediction of obesity using publicly available genetic profiles. In *2017 International Joint Conference on Neural Networks (IJCNN)* (pp. 2743–2750).

[24] Ahn, S. H., Wang, C., Shin, G. W., Park, D., Kang, Y. H., Joibi, J. C., & Yun, M. H. (2018, December). Comparison of clustering methods for obesity classification. In *2018 IEEE International Conference on Industrial Engineering and Engineering Management (IEEM)* (pp. 1821–1825). IEEE.

[25] Adnan, M. H. B. M., & Husain, W. (2012, June). A hybrid approach using Naïve Bayes and Genetic Algorithm for childhood obesity prediction. In *2012 International Conference on Computer & Information Science (ICCIS)* (Vol. 1, pp. 281–285). IEEE.

[26] Archana, R., & Rajathilagam, B. (2022). Comparative analysis of obesity level estimation based on lifestyle using machine learning. In *Intelligent Sustainable Systems* (pp. 101–114). Singapore: Springer.

[27] Parra, D., Gutiérrez-Gallego, A., Garnica, O., Velasco, J. M., Zekri-Nechar, K., Zamorano-León, J. J., … & Hidalgo, J. I. (2022). Predicting the risk of overweight and obesity in Madrid—a binary classification approach with evolutionary feature selection. *Applied Sciences*, *12*(16), 8251.

[28] Alhassan, A. M., & Zainon, W. M. N. W. (2021). Review of feature selection, dimensionality reduction and classification for chronic disease diagnosis. *IEEE Access*, *9*, 87310–87317.

[29] Kwak, G. H., & Hui, P. (2019). DeepHealth: review and challenges of artificial intelligence in health informatics. arXiv preprint arXiv:1909.00384.

[30] Wu, M., & Luo, J. (2019). Wearable technology applications in healthcare: a literature review. *Online Journal of Nursing Informatics*, *23*(3).

[31] Zerka, F., Barakat, S., Walsh, S., Bogowicz, M., Leijenaar, R. T., Jochems, A., … & Lambin, P. (2020). Systematic review of privacy-preserving distributed machine learning from federated databases in health care. *JCO Clinical Cancer Informatics*, *4*, 184–200.

[32] DiMaio, S., Hanuschik, M., & Kreaden, U. (2011). The da Vinci surgical system. In *Surgical robotics* (pp. 199–217). Boston, MA: Springer.

[33] Sung, G. T., & Gill, I. S. (2001). Robotic laparoscopic surgery: a comparison of the da Vinci and Zeus systems. *Urology*, *58*(6), 893–898.

[34] Beri, M., Kumar, B., Tiwari, S., Sharma, N., Vashishtya, H., & Chaudhary, P. (2022, April). IoT Based Health Monitoring System Built on ESP32. In *2022 2nd International Conference on Advance Computing and Innovative Technologies in Engineering (ICACITE)* (pp. 454–458). IEEE.

4 A Review of Deep Learning Applications in Modernized Healthcare Services

Umamaheswari Rajasekaran, M Bhagampriyal, A Malini, and Mohd Asif Shah

1 INTRODUCTION

"Good Health is above wealth" is the most appropriate proverb to begin this chapter. Today's contemporary lifestyle has had a substantial negative impact on human health, resulting in a number of chronic diseases. In the upcoming years, the risk of disease onset will increase as a result of shifting land-use patterns, dietary preferences, climate change and rapid industrialization. Sustaining a healthy lifestyle has become challenging in today's hectic work schedule. Think about a person who has had a terrible cough for two or more weeks. To determine whether he has a typical cough or tuberculosis, a diagnostic test is necessary. Deep learning (DL) is used for diagnosis assisting the patient in receiving the best care. For climatic changes, using contextual data provided to the model, DL can combat climate change by augmenting or changing technological systems to better utilize resources. The algorithmic development of DL related to disease diagnosis exemplifies the value of technology in healthcare profession. The definition of DL is that it is a subset of machine learning (ML) and it is series of algorithms developed in multiple layers based on artificial neural networks (ANN). These multiple layers are in charge of obtaining certain data. The physiological neural systems served as an inspiration for neural networks. Convolution gives more and accurate data which helps the physicians to notice the changes in their patients. Artificial intelligence (AI) in the form of DL has great potential for enhancing the precision and speed of medical imaging diagnostics. DL can be viewed as a pathway leading from large-scale medical data to enhanced human health care. Implementing DL into medical fields will have positive effects in improving health care. DL is used in health care because of its superior performance, ability to handle complex data and many other features [1]. DL is implemented in health care as it gives more accurate results based on image learning and voice recognition which will be used in treating various diseases. In fact, using DL,

DOI: 10.1201/9781003377818-4

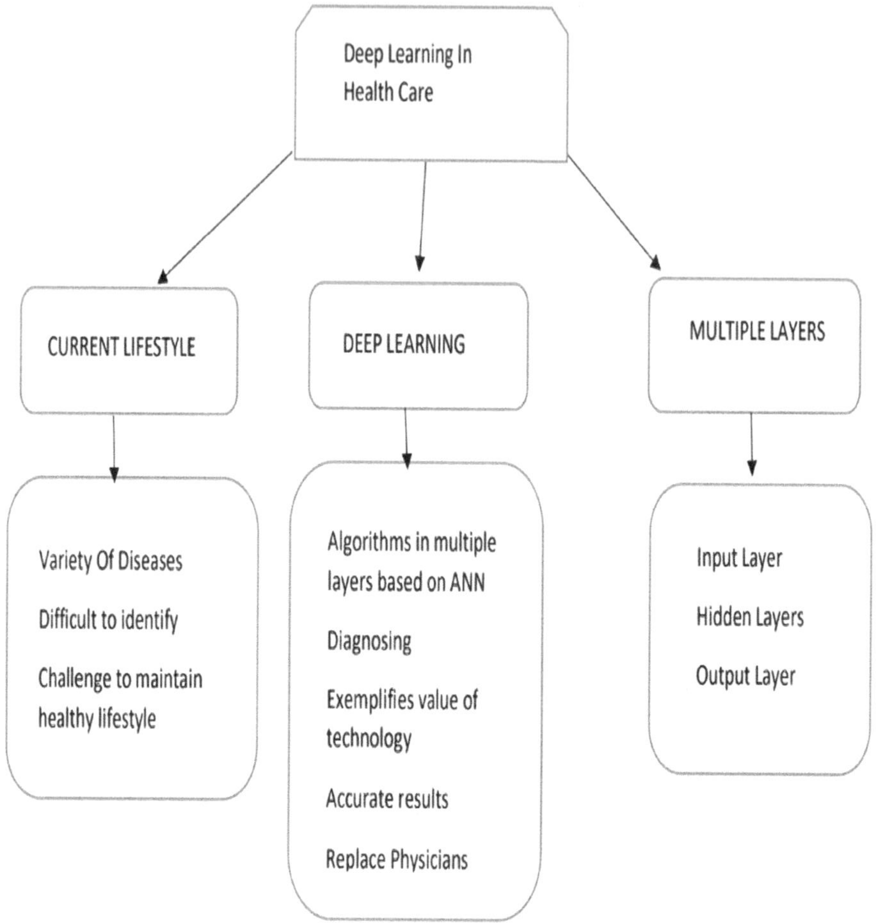

FIGURE 4.1 Deep Learning in Healthcare Industry

computer model built from several neural network processing layers can learn data representation with different levels of abstraction. Based on the input, each layer of DL builds a representation of observable patterns. The applications of DL technology, the overview of the technicalities are depicted in the Figure 4.1.

These layers are not designed by humans but they are learned from the general-purpose learning procedure. ANNs with multiple layers are known as deep neural networks. Every layer is in charge of obtaining some data, which is represented as a score times weight, and passing it to the following layer. The output is the total of all values associated with a certain input [2]. The input layer is responsible for gaining the input data, hidden layers are responsible for storing the associated weights, and the output layer produces the output results. DL algorithms can also replace medical professionals in fields. In the next generation, knowledge on ML and DL is essential for physicians to deal with close scrutiny of images of cells, radiology etc., In order to provide better healthcare, this paper will examine how DL is used in the medical field. This essay also discusses the

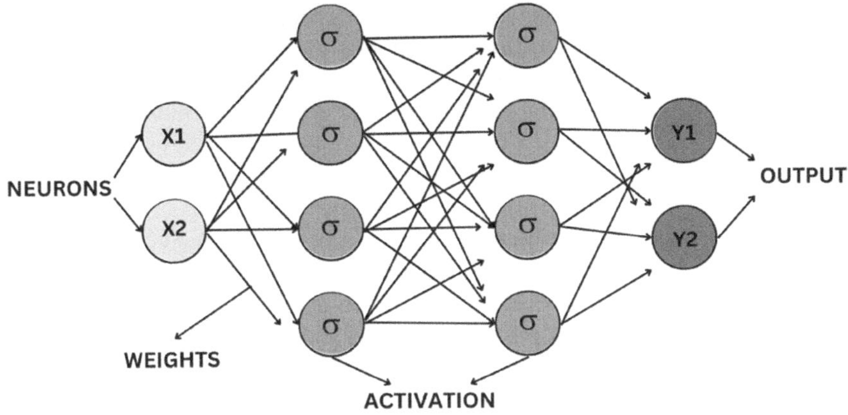

FIGURE 4.2   Neural Network Layers

difficulties that the modern medical industry faces and the most recent developments in DL technology [3].

In Figure 4.2, the input layer, which is utilized to feed the input, is made up of neurons. The layers between the input and output layers are known as the hidden layers. The network's output is created by the output layer. The output of each neuron serves as an input for every other neuron in the layer below. Therefore, the output of a single neuron won't matter to the following layer if it is not active or fired.

2   DL A REVOLUTION IN MEDICAL FIELDS

The medical field has already benefited greatly from DL. Medical data plays a more important role in treating a patient. "The appropriate treatment is provided to the appropriate patient at the appropriate time" with the help of sufficient data. As technologies advance, health care research faces additional difficulties. DL is playing a great role in natural language processing tasks, speech recognition, etc. [4]. DL can be used to introduce many new opportunities for health care. In DL medical fields is widely used in the areas of detection, genomics, drug development, electronic health record, and medical image. "Your well-being is your greatest wealth". ML doesn't need any prior introduction to learn anything. It will learn the relation between them through the data available [4]. Unlike ML, DL learns representation from raw data [5]. Computer models with several neural networks processing layers can learn embeddings with various levels of abstraction with the help of DL. ANNs have 3 layers of neural networks but DL architectures have multilayers.

The effective tuning of deep networks and extraction of deep structure from input to improve predictions is made possible by layer-wise unsupervised learning. Clinical success through DL includes skin classification, and diabetic retinopathy detection [2]. DL is used in genomics to capture the internal structures of high dimensional datasets. Energy Expenditure (EE) can be used to track the personal activity of a person which helps in chronic diseases such as diabetes, obesity, thyroid etc., with the help of CNN (Convulsion Neural Networks). DL can be used to introduce many new opportunities for health care. Google Deep Mind has a plan to improve health care [4]. In today's growing technology, wearable devices like smart watches monitor the physical activities of the individual and sends any alert or report to their mobile phones using DL methodology. Further, DL is also used to spot the errors in the prescription provided by the physician. In future, there are many possibilities for DL model to collaborate with medical professionals.

While everyone is aware of Internet of Things (IoT) many people are not aware of IoMTs. IoMT stands for Internet of Medical Things. IoMT refers to a network of networked electronic devices explicitly built to provide medical services. Examples include systems for remote and telemedicine care, illness, patient monitoring, conditioning, and abnormalities. The availability of wide range of medical data brings more opportunities and challenges in the field of health care. These challenges could be solved only with the help of ML. So, the advancement in medical fields is possible only with the help of computer technology. One of the most reliable sources of diagnostic data is medical imaging, but it relies on human interpretation and experiences of rowing resource problems. With the help of AI in the subfield of ML, it will be solved. The over-excitement in the research of DL field should not override the requirement for critical analysis. Medical fields have concerns of whether the study designs are biased or generalizable, whether it is performed in clinical environment, or silico [6].

As of now, 30 algorithms have been agreed to be brought into use by the US Food and Drug Administration. The first application of DL in health care data was on image processing. It is used to analyze the brain Magnetic Resonance Imaging (MRI). It treats Alzheimer's disease [4]. Strokes cause some brain parts to fail their functioning because of ischemic or bleeding death. Such malignant strokes can be detected using CT and MRI scans [7]. Heart diseases, cancers, and tumors are diagnosed using MRI scan, CT scan, and ECG with the help of DL. Maintaining an up-to-date document of a patient's health record manually is difficult. So, there DL techniques are used. DL is also capable of predicting risks [8]. DL plays a vital role in health insurance as it can predict the future trends and help the clients to escape from fraudulence. To clinical staff, DL algorithms have similar sensitivity and specificity. Data is required for any outcome of results for a given problem. Therefore, big data and DL are interconnected to each other and they rely on statistical models for the operation of data. The missing and inappropriate data can be predicted using Long Short-Term Memory-based DL. These types of data found to be missing are due to patient movement, wrong entry of data, faulty kits, etc. This Long Short-Term Memory (LSTM) is performed using Linear Regression and Gaussian Process Regression method. LSTM based on DL detects atrial fibrillation by using heart rate signals [9]. Internet and electronic applications are essential in the field of medical science. Therefore, MIoT (Medical Internet of Things) plays a crucial role in human life [3]. It is used in wearable sensor devices which detects the physical body condition and intimates if, any action is required.

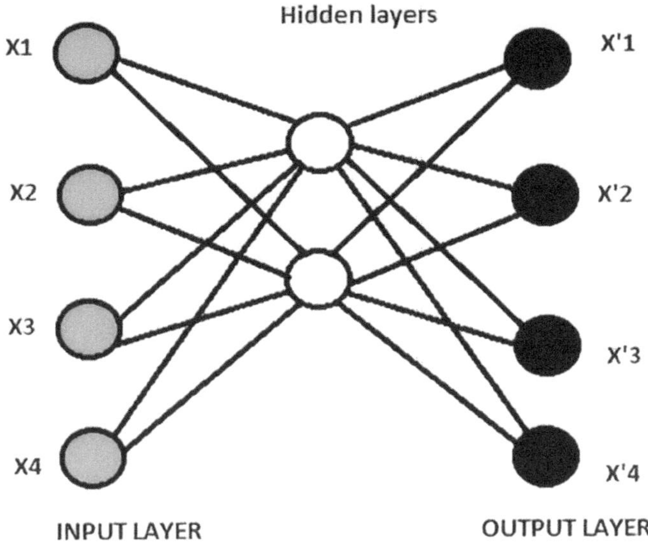

FIGURE 4.3   Auto Encoder Models

2.1   AUTO ENCODER MODELS

An unsupervised learning algorithm is the auto encoder. Both the input and output are the same. It reconstructs the output after compressing the input into a less complex code. The latent space representation is a term that is occasionally used to describe the code. It is the simplified method of compressing the data. Autoencoder consists of the following: encoder, code, and decoder. Autoencoder decreases dimension [10]. In Figure 4.3, encoder creates the code while compressing the input. The input is then rebuilt using only the code by the decoder. Autoencoder models find numerous application of data compression – they reduce dimensionality representation of data, etc. Autoencoders are one of the most important algorithms in DL that is used in image-based processing tasks, such as image inpainting, image generation, etc. Besides autoencoders, Generative Adversarial Networks are used widely for inpainting tasks. The trending models, such as DALL-E by OpenAI, StyleGAN-NVIDIA are most celebrated outcomes of Generative Adversarial Networks (Figure 4.4).

2.2   BOLTZMANN MACHINE MODELS

Restricted Boltzmann Machines (RBMs) are unsupervised ML algorithms. Boltzmann's machines are two-layered neural networks. The visible or input layer is layer one of the RBM, while the buried layer is layer two. Nodes can be linked among layers, but not within the same layer. Absence of communication between layers in an RBM is the restriction in RBMs. Input is processed at a node, which

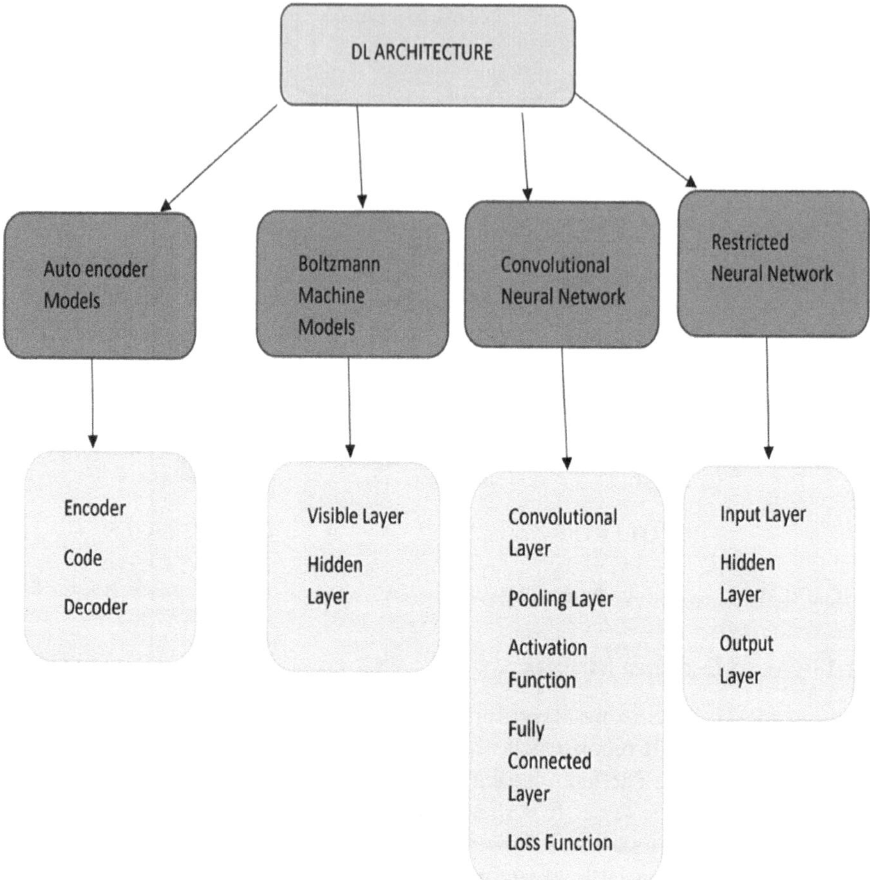

FIGURE 4.4 Types of Deep Learning Architecture

then makes a probabilistic choice about whether or not to transmit it [10]. The hidden layer is triggered when the input layer is taken into consideration utilizing the weights and biased concepts. It doesn't have an output layer. Thus, the input layer is rebuilt using the activated hidden state rather than computing the output layer. Through the active hidden neurons, the input layer is retraced. Following this, the input is reconfigured using the hidden state that has been activated. As shown in Figure 4.3, H1 and H2 hidden units are activated by the visible V1 unit, and the H2 and H3 hidden units are activated by the visible V2. Now that if any new visible unit V3 has entered the machine, V3 activates the H1 and H2 units as well. As a result, it is simple to trace back the hidden units and to determine that the new V5 neuron shares many properties with the V1 neuron. This is due to the earlier activation of the identical hidden unit by V1 (Figure 4.5).

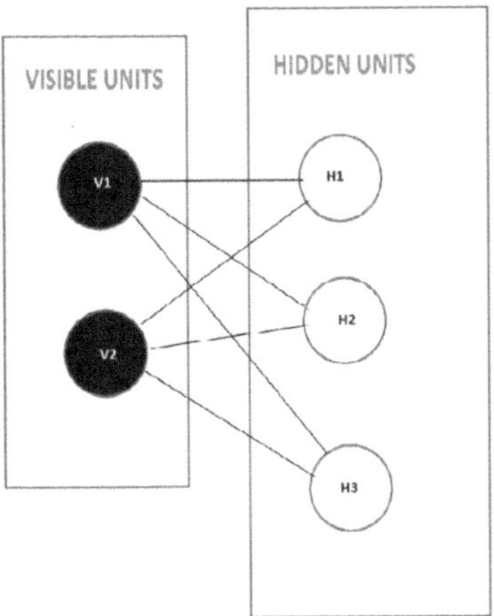

FIGURE 4.5   Boltzmann Machine Models

2.3   CONVOLUTION NEURAL NETWORKS (CNN)

A CNN is a supervised method that can take an input image, rank various items in the image according to importance, and then separate and distinguish the input image from others. CNN is primarily utilized in image classification and analysis, natural language processing, and video and image recognition. A CNN's job is to condense images into a format that is simpler to process. When utilizing the feature detector, some information from the image will be lost, but the essential features needed to obtain a reliable forecast won't be. CNN is employed to address image-related concerns, and hence it is able to address problems that may be presented as images [10]. The CNN architecture is made up of several layers.

2.3.1   Convolutional Layer

Convolutional layers are one of the important advancements of DL that enhanced the trend of image processing. The classical statistical approaches are replaced with neural network approaches in the field of image processing. Kernel, also called as the filter is the key element that performs the convolution operation within the neighborhood of the image pixels. Generally, the kernel is initialized randomly. The values may also be sampled from a pre-defined distribution like Gaussian distribution. During the training process, the values are adjusted so that it derives the correct estimate of the feature map. There can be multiple kernels used in a single convolutional layer, and the sizes of the kernels are generally estimated as 3x3, 5x5, 7x7, etc. There are 3 types of Convolutional Layers available in the Keras library, namely Conv1D, Conv2D, and Conv3D. The distinction between different types of layers lies in the dimensions of movement. Conv1D kernel moves in 1 dimension, Conv2D moves in 2 dimensions, and Conv3D moves in 3 dimensions. Stride specifies the degree of overlap between two adjacent applications of kernels. A stride value set to 1, moves the kernel by unit in every axis individually, stride set

$$\begin{bmatrix} 1 & 3 & 1 \\ 2 & 3 & 2 \\ 1 & 3 & 1 \end{bmatrix} X \begin{bmatrix} 1 & 4 & 1 \\ 2 & 3 & 1 \\ 2 & 3 & 2 \end{bmatrix} = 42$$

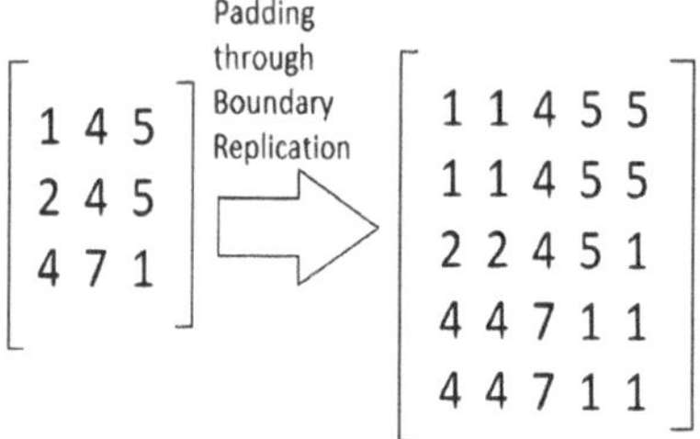

FIGURE 4.6 Convolution Operation between a 3×3 kernel and 3×3 Image

FIGURE 4.7 Padding through Boundary Replication

2 moves the kernel by 2 units in every axis. Padding specifies the additional pixels appended as the border pixels. The choice of adding additional pixels may be through zero padding (generally preferred) or through boundary replication process. The following figures demonstrate the convolution operation in 2 dimensions, padding process, and the stride operation (Figure 4.6).

In the above image, the left matrix represents a 3X3 kernel. Assuming the positions start with 0,0, the center pixel is chosen as 1,1 as shown by the yellow boundary. Convolution operation between a kernel and an image is the sum of the multiples of every (i,j) pixel of the kernel with the (i,j) pixel of the image. Hence the result is, 1*1 + 3*4 + 1*1 + 2*2 + 3*3 + 2*1 +1*2 + 3*3 + 1*2 = 42 (Figures 4.7 and 4.8).

The above 2 figures demonstrate the padding operation. Generally, padding is done so that every pixel in the image can be acted upon (as the center pixel of the kernel). We can see from the above figure that, in order to use the 0,0 pixel and the 2,2 pixel as the center pixels of the kernel, 3x3 image slice has been padded to 5x5 dimension using different techniques of boundary replication and zero padding. Other than these 2 techniques, some constants can also be used (Figure 4.9).

In the above figure, assuming 0,0 as the starting position, pixel (8) at (0,1) is taken as the center pixel. 8+4+1=13 which is at (0,0) of the output frame, Then, the very adjacent pixel (4) at (0,2) is taken as the center pixel followed by pixel(2) at (0,3). The above image demonstrates convolution operation using a 1x3 kernel on 1x5 input images. It demonstrates a convolutional operation in 1 dimension. The same procedure will be followed for convolution operation in 2 dimension and 3 dimensions.

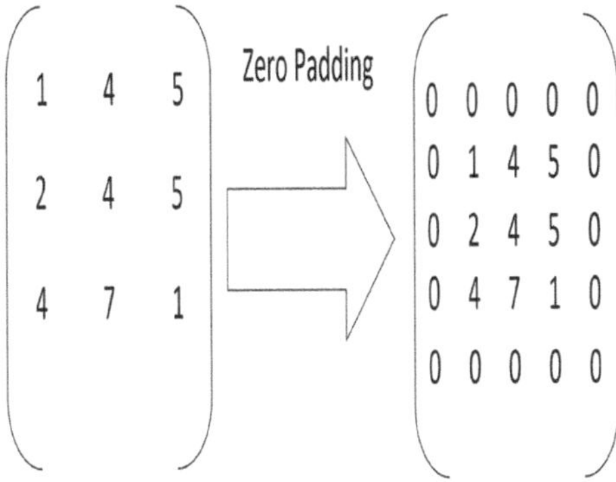

FIGURE 4.8   Zero Padding

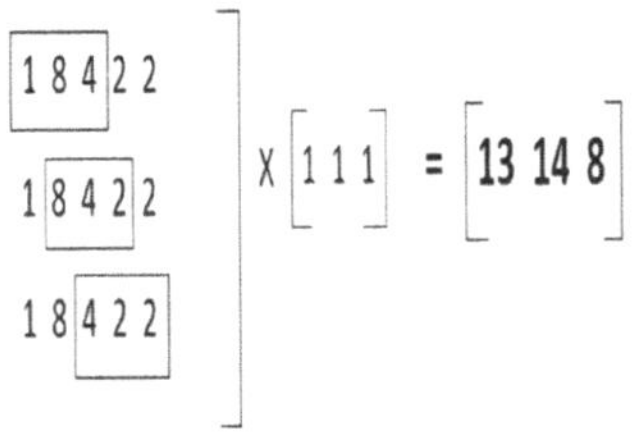

$$\begin{bmatrix} 1\ 8\ 4\ 2\ 2 \\ 1\ 8\ 4\ 2\ 2 \\ 1\ 8\ 4\ 2\ 2 \end{bmatrix} \times \begin{bmatrix} 1\ 1\ 1 \end{bmatrix} = \begin{bmatrix} 13\ 14\ 8 \end{bmatrix}$$

FIGURE 4.9   Stride Operation With a Stride of 1

2.4   RECURRENT NEURAL NETWORKS

The Recurrent Neural Network (RNN) is also a kind of ANN. The only kind of neural network that has internal memory is this one. RNNs are able to recall crucial details about the input they receive as a result. An RNN model is trained to identify sequential patterns in data and utilize those patterns to make extremely accurate predictions about the future. The decision is based on the current input and the previous input. Typically, RNNs have a short-term memory. They possess long-term memory when coupled with LSTM [10].

In Figure 4.10, a single layer of recurrent neural networks is created and the nodes from several layers of the neural network are compressed. The network's parameters are A, B, and C.

2.5   LONG SHORT-TERM MEMORY

An ANN called LSTM is employed in DL and AI. LSTM features feedback connections as opposed to typical feedforward neural networks. Such an RNN may analyze whole data sequences (video) in addition to single data points (image). Because of this quality, LSTM networks are perfect for handling and making predictions about data. A cell, an input gate, an output gate, and a forget gate make up a typical LSTM unit. By assigning a value between 0 and 1 to a previous state

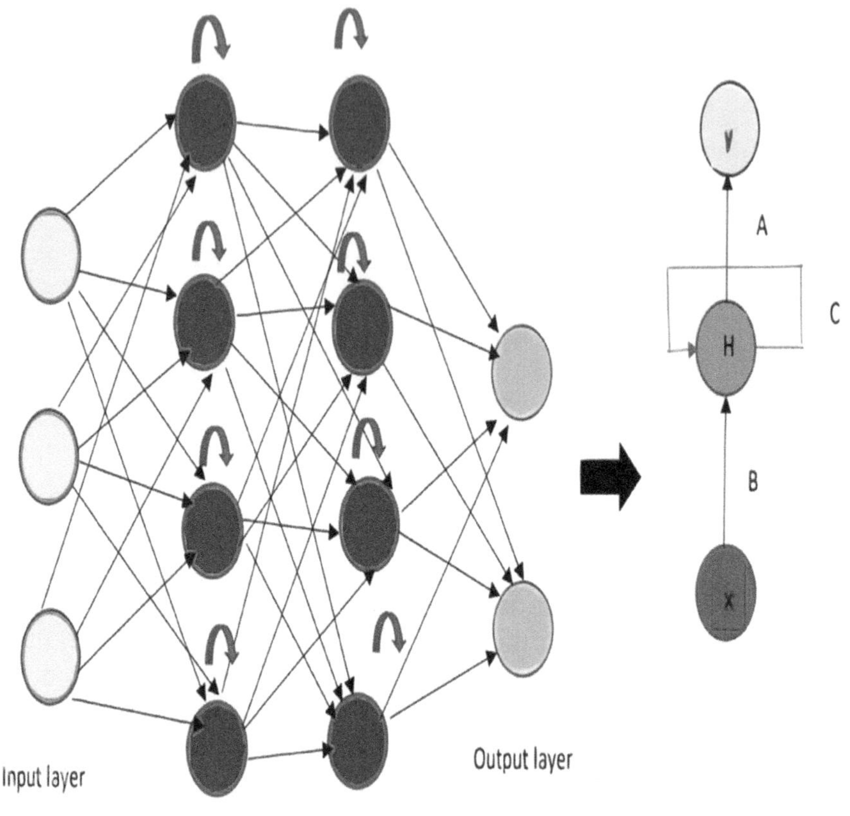

FIGURE 4.10　Recurrent Neural Networks

in comparison to a current input, forget gates choose which information from a previous state to discard. A number of 0 signifies to throw away the information, whereas a value of 1 means to maintain it. Input gates decide which brand-new pieces of data are to be kept in the existing state. By giving each piece of information in the current state a value between 0 and 1, output gates can decide which information to output while taking into account both the past and current states. The LSTM network can preserve valuable, long-term dependencies to make predictions, both in present and future time-steps, by selectively outputting relevant data from the current state (Figure 4.11).

This image shows that by gathering the necessary information and processing the data, missing data may be anticipated using LSTM-based DL [9].

DL is built on a foundation of artificial neurons that relates closely to those found in the human brain. A perceptron is also called an artificial neuron. By using a series of inputs, with each having a specific weight, it mimics the function

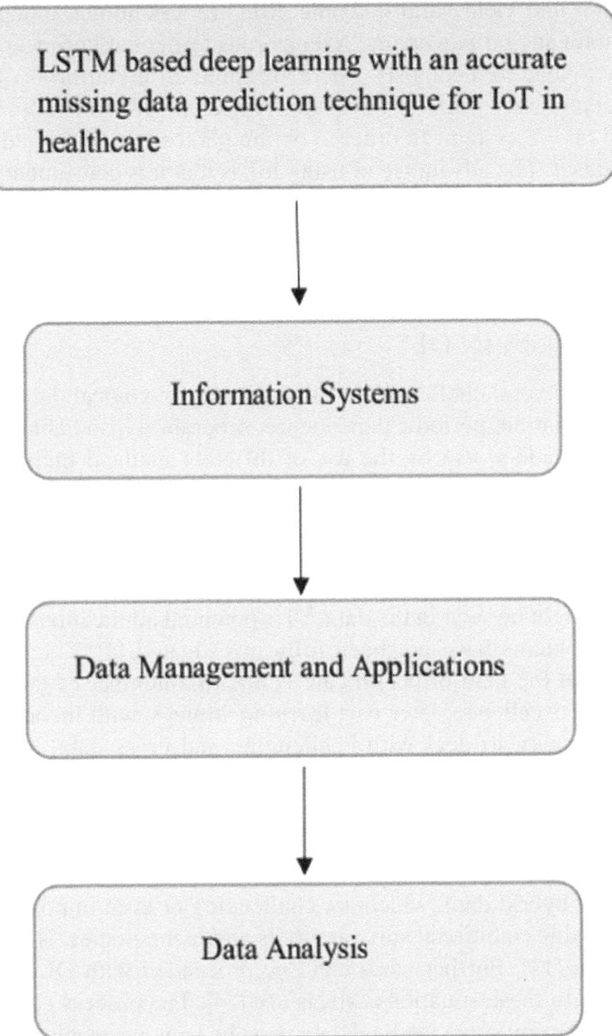

FIGURE 4.11 Missing Data Prediction

of a neuron based on these weighted inputs, the neuron does some computation and generates an output. N inputs are given to the neuron. It adds the inputs, makes a change (activation), and produces the result. The weight of a specific input shows its strength. It enables the model to have the best suitable fit to the data. Inputs are transformed into outputs via an activation function. CNN can be used in an IoT framework to categorize strokes through CT scans and identify whether the brain is healthy, the stroke is ischemic, or it is caused due to bleeding. Similarly, lung cancer poses a great threat to humans. Lung tumor is of 2 types, namely malignant and benign. Here, deep reinforcement learning can identify the type of tumor and yield valid outcome. IoTs are less human independent and it doesn't contain any human errors. A dangerous form of skin cancer, melanoma is more likely to lead to melanosis. There are three different forms of melanocytic lesions: melanomas, common nevi, and typical nevi. Skin lesions are categorized based on IoT system. In order to obtain photos, the suggested method used CNN on dataset. The advantage of using IoT is that it is convenient and usable in all situations. Its drawback is that it requires internet accessibility. Stable internet connection is necessary for sending photos and connecting to LINDA API (Application Programming Interface).

3   CHALLENGES IN DL

There are still several challenges to fully utilizing biological data due to its high complexity, variation, periodic dependence, separability, and abnormality. These problems are made worse by the use of different medical ontologies' versions to generalize the data (example : SNOMED-CT, UMLS, ICD-9) SNOMED-CT stands for Systematized Nomenclature of Medicine-Clinical Terms, UMLS stands for Unified Medical Language System, and ICD-9 stands for International Classification of Disease-9th. Sometimes, several ways of expressing the same clinical trait might be seen in the data. DL's potential applications to a wide range of medical problems have not been fully investigated [4]. The primary reason for using DL in the field of health care is due to a number of factors, including its operational excellence, later part learning strategy with incorporated feature extraction, capacity to deal with challenging and cross data, and others. [11]. Despite the encouraging outcomes produced by deep architectures, there are still a number of issues that need to be resolved before DL in healthcare may be used clinically. DL techniques can't be used all the time because they need a lot of data. The exponential growth and widespread availability of discrete, continuous, categorical, or hybrid data, which are challenging or even impossible to manage and analyze using traditional software tools and technologies, is what is referred to as big data. [12]. Further steps can't be proceeded with DL if the detection data is sparse. In these situations, ML is used [4]. The process is costly, difficult, and time-consuming since medical data must be kept electronically as electronic medical records in the universal structured form in use by SNOMED, ICD-10, and other systems. Only when medicare data is organized in accordance with global standards can it be most effectively assessed and interpreted globally [13].

Studies testing DL models generally use a variety of methodologies and communicate their findings insufficiently. To guarantee the caliber and interpretability of upcoming investigations, new worldwide standards for study protocols and reporting are required, which recognizes the particular challenges of DL [14]. Though many DL architectural variants have made an effort to address this issue, more work needs to be done in order to effectively analyze large-scale, rapidly changing streaming data. These concerns include memory usage, feature selection, and missing data. Analyzing the medical big data is one of the biggest challenges. The size of the data is critical. Furthermore, it is crucial that the data contain crucial and necessary properties for the training. Due to the difficulties in producing or acquiring data, as well as the need occasionally for domain specialists to label data, some medical fields that desire to benefit from DL are constrained. The heart of the DL technique can only handle numerical input data since it is ultimately simplified to sequences of ones and zeros for the computer system [5]. Some qualitative data cannot be quickly transformed into a format that is usable, and processing can occasionally become challenging. To accurately express analogous processes and circumstances in DL, a great number of encoding, thorough math formulations in DR, and transition are required [12]. DL models with generally good performance occasionally commit catastrophic errors [15]. Patients and healthcare providers must have faith in the results of DL models for DL to have the maximum influence on healthcare delivery. Gaining public trust is another hurdle for DL models [2]. There are three main blocks faced in the development and implementation of DL. It is quite difficult to get access to massive, carefully curated, and accurately labeled datasets. There is a need for highly specialized computing resources and at last to create DL models, one needs specialized technological know-how and mathematical understanding [14]. One strategy to overcome these challenges is the growingly well-liked method of transfer learning, which makes use of a model created for one job as the basis for training on another [2].

4 ANALYSIS

Smartphones and wearable technology are used in this analysis to identify human activity. These devices have access to a variety of sensors, including microphones, proximity and light sensors, accelerometers, gyroscopes, magnetometers, Bluetooth, Wi-Fi, and microphones all of which can be used to refer details of the activity. DL technique is classified into two. Generative feature extraction techniques include Deep Belief Network (DBN), Deep Boltzmann Machine (DBM), sparse coding and discriminative feature extraction includes CNN, RNN, and hybrid methods that combine generative and discriminative DL algorithms which makes up the subsets of the DL technique [16]. Dimensionality reduction reduces the dimension of the extracted features to speed up computation. Principal component analysis (PCA), linear discriminate analysis (LDA), and empirical cumulative distribution functions are the dimensionality reductions frequently employed in ECDF. Still this remains as an open research challenge [16].

Studies evaluating the accuracy of DL algorithms and physicians in using medical imaging to diagnose any condition were taken into consideration. Research using electrocardiography, a medical wave graphics, was left out of the study because it focuses more on the accuracy of image segmentation than disease classification. Information on binary diagnostic performance is obtained at the predetermined levels and produced contingency tables. Sensitivity and specificity were determined using contingency tables, which included true-positive, false-positive, true-negative, and false-negative data. It is assumed that multiple contingency tables that were provided by a study for either the same algorithm or for other algorithms were independent from one another. Statistical distributions are involved in the hierarchical model at two separate levels. Binomial distributions are utilized to define the number of cells counted that makes up the contingency tables at a more primitive level [5]. The diversity between researches, often known as heterogeneity, is modeled at a higher level. This investigation sought to determine whether internal validation alone overstates diagnostic accuracy [17]. As a result, the meta-analysis included diagnostic classifications for a variety of medical specialties, including ophthalmology (six studies), breast cancer (three studies), lung cancer (two studies), dermatological cancer (three studies), trauma and orthopedics (two studies), respiratory disease (two studies), gastroenterology or hepatology (one study), maxillofacial surgery, thyroid cancer, neurology, and nasopharynx. The pooling sensitivity for DL outperforms medical professionals when studies are averaged. It is discovered that DL algorithms are as sensitive and precise as medical experts. [5]. DL algorithms approximate the accuracy of clinicians, although there are some methodological flaws that should be taken into account throughout most included experiments. It is acknowledged that flawed study design does not always equate to poor reporting, and vice versa; similarly, poor study design does not always correspond to poor DL algorithm. As a result, the predictions of clinical outcomes given in our exploratory meta-analysis are surrounded by a lot of ambiguity [5]. However, the only studies that can generate trustworthy predictions of the performance levels are those that are well-conceived, well-executed, reduce bias, and give complete, transparent reporting. This exploratory meta-analysis shows that DL techniques are as reliable as medical professionals, while also recognizing the need for additional research on the application of such algorithms in practical contexts. Studies on DL treatments have reached a level of quality that allows us to judge how effectively these DL algorithms perform in real-world settings in a way that benefits patients and healthcare systems [18].

Methods of detecting uncertainty may be useful in preventing DL systems from making big but rare misclassifications. This study uses medical databases gathered from various organizations to predict the uncertainty. The goal is to develop a conceptual framework for defining the confidence of DL predictions while critically analyzing approaches for measuring uncertainties in DL for healthcare systems [18]. Doubt in DL can be characterized as either epistemic (caused by uncertainty about model parameters or ignorance) or aleatoric (i.e., attributable to stochastic variability and noise in data). By including additional training instances, epistemic ambiguity may be thought of as an insufficient knowledge about the best model—can be diminished [12]. In stochastic models, predicted parameters also become more constant with more training data. Convolutional neural networks are used in all medical imaging application models to anticipate uncertainty. Utilizing the Gaussian approach, uncertainty is quantified. Studies showed that uncertainty estimations were helpful. This review found that for use in medical imaging, Monte Carlo dropout methods on convolutional neural networks are most commonly utilized to evaluate the uncertainty in DL predictions. Applications of imaging for non-medical purposes had scattered and diverse estimates of uncertainty. Monte Carlo dropout methods accurately estimate uncertainty for convolutional neural network predictions on medical images. A general lack of data implies that using too many uncertainty estimating techniques can enhance prediction outcomes for non-medical imaging techniques. By spotting rare but potentially important classification errors made by DL models, uncertainty estimations are positioned to improve clinical applicability both for the imaging and non-imaging applications. Developing agreement on performance and uncertainty assessments and standard reporting standards could help the rapid expansion of DL ambiguity predictions in medical literature [18].

Clinicians without coding expertise can use automated DL to develop algorithms that accomplishes clinical classification tasks on par with traditional DL models [2]. ANNs can adjust to their inputs and grow as a result of their capacity to fine-tune depending on experience. They are effective tools for pattern recognition, classification, and forecasting since these features aren't specified by human engineers instead by the patterns that they have automatically mastered from input data. Physicians without coding skills are also able to use the automated DL to construct algorithms for clinical categorization tasks to the same extent as traditional DL models [2]. Because the search space for all feasible model architectures might be indefinitely huge, DL requires time and experimentation. The scientists automatically developed DL models for the identification of diseases using datasets including medical photographs. They trained and fine-tuned a DL model using a dermatology image set and evaluated its effectiveness using a second dataset of skin lesion images. Automated model selection or hyper parameter optimization techniques are often referred to as automated ML. Building and choosing model architecture requires time and experimentation because the search space for all conceivable model architectures in DL might be exponentially vast [2]. Duplicate photographs were automatically identified and excluded using the API. Reinforcement learning or evolutionary algorithms were used to simplify this. In that situation, automated DL learning models' poor performance might be attributed to peculiarities in the datasets that were used to train the models. Due to the API's inability to provide saliency maps, it's unable to query the model for the image regions it believed were most important for its forecast. [15]. Splitting test and training when done on a per-patient or per-test set basis could have a major negative impact on model accuracy because the quality of the results acquired using DL models heavily rely on the quality of the dataset utilized in the model development. Other APIs can lack this capability and produce fictitious evaluation metrics. Due to their easy access to patient data and photos within their own facilities, researchers and clinicians may be able to construct automated ML models for internal research, triage, and the delivery of tailored care. Before these models might be applied in clinical practice, there must be regulatory guidelines for both clinical and medical DL. The findings of this investigation cannot yet be generalized into clinical practice, despite the fact that our strategy appears reasonable in this preliminary assessment [2] (Figure 4.12).

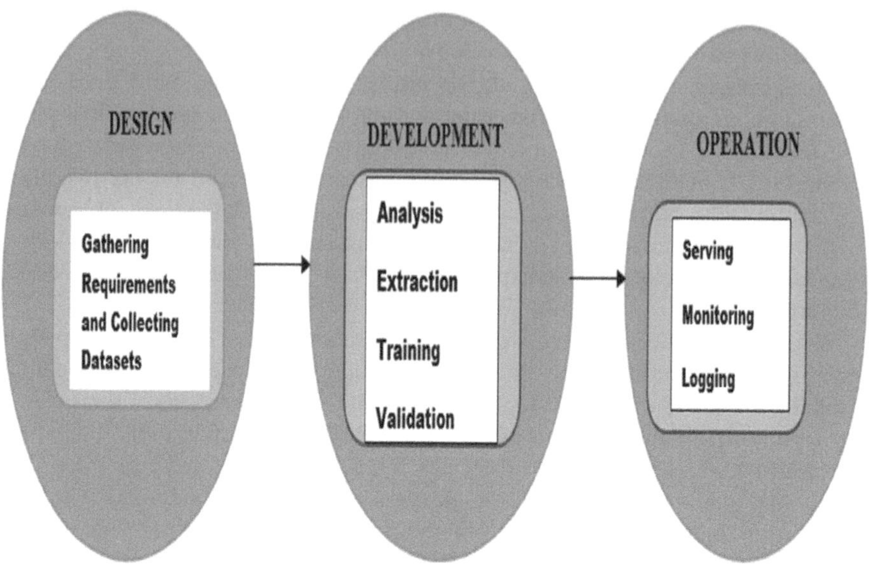

FIGURE 4.12   Deep Learning Process

The above diagram depicts the process of DL technique. It involves the process of design, development and operation.

The symptoms of pneumonia, a lung infection, can vary greatly in severity in people of all ages. It is the greatest cause of infection-related death in children under the age of five throughout the world. The neural network architecture was created especially for challenges involving the classification of images of pneumonia. The suggested method is based on the CNN algorithm and uses a network of neurons to interpolate a picture and identify key details from it. CNN-motivated DL systems have recently taken over as the industry standard for classifying medical images [14]. The original dataset [8] is made up of two subfolders holding images of normal (N) and pneumonia (P) chest X-rays, respectively, and three main folders (training, testing, and validation). A CNN model with two main components—feature extractors, a classifier—is used. The output of the immediately preceding layer is supplied as input to the next layers in the feature extraction layer, which each layer in turn uses as an input. In the CNN model that has been presented, the classifier is located at the very end. It is merely a dense layer, often known as an ANN. The trial is carried out for 10 times each for three hours in order to assess and confirm the efficacy of the suggested technique. CNN is used for classifying and identifying medical images. Since CNN is highly effective, the accuracy obtained is higher than other models [14]. The training and validation datasets are changed and still the outcomes were remarkably similar in order to validate the trained model's performance on various sizes of chest X-ray pictures. Significant improvements can be realized by expanding data availability and training the model using patient's and no patient's radiological data around the globe [14].

Big data gives health policy experts, medical professionals, and healthcare organizations the chances of making data-driven judgments that improve patient care, disease control, and healthcare choices. Big data can only be used to a small degree by conventional ML approaches and algorithms, and in most circumstances, this results in unsatisfactory and complex solutions. A promising answer to this problem is offered by DL. To attain high quality performance and outcomes, more regions and domains are turning toward DL. The necessity to resolve data issues of the type and shape that only these DL approaches can handle successfully explains why RNN and CNN are two of the most often employed DL algorithms. In addition, the majority of typical facts are temporally or visually dependent. RNN relies on the idea of preserving the previous layer outcome and transmitting this again to the input in order to anticipate the outcome of the present layer, in contrast to CNN, which only allows information to flow in one direction (forward) [19]. DL methods performed well at early-stage COVID-19 case detection. A unique COVID-19 identification method based on a CNN and ConyLSTM was recently proposed by Sedik et al. [20]. The proposed method uses DL algorithms to compare the chest X-rays of normal patients with those of COVID-19 patients. The suggested method provides an accuracy of 99%.

Heart disease is difficult to diagnose, and frequently patients are not even aware that a serious condition is going to affect them until heart-related issues like tachycardia or stroke is experienced. In order to diagnose a patient with a heart disease, a skilled doctor must study the patient in order to recognize the typical signs of cardiac condition. Practically, this is daunting since there are insufficient physicians and majority of countries continue to deny that computers are capable of logically and properly diagnosing heart problems. In order for patients to receive the results by the deadline, preconfigured systems for processing patient data are connected by established healthcare systems. These systems are created using cloud or fog computing platforms that are IoT-driven. The health fog model is an IoT based fog-enabled cloud computing model for healthcare that effectively manages the data of heart patients and assesses the patient's well-being condition to determine the level of risk of heart disease. With the assurance of the claim, the fog computing model receives data of cardiac patient from the sensors and returns outcomes that include whether the patient has cardiovascular disease or not. Python was used to implement the pre-processing technique and ensemble DL components. Based on the distribution of the maximum and minimum field parameter values in the dataset, the pre-processing module normalizes the data. The model has been utilized for quickly identifying heart abnormalities in patients combining cutting-edge DL methods and computing methods based on fog [21].

5 CONCLUSION

Finally, despite the potential of DL, academics in the field of healthcare should not become excessively excited. DL is not appropriate for all issues involving clinical data, despite being very helpful for some tasks like identifying medical images.

The provision of healthcare as a free service is a massive undertaking. This article has discussed the various medical fields in which DL has been employed and how it is applied as a solution to those diseases. This chapter gave a survey of popular DL methods, including auto encoders, convolutional neural networks, RBMs, and recurrent neural networks. It is also discussed that physicians having no knowledge of coding also can use DL algorithms. This article also deals with how big data, IoT, and cloud computing can be used in integration with DL for medical healthcare. For large and diverse datasets, DL outperforms traditional analysis and machine classification techniques. DL algorithms attempt to build the model utilizing every available piece of data. From this chapter, it is concluded that DL algorithms feature many hidden layers, making them more effective in classifying data. However, this also means that they use more resources and need a lot more data to train on. An excessive reliance on DL without comparison to other approaches can hinder the development of AI in therapeutic contexts.

6　FUTURE WORKS

Research is still needed in a number of areas, including sensor technology, actual and on-board deployment on mobile and wearable devices, gathering of big datasets, data pre-processing and review, and imbalanced class problems. A major challenge is getting the general public to trust the development and use of DL. Further advancements can only be made with their support, making it helpful for higher order disease diagnosis. Therefore, a solution must be found in the next years.

REFERENCES

[1] Kaul, D., Raju, H., & Tripathy, B. K. (2022). Deep learning in healthcare. In *Deep Learning in Data Analytics* (pp. 97–115). Springer, Cham.

[2] Faes, L., Wagner, S. K., Fu, D. J., Liu, X., Korot, E., Ledsam, J. R., … Keane, P. A. (2019). Automated deep learning design for medical image classification by health-care professionals with no coding experience: a feasibility study. *The Lancet Digital Health*, *1*(5), e232–e242.

[3] Bolhasani, H., Mohseni, M., & Rahmani, A. M. (2021). Deep learning applications for IoT in health care: a systematic review. *Informatics in Medicine Unlocked*, *23*, 100550.

[4] Miotto, R., Wang, F., Wang, S., Jiang, X., & Dudley, J. T. (2018). Deep learning for healthcare: review, opportunities and challenges. *Briefings in Bioinformatics*, *19*(6), 1236–1246.

[5] Tobore, I., Li, J., Yuhang, L., Al-Handarish, Y., Kandwal, A., Nie, Z., & Wang, L. (2019). Deep learning intervention for health care challenges: some biomedical domain considerations. *JMIR mHealth and uHealth*, *7*(8), e11966.

[6] Liu, X., Faes, L., Kale, A. U., Wagner, S. K., Fu, D. J., Bruynseels, A., … Denniston, A. K. (2019). A comparison of deep learning performance against health-care professionals in detecting diseases from medical imaging: a systematic review and meta-analysis. *The Lancet Digital Health*, *1*(6), e271–e297.

[7] Zhao, R., Yan, R., Chen, Z., Mao, K., Wang, P., & Gao, R. X. (2019). Deep learning and its applications to machine health monitoring. *Mechanical Systems and Signal Processing*, *115*, 213–237.

[8] Srivastava, S., Soman, S., Rai, A., & Srivastava, P. K. (2017, September). Deep learning for health informatics: recent trends and future directions. In *2017 international conference on advances in computing, communications and informatics (ICACCI)* (pp. 1665–1670). IEEE.

[9] Verma, H., & Kumar, S. (2019, January). An accurate missing data prediction method using LSTM based deep learning for health care. In *Proceedings of the 20th International conference on Distributed Computing and Networking* (pp. 371–376).

[10] Abdel-Jaber, H., Devassy, D., Al Salam, A., Hidaytallah, L., & EL-Amir, M. (2022). A review of deep learning algorithms and their applications in healthcare. *Algorithms, 15*(2), 71.

[11] Navamani, T. M. (2019). Efficient deep learning approaches for health informatics. In *Deep learning and parallel computing environment for bioengineering systems* (pp. 123–137). Academic Press. https://www.sciencedirect.com/book/9780128167182/deep-learning-and-parallel-computing-environment-for-bioengineering-systems#book-description

[12] Hullermeier, E., & Waegeman W. (2021). Aleatoric and epistemic uncertainty in machine learning: an introduction to concepts and methods. *Machine Learning, 110*(3), 457–506.

[13] Shafqat, S., Fayyaz, M., Khattak, H. A., Bilal, M., Khan, S., Ishtiaq, O., ... Chatterjee, P. (2021). Leveraging deep learning for designing healthcare analytics heuristic for diagnostics. *Neural Processing Letters*, (2023), 1–27.

[14] Stephen, O., Sain, M., Maduh, U. J., & Jeong, D. U. (2019). An efficient deep learning approach to pneumonia classification in healthcare. *Journal of Healthcare Engineering, 2019.*

[15] Oakden-Rayner, L. (2019). Explain yourself, machine. Producing simple text descriptions for AI interpretability.

[16] Nweke, H. F., Teh, Y. W., Al-Garadi, M. A., & Alo, U. R. (2018). Deep learning algorithms for human activity recognition using mobile and wearable sensor networks: state of the art and research challenges. *Expert Systems with Applications, 105*, 233–261.

[17] J. Melendez, G. B. Van, P. Maduskar, Philipsen, R. H. H. M., Reither, K., Breuninger, M., O Adetifa, ... Sanchez, C.I. (2015). A novel multiple-instance learning-based approach to computer-aided detection of tuberculosis on chest x-ray. *IEEE Transactions on Medical Imaging, 34*(1), 179–192.

[18] Loftus, T. J., Shickel, B., Ruppert, M. M., Balch, J. A., Ozrazgat-Baslanti, T., Tighe, P. J., ... & Bihorac, A. (2022). Uncertainty-aware deep learning in healthcare: a scoping review. *PLOS Digital Health, 1*(8), e0000085.

[19] Tobore, I., Li, J., Yuhang, L., Al-Handarish, Y., Kandwal, A., Nie, Z., & Wang, L. (2019). Deep learning intervention for health care challenges: some biomedical domain considerations. *JMIR mHealth and uHealth, 7*(8), e11966.

[20] Sedik, A., Hammad, M., El-Samie, A., Fathi, E., Gupta, B. B., El-Latif, A., & Ahmed, A. (2022). Efficient deep learning approach for augmented detection of Coronavirus disease. *Neural Computing and Applications, 34*(14), 11423–11440.

[21] Tuli, S., Basumatary, N., Gill, S. S., Kahani, M., Arya, R. C., Wander, G. S., & Buyya, R. (2020). HealthFog: an ensemble deep learning based smart healthcare system for automatic diagnosis of heart diseases in integrated IoT and fog computing environments. *Future Generation Computer Systems, 104*, 187–200.

5 An Empirical Evaluation of Learning Models for the Classification of Fall Detection Dataset

Monika and Sakshi Sinha

ABBREVIATIONS:

ADL (Daily Life Activities); ANN (Artificial Neural Network); KNN (K- Nearest Neighbor); WHO (World Health Organization)

1   INTRODUCTION

The number of elderly people in our world is increasing and so there is a need for studying issues related to their health and making their life easier and simpler. The main issue which the elderly people have to deal with daily is related to health [1]. Thus, it can be seen as an area of multidisciplinary research. The most important cause of health issues in elderly people is their falls. The elderly people the authors are referring to here are of the age 65 years and above.

Falls are the main cause of disability and illness in elderly people. More than one-third of the people who are above the age of 65 experience fall each year [2]. And the more pressing matter above it is that in half of these cases the old people not only fall once. Rather, it is a recurrent phenomenon in their cases. This is a matter of grave concern. And if the person has a case of impairment, then the risk can be twice or thrice as high as compared to the normal case. In Canada, falls are the most common cause (85%) of injury-related hospital admissions among those aged 65 years or older [3].

Most of the people think that falls lead to the risk of fracture or possibly a muscle strain or pull [4]. But they forget the fact that it can lead to other irreversible physical, mental as well as emotional injuries and economic effects [5]. The currently available studies and gadgets or systems which are being developed for the identification of the falls in the elderly people should be accurate in observing and analyzing activities of daily life such as standing, sitting, lying down, walking, ascending/descending stairs, and most importantly, events such as falls

    DOI: 10.1201/9781003377818-5

[6] According to the WHO, a fall is defined as an event which results in a person coming to rest inadvertently on the ground or other lower level [7]. A fall can occur when the center of mass of a person suddenly changes, which leads to loss of balance and hence leads to the falling of a person [7].

Daily life activities and falls need to be considered together, as they are like the two faces of the coin. Falls occur unexpectedly while performing daily life activities [8]. A fall is never pre-planned; it is sudden and occurs mostly during performing the basic day-to-day activities of our life [9]. It leads to a sudden and rather drastic change in the vitals of a person like lowering of BP [10] and also increase in the brain activities which leads to an increase of EEG [11]. Falls are generally not treated as serious and hazardous health injuries, but they should be, especially with the steep rise of elderly people who live alone or in an old age home [12].

Falls are a public health problem and a health threat, especially for adults of age 65 and older [13]. Statistics indicate that one in every three adults age 65 or older experiences at least one falls every year [11]. Besides the elderly, children, disabled individuals, workers, athletes, and patients with visual, balance, gait, orthopedic, neurological, and psychological disorders also suffer from falls [5]. The intrinsic factors associated with falls are aging, mental impairment, neurological and orthopedic diseases, vision, and balance disorders [6]. The normal maturing process frequently puts more seasoned grown-ups at an expanded danger of having a fall. Falls are atypical and frequently disregarded reason for injury in the older [14]. There are three principal reasons why more established individuals are bound to have a fall. These are:

- Interminable well-being conditions, for example, coronary illness, dementia, and low circulatory strain (hypotension), which can cause unsteadiness hindrances, for example, poor vision or muscle shortcoming diseases that can influence balance, for example, labyrinthitis (aggravation of the fragile equalization managing portions of the ear) [15]. Constant well-being conditions, for example, those recorded above, can here and there cause lost equalization, a concise loss of cognizance or blacking out, or an unexpected sentiment of dazedness, all of which could add to a fall [16], [17].
- Typical changes in our bodies as we age likewise make falls almost certain. Visual disability or muscle shortcoming may likewise make it increasingly hard for a more established individual to forestall a fall. More seasoned individuals may likewise have more vulnerable muscles and stiffer joints or may lose a portion of the inclination in their feet and legs. They're likewise slower to respond and may experience issues focusing on more than one thing as they age. Among more established grown-ups, the most well-known purposes behind unintentionally falling or slipping include: wet or as of late cleaned floors, for example, in a restroom; diminishing lighting; floor coverings or rugs that are not

    appropriately made sure about going after capacity regions, for example, pantries steps.
- Another normal reason for falls, especially among more seasoned men, is tumbling from a stepping stool while doing home upkeep work. For individuals who have osteoporosis (diminishing and debilitating of the bones), falling can be especially perilous as there is more danger of a messed-up bone.

The typical changes of maturing, similar to poor visual perception or poor hearing, can make you bound to fall. Sicknesses and states of being can influence your quality and parity. Poor lighting or carpets in your home can make you bound to outing or slip. The symptoms of certain meds can disturb your parity and make you fall. Drugs for wretchedness, rest issues, and hypertension regularly cause falls. A few medications for diabetes and heart conditions can likewise make you precarious on your feet. The elderly might be bound to fall on the off chance that you are taking at least four drugs. You are additionally prone to fall in the event that you have changed your medication inside the previous 14 days. Falls are a marker of delicacy, fixed status, and intense and ceaseless well-being hindrance in more established people. Falls thus decrease work by causing injury, action confinements, dread of falling, and loss of portability. Most wounds in the old are the aftereffect of falls; breaks of the hip, lower arm, humerus, and pelvis as a rule result from the joined impact of falls and osteoporosis.

Counteraction of falls must traverse the range of ages and well-being states inside the more established populace and address the decent variety of reasons for falls without pointlessly trading off personal satisfaction and autonomy. Inborn hazard factors for falls have been found in controlled examinations, which permit the recognizable proof of those in danger and recommend potential preventive intercessions. Old people with various well-being disabilities are at most serious hazard; however, numerous solid more seasoned people likewise fall every year. Current comprehension of the etiology of postural flimsiness and falling is restricted, and there is little data about the adequacy of intercessions to forestall falls.

A fall is an unexpected happening that outcomes in the individual stopping on the ground or another lower level. A total of 56 falls can be portrayed regarding three stages. The main stage is a starting occasion that uproots the body's focal point of mass past its base of help. Starting occasions include extraneous factors, for example, natural dangers; characteristic factors, for example, unsteady joints, muscle shortcoming, and temperamental postural reflexes; and physical exercises in progress at the hour of the fall. The second period of a fall includes a disappointment of the frameworks for keeping up an upstanding stance to recognize and address this removal so as to stay away from a fall. This disappointment is common because of components characteristic for the individual, for example, loss of tangible capacity, hindered focal preparing, and muscle shortcoming. The third stage is an effect of the body on ecological surfaces, normally the floor or ground, which brings about the transmission of powers to body tissues and organs. The potential for injury is a component of the extent and heading of the powers and the powerlessness of tissues and organs to harm. A fourth stage, in spite of the fact that not part of a fall, concerns the clinical, mental, and medicinal services sequelae of the fall and chaperon wounds. These sequelae influence the level of harm and handicap coming about because of the fall. Ways to deal with forestalling falls and their outcomes should concentrate on factors identified with every one of these stages.

Falls with certain starting qualities (e.g., loss of awareness, stroke, overpowering outer power from an engine vehicle mishap, or savagery) are regularly ejected from the meaning of falls in more seasoned people. The physical changes intrinsic to maturing can diminish self-sufficiency and useful freedom, which may straightforwardly or in a roundabout way lead to falls. Falls are coded as E880–E888 in the International Classification of Disease-9 (ICD-9) and as W00–W19 in ICD-10; they are ordinarily characterized as "incidentally stopping on the ground, floor or other lower level, barring a deliberate change in position to rest in furniture, divider or different items". Approximately one-third of individuals aged over 65 experience at least one indoor fall annually, with around half of this demographic experiencing recurring falls. Among the older, falls are one of the primary drivers of wounds, physical inadequacy and even passing. Every year, around 37.3 million falls among the old will require human services, and around 424,000 lead to the passing of the faller. Falls are occasions that rely upon different factors and can be identified with the nearness of pathologies. The pathologies innate to the way toward maturing, which may prompt fall in the older populace, are various and differing. Along these lines, four classifications were thought of: neurological, musculoskeletal, cardiovascular, and different pathologies. The neurologic and musculoskeletal pathologies were the most referenced in the broke down writing. The cardiovascular pathologies additionally had a significant rate of references, albeit little when contrasted and the previous [18].

In the most recent decade, populace maturing has been enlisted as a worldwide marvel. A connection exists among falling and maturing, since falling recurrence increments altogether with age. To tell the truth, one out of every three more seasoned grown-ups falls every year. Albeit maturing is conventionally connected with lessening and degeneration of mental and physical capacities, it is as yet not regular for the right recognizable proof of hazard elements to prompt clinical anticipation of the senior being in danger of falling. Accordingly, the objective of this audit article is to recognize, arrange, and investigate ordinary maturing and fall factors referenced in the writing just as to measure the occasions they were referenced. The exploration thought about many distributions, yet examination was then confined to the 87 most appropriate articles written in English and distributed in diaries or logical magazines somewhere between 1995 and 2010. We presumed that falls among more seasoned grown-ups can be portrayed by the following factors: anatomic qualities and physiological outcomes of maturing; the pathologies that prompt falls, which can be neurological, musculoskeletal, cardiovascular, and different maladies; causes and hazard components of falls that can be conduct, organic, ecological, or financial; kind of physical results of falls, including breaks, wounds, or other physical results; and procedures to forestall, alleviate, or restore, which can be of a physical, natural, or social nature [19].

This chapter aims at classifying falls on the basis of the body vitals, and identifying the fall of a person while performing daily life activities. It will help us in categorizing the activity as "Fall" or "No Fall" as shown in Figure 5.1. This chapter will provide an empirical study of various classification algorithms based on machine learning.

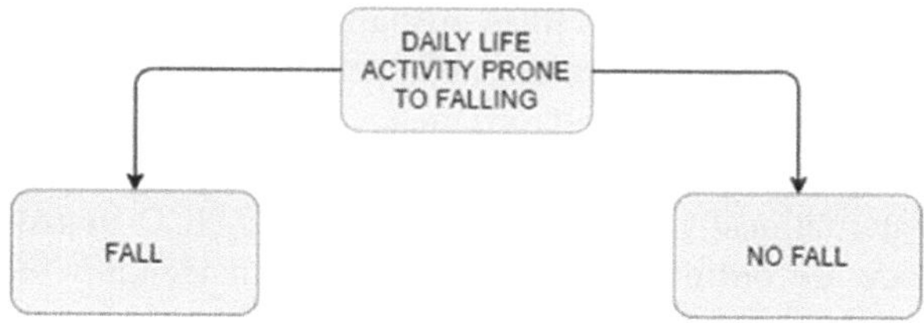

FIGURE 5.1   Visualization of Classification of Daily Life Activity as Fall or No Fall

2   MATERIALS AND METHODS

The general methodology and process by which the experimental study has been performed is shown Figure 5.2.

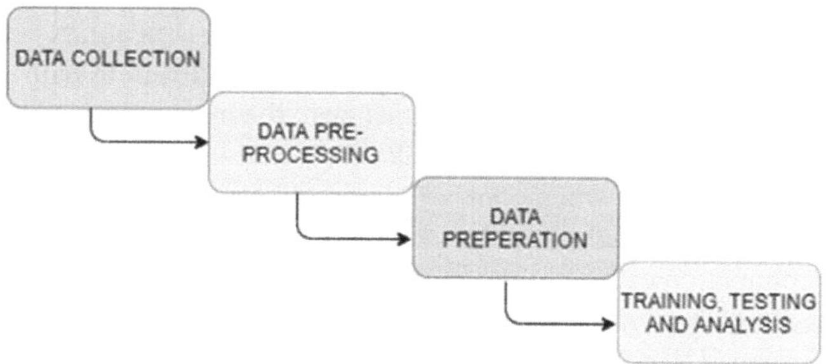

FIGURE 5.2   Major Steps of Proposed Method

2.1   COLLECTION OF DATA

In this study, the authors are using a dataset 0 which has been gathered from individuals with the help of gadgets which has sensors in them. The dataset has the dimension 16382x7. The gadgets which have been used on them have motion sensors and works on the principle of three dimensions for accurate and better results. The devices which are embedded in the gadget are also tri-axial, meaning that they consider the 3-D coordinates of the surrounding. The devices used for this purpose are accelerometer, gyroscope, and compass. The focus on the raw data for each sensor is in a 4s time window around the point of peak total acceleration of the waist sensor, and then perform feature extraction and reduction. The dataset has been formed while doing normal daily life activities and falling during performing those activities. This is done based on the fact that most of the falls and the related injuries occur at the time of performing normal activities. In total six activities of daily life are considered in this dataset, which broadly covers the activities elderly people perform in daily life. The activities and the parameters have been recorded in this dataset.

2.2 DESCRIPTION OF DATA

The columns that are present in the dataset have been mentioned here. There are totally seven columns. A snippet of data being used is presented in Figure 5.3.

Activity. The activities which have been captured in this dataset are given in Table 5.1 along with label numbers.

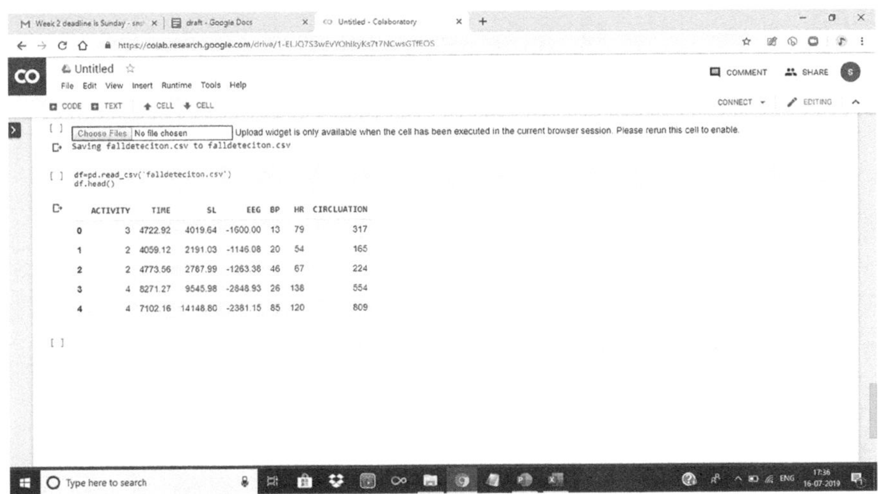

FIGURE 5.3 Snippet of the Head of Datafile Being Used

TABLE 5.1

The Activities for Which Data Has Been Recorded with Their Labels

Activity	Label
Standing	0
Walking	1
Sitting	2
Falling	3
Cramps	4
Running	5

The numerical values which have been mentioned in Table 5.1 are the label values given to these activities in the dataset. The frequency of these activities has been shown with the help of the graph given below in Figure 5.4.

Time. The time distribution graph which has been shown in Figure 5.5 represents the time spent on various activities. From the graph, we can observe that most amount of time is spent standing by elderly people.

Sugar Level. The graph given in Figure 5.6 shows the sugar level of the elderly people while performing various activities.

EEG. The graph given in Figure 5.7 shows the variance of the EEG, which is simply the measure of brain activity with various activities.

Blood Pressure. The blood pressure is the measure of the flow of blood through our blood veins. The narrower the arteries are, the more the blood pressure rate will be. It also symbolizes that the person may be suffering from restlessness or anger issues, or some other physical problem which can lead to the variance of

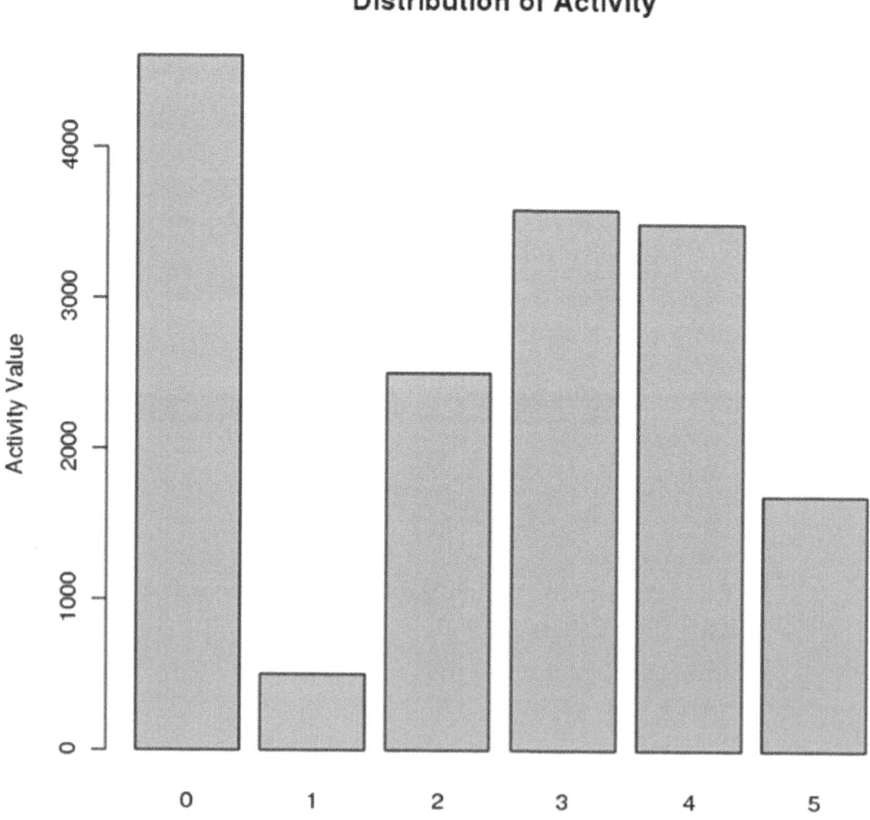

FIGURE 5.4 Numeric Distribution of the Data in Dataset on the Basis of Activity Being Performed

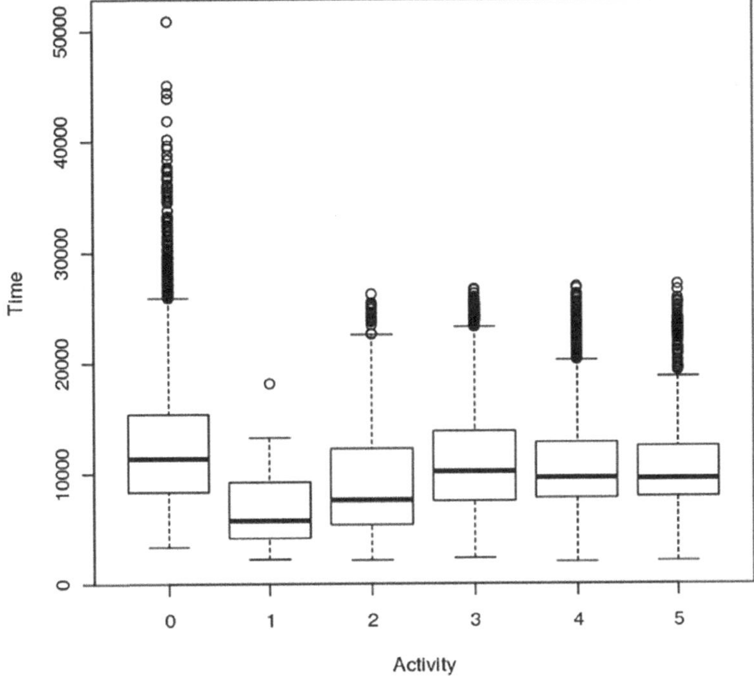

FIGURE 5.5   Distribution of Variance of Time with Activity

blood pressure. The distribution of blood pressure in accordance to the activity has been shown in Figure 5.8.

Heart Rate. The graph in Figure 5.9 shows the heart rate of elderly people varying for the six different activities.

Blood Circulation. The graph in Figure 5.10 shows the rate of blood circulation with respect to the different activities performed by the elderly people.

2.3 ALGORITHMS USED

The authors are using various classification algorithms on the given dataset for identifying whether a person is falling or not when doing the daily life activities in Figure 5.11.

In the dataset, various body vitals such as sugar level, EEG, blood pressure, heart rate, and the activities they are performing with a duration of time are given in [20], [21]. The authors are classifying the activities as Fall or No Fall by thresholding these vital values. After assigning the label value as fall or no fall to each set of input, the authors are classifying them using different machine learning classification algorithm. The algorithms which the authors are using are mentioned in Figure 5.11.

Logistic Regression. The classification algorithm of Logistic Regression is a tool of statistics which is used to analyze the data based on one or more variables

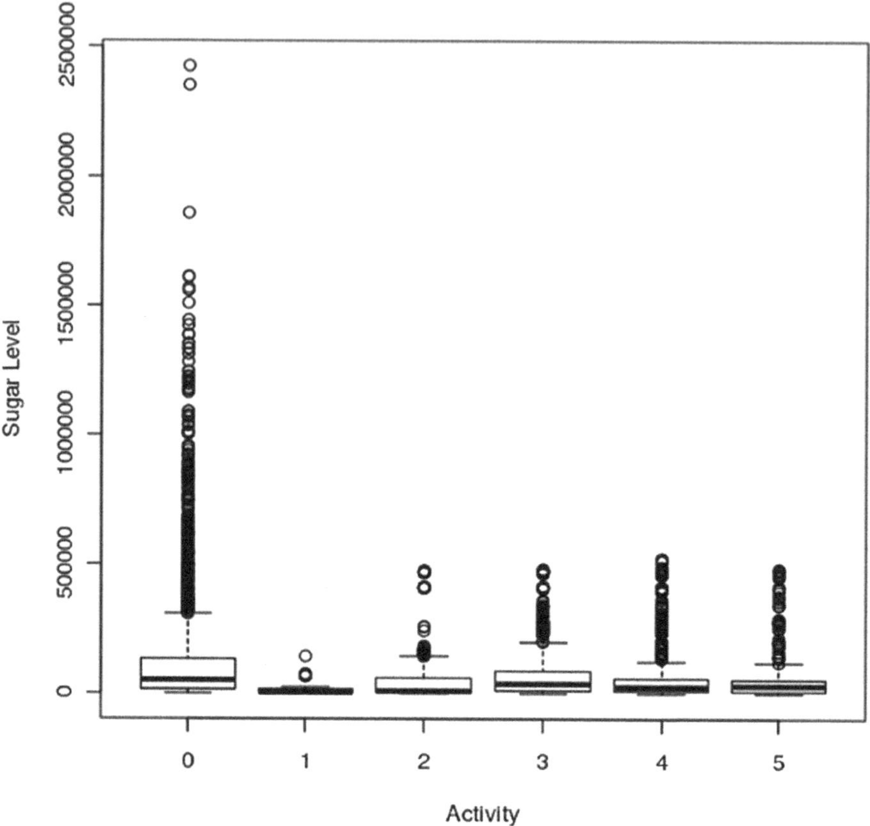

FIGURE 5.6	Distribution of Variance of Sugar Level with Activity

which are independent. It works on various independent parameters of the dataset and gives a single outcome. The outcome of the dataset is measured as a binary outcome, like true or false, i.e. 0 or 1. So if the given condition is satisfied the tuple will be encoded as 1, otherwise, it will be encoded as 0. It has been graphically represented in Figure 5.12, which has been studied from [14].

KNN Classifier. KNN refers to the K Nearest Neighbor Algorithm. What it does is that it will start forming group(s) with the values which are more alike and soon the data is classified into multiple groups depending on which value is more similar in features to which group. So, the data is classified in a pattern recognized manner. The classes are labeled as 0, 1, 2, and so on depending on the number of classes they need to be categorized in. For the purpose of this experimental study, the authors have used the value of K=1 [22]. A graphical representation of KNN algorithm is shown in Figure 5.13.

Random Forest. Random Forest algorithm is a supervised classification algorithm. As the name suggests, this algorithm creates the forest with a number of trees. In general, the more the number of trees in the forest, the more robust the

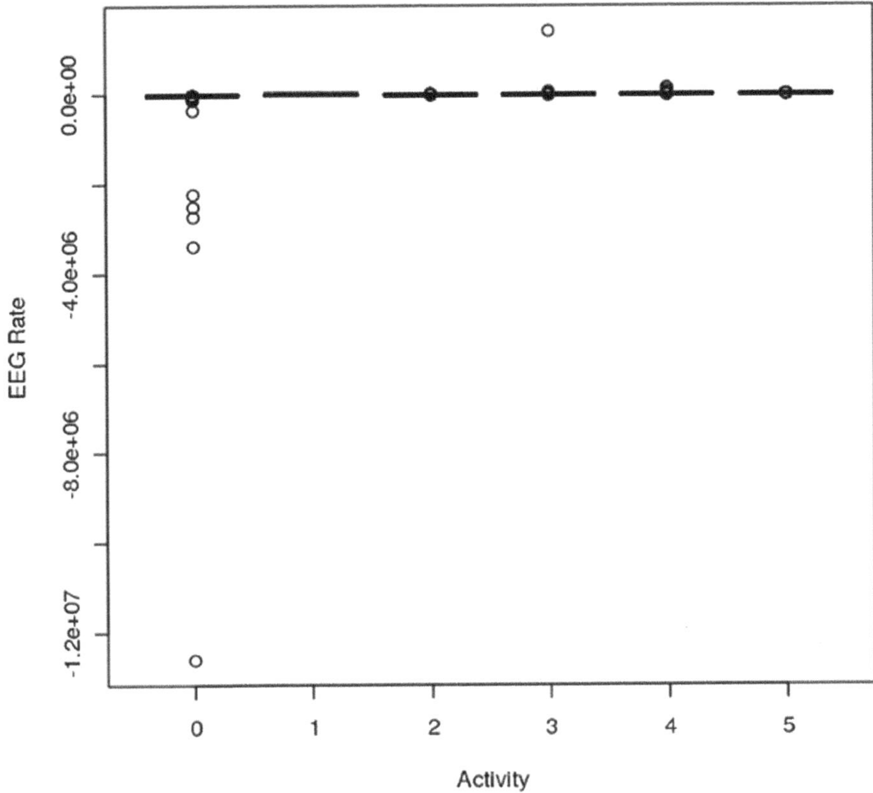

FIGURE 5.7   Distribution of Variance EEG Monitoring Rate with Activity

forest looks like. Similarly, the authors can say that when the authors use the Random Forest classifier, the higher the number of trees in the forest gives the higher accuracy results. These trees are mostly used for the purpose of making decisions, hence are called decision trees as well. The graphical representation of the tree which is being used in this study has been shown in Figure 5.14.

Ridge Regression. Ridge Regression is a very good technique of regression in comparison to that of Linear Regression because it reduces the parameters of the given dataset thus downsizing to it absolutely what is needed of that dataset and no additional parameters. And, it reduces the model complexity by coefficient shrinkage. Also, it uses the L2 regularization technique.

ANN Classifier. ANN classifier is the abbreviated form for artificial neural networks. It can also be called as connectionist systems. As the name suggests it is a neural network which has been developed artificially [23]. It works like a synthetic brain, and the results produced from these are many a time shockingly close to human thinking yet more precise. Thus, they can be inferred as a synthetic brain. Such systems "learn" to perform tasks by considering examples, generally without being programmed with any task-specific rules.

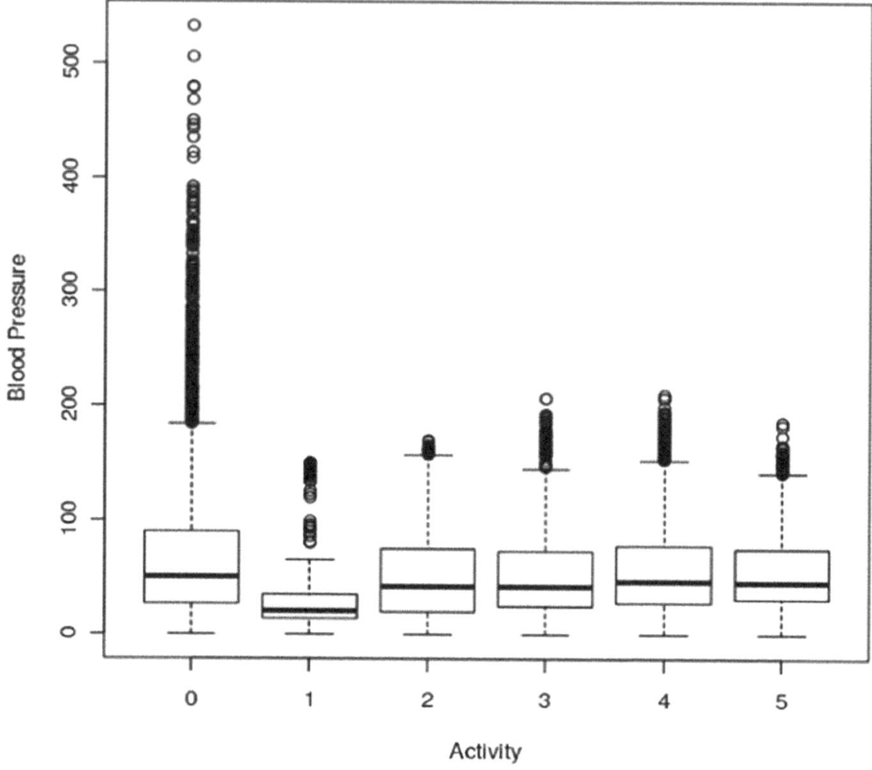

FIGURE 5.8   Distribution of Blood Pressure

In our neural network the authors have used 6 inputs, 7 hidden layers, and one output line. The activation function used in our network is ReLu as the activation function. The graphical representation of the ANN model being used in this study is shown in Figure 5.15.

2.4   METHODOLOGY

The authors have threshold the value of the body vitalities which varies drastically at the time of the fall of a person, i.e. the activities of the brain and the functioning of the heart. So, it means that the authors have threshold the values of heart rate, circulation, EEG, and blood pressure. If a person is going to fall these are the most important parameters that will vary in the person, whether young or old. However, the range of these values differs from age to age. The authors have found and studied the values of these body vitals for the age of 65 and above. The data for thresholding the values of circulation rate, blood pressure, heart rate, and

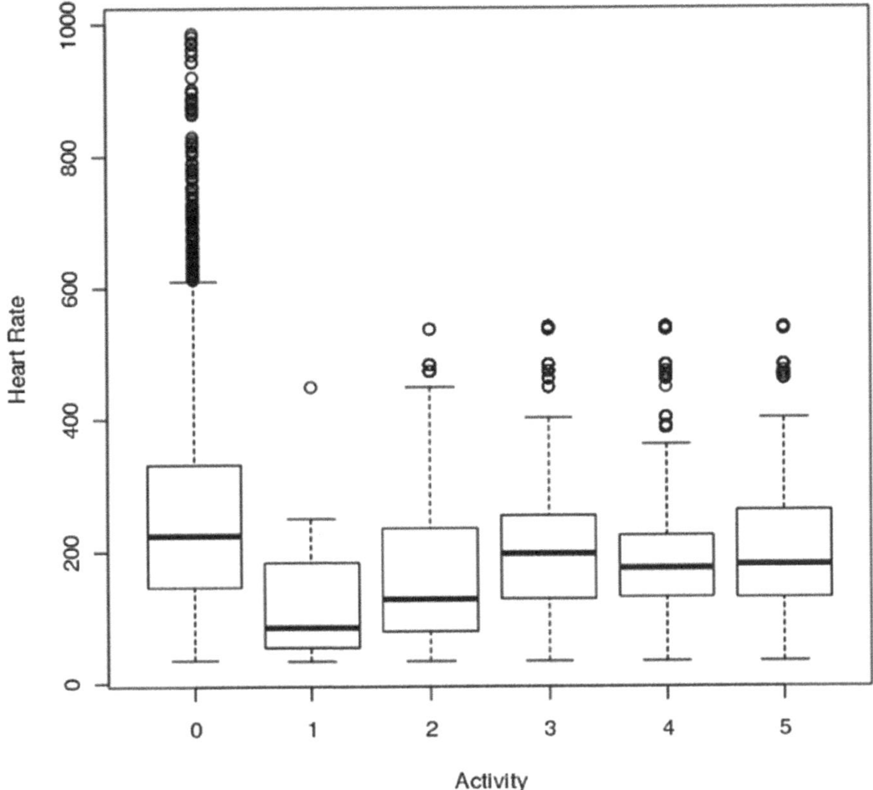

FIGURE 5.9   Distribution of Heart Rate

EEG have been gathered and reference from various medical research papers and medical websites. After this, the various classification algorithms are applied to the given dataset and accuracy value for each algorithm, namely Logistic Regression, Ridge Regression, Random Forest, KNN, and ANN is found.

2.5   SOFTWARE USED

The various algorithms which have been mentioned above are performed on the given dataset and after that accuracy for each of the algorithms is calculated. All these machine learning algorithms have been executed and their accuracy is found on the platform of Python. The software used for this study is Jupyter Notebook 5.7.8, with the support of Python 3.6. For the algorithms to be implemented Scikit learn version 0.21.2 has been used. Scikit learn is a tool which is used for data mining and data analysis. For the graphs, matplotlib version 3.1.0 has been used.

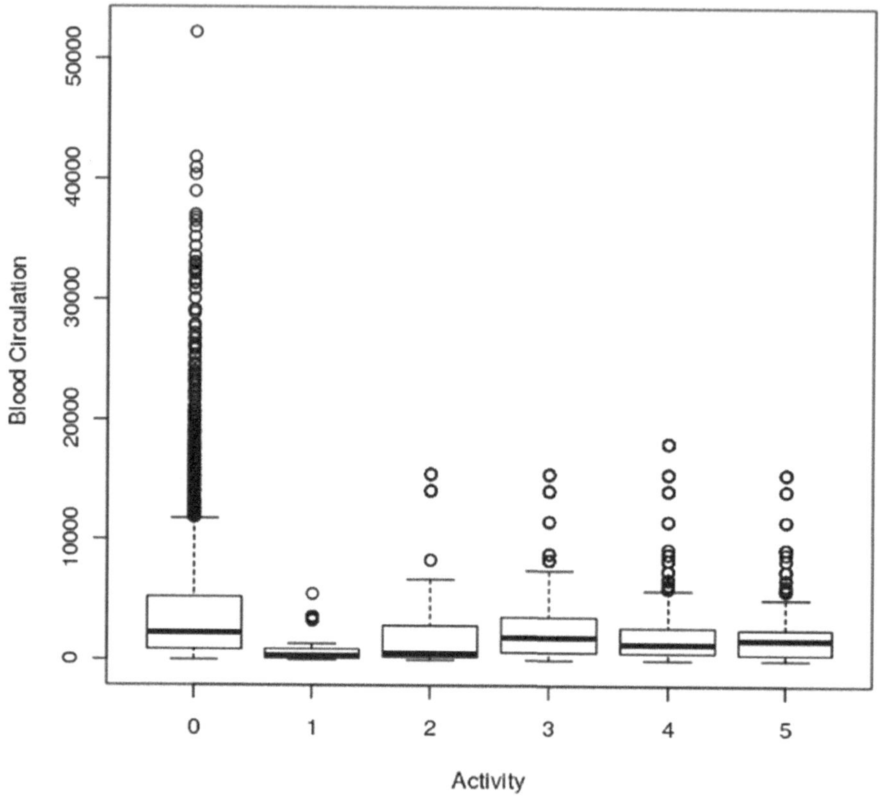

FIGURE 5.10 Distribution of Variance of Circulation with Activity

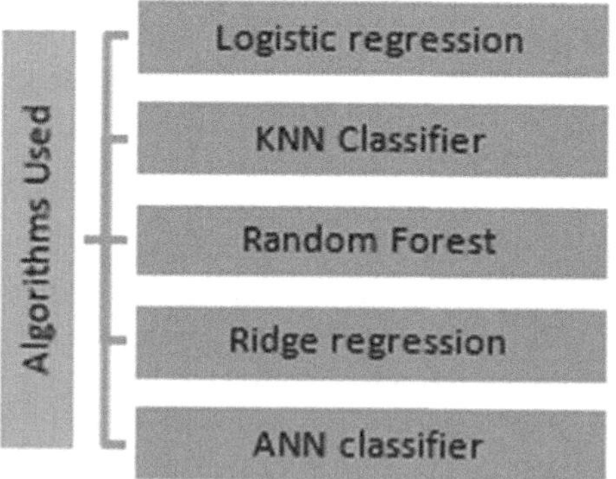

FIGURE 5.11 Algorithms Used in this Experimental Study

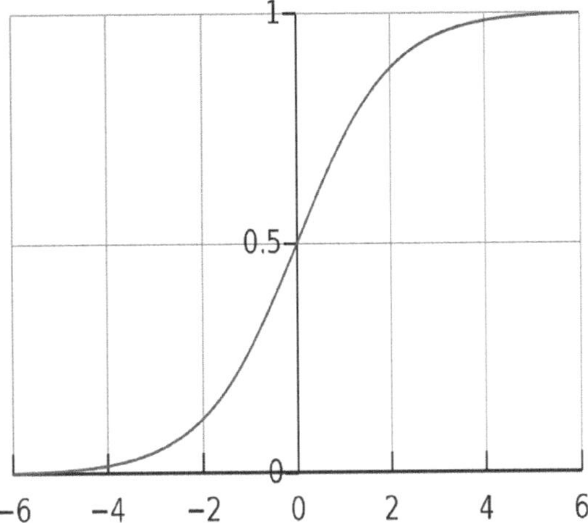

FIGURE 5.12 Graphical Representation of Logistic Regression

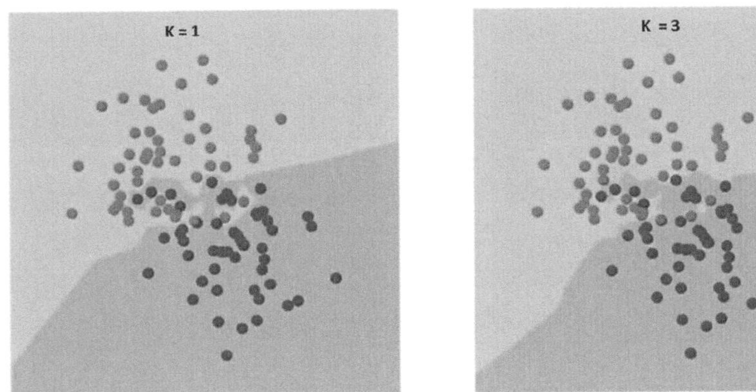

FIGURE 5.13 Graphical Representation of KNN Algorithm when K=1

3 RESULTS AND DISCUSSION

The accuracy for both the train and test split test cases have been observed through Table 5.2. From Table 5.2 and Figure 5.16, it can be clearly seen that the train accuracy of the algorithms is better than the test accuracy as training will always yield a higher accuracy and thus provide most precise results. The best result has been obtained from the Random Forest as the test accuracy for this algorithm is 99%.

The scores of the different algorithms have been calculated using F-Score. It provides mathematical formula to calculate the accuracy of a certain algorithm

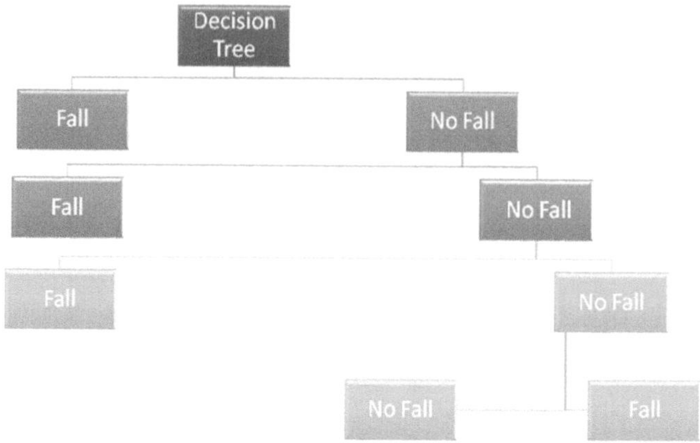

FIGURE 5.14   Graphical Representation of Random Forest

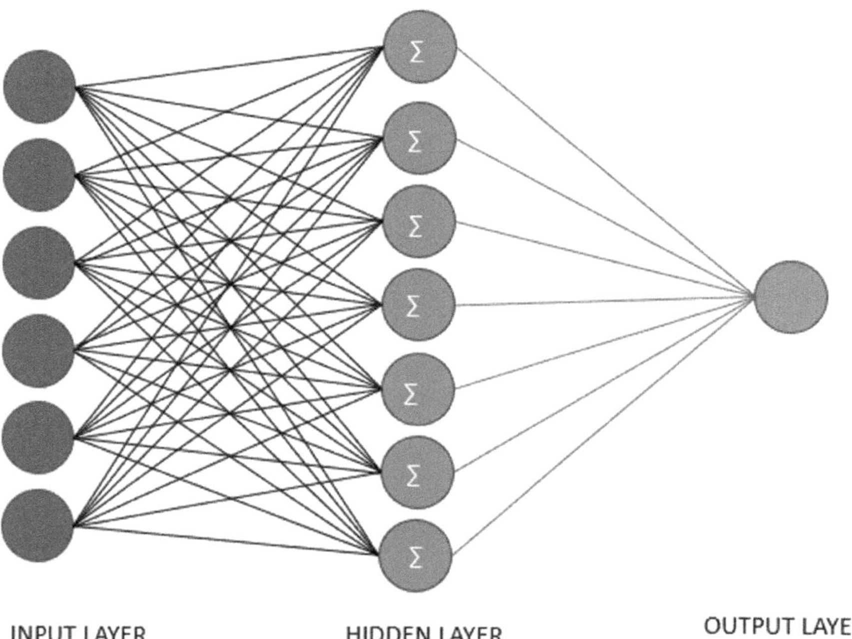

FIGURE 5.15   Graphical Representation of the ANN Classifier in Our Study

on a data set. Through the insights which we have obtained using this school we can clearly see that the Random Forest has the highest efficiency in both test and train duration.

So, the result which we have obtained is that for predicting the chances of fall of an elderly person during a certain daily life activity, Random Forest is the most suited algorithm to be calculated. These are all are classification algorithms which have calculated the fall of an elderly person and further study can be concluded on the basis of these results.

The comparison of the accuracy of the test and the train data of the abovementioned algorithms have been shown through Figure 5.16.

TABLE 5.2
Accuracy of Test and Train Data

Algorithm	Test Data Accuracy	Train Data Accuracy
Logistic Regression	0.73	0.73
KNN Classifier	0.92	0.83
Ridge Regression	0.99	0.97
ANN Classifier	0.99	0.98
Random forest	1.00	0.99

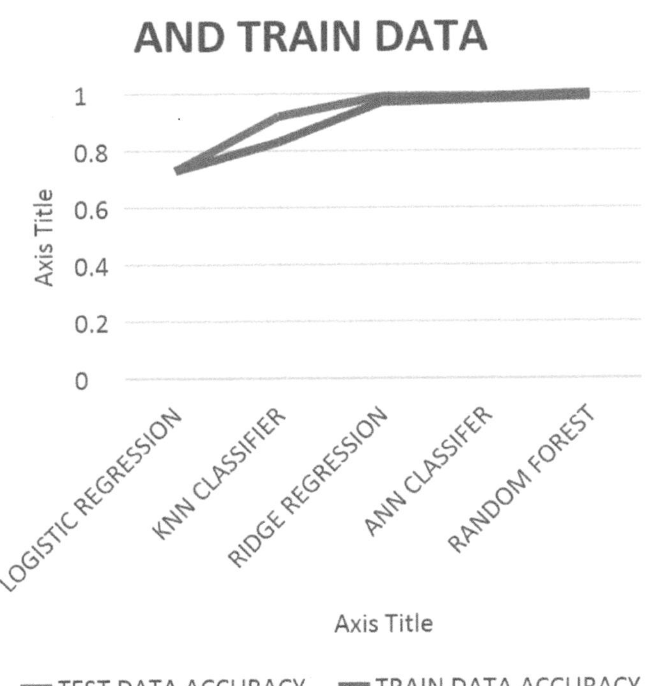

FIGURE 5.16   Graphical Comparison of Test and Train Data Accuracy for the Used Algorithms

4 CONCLUSION

This experimental study has been conducted to find out the best suited algorithm for the purpose of categorizing the activities of aged people as fall or no fall. This study will be helpful for the development of newer ways to prevent falls in elderly people. The accuracy rate for various algorithms has been listed in Table 5.2. The accuracy for the test and train data has been plotted as shown in Figure 5.16. From the observation of the values of accuracy for the algorithms used for the classification of the falls in elderly people, the authors can conclude that Random Forest Algorithms is the most efficient algorithm. The classical comparison of the classification algorithms in terms of their classification efficiency can be observed through Figure 5.17. For determining the falls in elderly people on the basis of thresholding the vital values of the body associated with heart and brain, after Random Forest, ANN Classifier yields the second-best output followed by the Ridge Regression, then KNN Classifier, and then Logistic Regression.

So, the most efficient algorithm turned out to be Random Forest followed by ANN classifier then Ridge Regression and after that comes KNN Classifier, which is then followed by Logistic Regression.

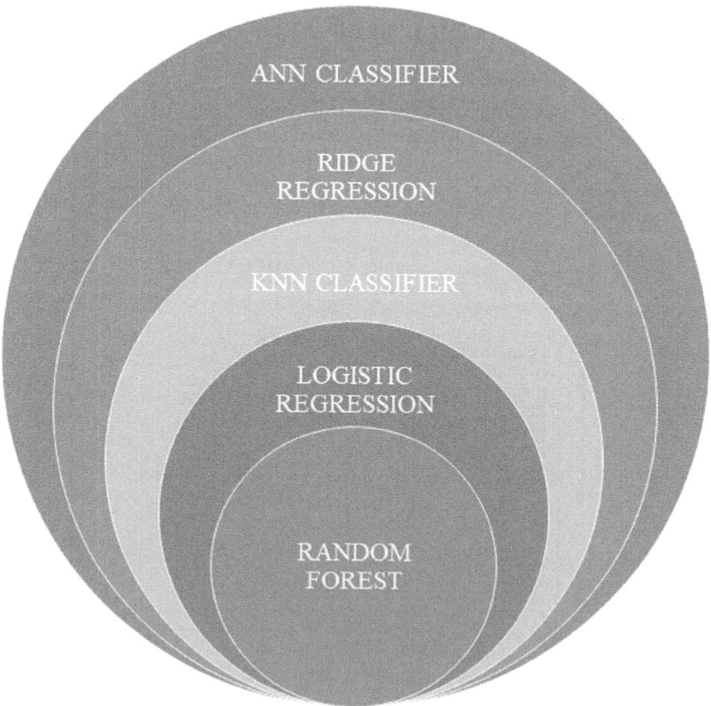

FIGURE 5.17 Graphical Representation of the Algorithms Used in Increasing Order of Accuracy

5 FUTURE SCOPE

The trials and testing of this chapter can be used to help build an accurate algorithm for the development of devices that can be developed for predicting as well as predicting fall of elderly people. This will be tremendously helpful as most of the injuries in elderly people are due to them falling while performing daily life activities. If according to their body vitals the fall is predicted beforehand, then it could be prevented and they can be effectively saved from serious injuries.

REFERENCES

[1] Al-Aama, T. "Falls in the elderly spectrum and prevention." *Canadian Family Physician* 57.7 (2011 Jul): 771–776.

[2] Rubenstein, L. Z., and Josephson, K. R. "Falls and their prevention in elderly people: what does the evidence show?" *Medical Clinics* 90.5 (2006): 807–824.

[3] Blake, A. J., et al. "Falls by elderly people at home: prevalence and associated factors." *Age and Ageing* 17.6 (1988): 365–372.

[4] Robbins, A. S., et al. "Predictors of falls among elderly people: results of two population-based studies." *Archives of Internal Medicine* 149.7 (1989): 1628–1633.

[5] Tinetti, M. E. "Preventing falls in elderly persons." *New England Journal of Medicine* 348.1 (2003): 42–49.

[6] Moiz, J. A., et al. "Activities-specific balance confidence scale for predicting future falls in Indian older adults." *Clinical Interventions in Aging* 12 (2017): 645.

[7] Available online: https://www.who.int/violence_injury_prevention/other_injury/falls/en/

[8] Al-Aama T. Falls in the elderly: spectrum and prevention [published correction appears in Can Fam Physician. 2014 Mar;60(3):225]. *Canadian Family Physician* 57.7 (2011): 771–776.

[9] Balzer, K., Bremer, M., Schramm, S., Lühmann, D., and Raspe, H. GMS Health Technology Assessment 8.Doc01 (2012): Epub 2012 Apr 12.

[10] Das, C. P., and Joseph, S. Falls in elderly. *Journal of Indian Medical Association* 103.3 (2005 Mar): 136, 138, 140 passim.

[11] Cumming, R. G., et al. "Medications and multiple falls in elderly people: the St Louis OASIS study." *Age and Ageing* 20.6 (1991): 455–461.

[12] Tinetti, M. E. "Preventing falls in elderly persons." *New England Journal of Medicine* 348.1 (2003): 42–49.

[13] Yardley L. et al. Recommendations for promoting the engagement of older people in activities to prevent falls. *Quality and Safety in Health Care* 16.3 (2007): 230–234.

[14] Patidar, A. B., et al. "Contributing factors and safety related lifestyle changes among older persons with history of falls." *International Journal of Nursing Care* 1.2 (2013): 7.

[15] Skelton, D., and Todd, C. What are the main risk factors for falls amongst older people and what are the most effective interventions to prevent these falls? Copenhagen, WHO Regional Office for Europe, Health Evidence Network report, 2004. Available online: http://www.euro.who.int/document/E82552.pdf (accessed on 27 August 2007).

[16] Yardley, L., et al. Older people's views of advice about falls prevention: a qualitative study. *Health Education Research* 21 (2006): 508–517.

[17] Yardley, L., et al. Older people's views of falls-prevention interventions in six European countries. *The Gerontologist* 46 (2006): 650–660.

[18] Institute of Medicine (US) Division of Health Promotion and Disease Prevention, Berg, R. L., and Cassells, J. S., editors. *The Second Fifty Years: Promoting Health and Preventing Disability*. *National Academies Press (US)*: Washington (DC), 1992. 15, Falls in Older Persons: Risk Factors and Prevention. Available online: https://www.ncbi.nlm.nih.gov/books/NBK235613/.

[19] Terroso, M., et al. Physical consequences of falls in the elderly: a literature review from 1995 to 2010. *European Review of Aging and Physical Activity* 11 (2014): 51–59. https://doi.org/10.1007/s11556-013-0134-8.

[20] Ludwig, W., Wolf, K. -H., Duwenkamp, C., Gusew, N., Hellrung, N., Marschollek, M., Wagner, M., Haux, R. Health-enabling technologies for the elderly—an overview of services based on a literature review. *Computer Methods and Programs* 106 (2012): 70–78.

[21] Liu, J., Lockhart, T. E. Automatic individual calibration in fall detection—an integrative ambulatory measurement framework. *Computer Methods in Biomechanics and Biomedical Engineering* 16 (2013): 504–510. University of Irvine Machine Learning Repository. Available online: http://archive.ics.uci.edu/ml/ (accessed on 15 June 2014).

[22] K neighbours Algorithm clustering. Available online: https://www.analyticsvidhya.com/blog/2018/03/introduction-k-neighbours-algorithm-clustering/

[23] Haykin, S. *Neural Networks and Learning Machines*; Prentice Hall: Upper Saddle River, NJ, USA, 2009.

6 Review in Healthcare Using Augmented Reality/Virtual Reality

An IoT perspective

Manisha Rajput, Rajan Kumar Dudeja, and Shubham Gargrish

1 INTRODUCTION

All facets of human existence and social well-being, such as self-gratification, employee's productivity, and economic expansion, are positively impacted by good health. Acknowledging the significance of healthcare, the United Nations' new sustainable development goals (SDGs) have already made ensuring accessible universal access to healthcare a key priority [1]. In order to bring together patients, medical personnel, apparatus, and other stakeholders for information exchange in this rapidly expanding healthcare sector's growing number of remote-end applications, a robust computer network is needed [2]. Traditional medicine is an approach in which physicians and other medical professionals such as therapists, pharmacists, and nurses are employed. They treat symptoms and illnesses by using radiation, surgery, or medicine. For a number of years, this element of development in the healthcare business has been one of the most revolutionary. The previously exclusive domain of doctors and patients now includes only one-third of them because of technology. While it has already found a place in the practice of medicine, information and communication technology currently plays a noteworthy role and dominates patient-level healthcare segment [3].

The development of Augmented Reality (AR) and Virtual Reality (VR) can be traced back to Charles Wheatstone's invention of the stereoscope in 1838, which gave the spectator a 3D image by using an image for each eye [4]. AR adds virtual content to the actual environment. Most of the time, it involves superimposing supplementary multimedia information on real-time photos and movies. VR, in disparity, only employs manufactured, computer-generated scenes that have no connection to reality [5]. Internet of Things (IoT) aims to improve the communication channels available to us right now.

DOI: 10.1201/9781003377818-6

Device-to-device communications will soon surpass people-to-people ones as the dominant form of communication. In fact, IoT paradigm is predicted to incorporate a huge number of smart devices with actuation, sensing, and processing capabilities [6].

IoT revolution is a cutting-edge technique that provides a broad range of applications in cities with smart technologies, emergency services, security, retail, industrial driven, waste management, and in logistics. Above and beyond all other considerations, IoT is regarded as alluring technique that has great potential to completely transform the way healthcare is delivered today through a range of innovative and personalized way out. The options incorporate tele-auscultation, telediagnostics, chronic illness management, remote health monitoring, independent senior care, and many more [1]. A health monitoring system was built on ESP 32, which monitors levels of oxygen and other gases in user's blood and send these details to the doctor through internet. [7].

Protection of medical information is especially important because cutting-edge medical technology, like VR and AR, is widely employed in surgery and medical education [8].

2 DIGITIZATION USED FOR THE IMPROVEMENT IN HEALTHCARE SYSTEM

2.1 Augmented Reality (AR)/Virtual Reality (VR)

AR glasses help the surgeon through a variety of surgical operations, from giving important information regarding the patient's condition to giving useful information for the surgery. Surgery simulation training in VR is particularly beneficial for health care providers. A typical 360° VR video stream needs to have a data rate of at least 2.5 Gbps and a minimum bit rate of 10 bits per pixel. Additionally, with 5G in place, the sophistication of haptic and tangible communication may be reaped more consistently and in ultra-real time [2].

2.2 Internet of Things (IoT)

The pharmaceutical and healthcare industries hold enormous application possibilities for the IoT technologies. By digitally gathering, storing, handling, transferring information, personnel information, prescription information, equipment information, sharing medical information, and management of information inside hospitals, it aids hospitals to implement smart medical treatment and management so as to achieve their objectives for digitized medical care and processing of data, humanized customer service, and communication. Additionally, it can more effectively address the requirement for efficient monitoring and management of healthcare information, medical tools supplies, and public health security to assist in resolving current issues with medical platform development, the level of services in the medical field, and the safety of medical production [9].

2.3 TELEMEDICINE

In 2015, there were over a million telehealth patients registered. This number increased to 7.5 million in 2018 with good cause. Today's telesanitary techniques allow patients to receive lifesaving diagnostics and access high-quality healthcare even in the most remote areas of the world [10]. Can't allow leading cancer experts to travel the nation by plane? It makes no difference. To ensure that you never miss a step in your treatment, this specialist may digitally link with your primary care physician. Telemedicine somewhat provides to level the things financially and geographically, enabling everyone to have the best medical treatment whenever they need it [11].

2.4 ARTIFICIAL INTELLIGENCE (AI)

By performing duties often performed by person but by fraction of a price and in a fraction of the time, AI simplifies the lives of patients, doctors, and hospital administrations. According to estimates, the global market for AI would expand from 600 *million in* 2014 *to* 150 billion by 2026. By utilizing technology that can forecast, thoroughly learn, and act, AI reinvents and revitalizes current healthcare, either it is employed to find new connections among gene or to control robots [11].

2.5 BLOCKCHAIN

A medical blockchain is a system that gives people access to their own comprehensive personal medical records and guarantees the safe, secure, and reliable storage and exchange of health information among patients, healthcare organizations, and third-party providers in the system. The ideal attributes of a medical blockchain include patient ownership, data storage, privacy, and easy and convenient interoperability. A distributed and open method of storing and managing medical data is offered by health blockchain [11].

3 ROLE OF AR/VR IN HEALTHCARE FIELDS – AN IOT PROSPECTIVE

In healthcare system AR/VR and IoT is applied in various fields like depression diagnostics and control, dental, rehabilitation, human anatomy, neurosurgery, nursing, theater, mental health etc.

3.1 DEPRESSION DIAGNOSTICS AND CONTROL

In today's world, depression is a condition that is getting progressively worse. Victims with anxiety disorder and depression need to be treated with the maximum care and support in order to recover and return to normal, but this is rarely the case. Depression will cause a person to feel down and uninterested in their

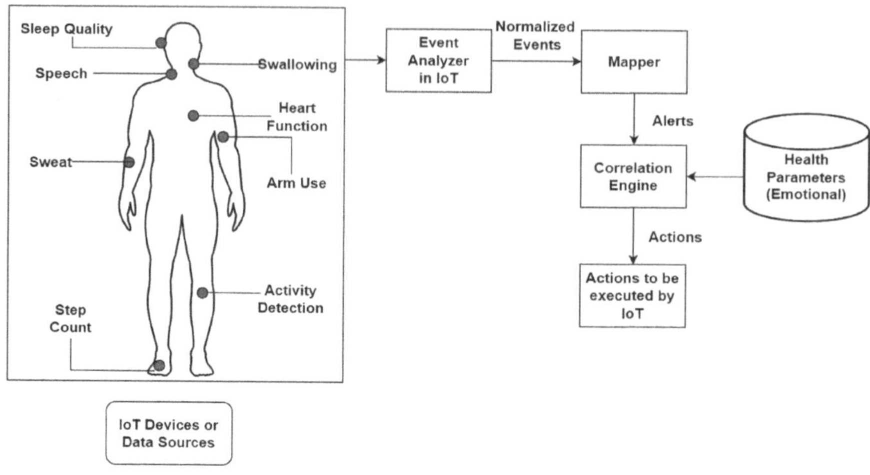

FIGURE 6.1　Depression Detection Mechanism

activities, which can be seen in a change in behaviour or behaviours. Most sufferers never notice that they have a problem inclination; if found early, few might be treated depending on their level of depression, few might die by suicide, and few could receive treatment continuously for the rest of their lives. Therefore, it is crucial for the individual to receive an early diagnosis and prompt treatment in order to avoid progressing to a serious stage of depression [12].

Therefore, early detection of any mental health concerns in individuals is essential. By observing their behavioural changes without engaging in human interaction, IoT devices can be used to identify and track depression symptoms. Instead of observing the patient's behaviour in the setting of a mental institution or when he is accompanied by family or friends, it might be beneficial to examine it when the patient is alone. The mechanism used for diagnosis must be trained first with the victim's typical behaviour in order to be able to recognize the behavioural switch and alert the patient at a very initial phase [13].

Figure 6.1 shows the diagnostic mechanism for depression. This figure is explained as: by using IoT devices, data will be collected through various sensors that are attached to the patient's body. This data is sent to an event analyzer in IoT for analysis. Then, this analyzed information is passed as normalized events to the mapper (Event to Alert mapper). Alerts will be generated. Generated alerts and health parameters such as emotions are sent to the correlation engine. Then, this engine will suggest some actions which will be performed by IoT.

In an experiment, the patients' mood and cognitive patterns were examined. Based on this information, it was necessary to teach the patients CBT (cognitive behavioural treatment) techniques. They were more suited by this therapy than other mechanisms to the established AI-based methodology. We need better wearable instruments to track our vital statistics since it is challenging to quantify mental wellness. IoT-driven smart ideas backed by algorithms benefit both rural residents' health and their doctors' ability to accurately diagnose illnesses before they spread. These programs or systems have a great chance of saving a great deal of lives. AI and ML, for example, might learn from the signs and results of a particular ailment as well as provide the doctor insights that would be challenging to foresee as a human.

IoT devices have been used to track and monitor mental wellness because it is crucial to treating depression in patients. A perfect mechanism for this ought to be able to assess the facts or the data produced by VR and IoT devices in order to determine severity of the patient's sadness before generating suggestions for how to assist them get well.

The person's actions and emotions can be tracked by this system, and the information can be utilized to identify any mental disorders. The merits of this mechanism include the ability to continuously monitor patients and provide reports to physician-family members along with the suggestions created on the patient's level of mental condition. Every day, new wearable technology is released onto the market. These gadgets can be used to track all emotions and, using the data, identify the symptoms. By integrating IoT systems with AI and ML algorithms, it could be further enhanced to offer decent experience. IoT could be linked with various new technologies, such as augmented reality or virtual reality (VR), to offer an AR juncture, a trustworthy self-evaluation service based on the knowledge of actual practitioners, an uninterrupted route to readdress the relevant psychiatric ill health sources, as well as individualized assistance and interventions. As a result, IoT systems can produce superior results when integrated with AI, ML, or AR/VR dramatically reducing the death rate [13].

3.2 PHYSICAL REHABILITATION OF STROKE PATIENTS

Patients must perform the physical therapy exercises advised in physical therapy clinics as well as at home to shorten the length of their rehabilitation, which will aid them to enhance their mental state. Patients must also practice the exercises to boost their motor state. Additionally, current research indicates that early and comprehensive rehabilitation may result in the capacity for motor function to recover. Combining, mobile devices and smartphone apps, serve as a platform for computation, communication, and the GUI for sufferers as well as for medical professionals. The one particular goal of this study is to improve physical therapy treatments while cutting costs in light of the demand for services brought on by the aging phenomenon [14]. The normal process of aging is typically followed by a decline in daily motor function that is linked to musculoskeletal problems and may also follow stroke occurrences. Another group of individuals that needs physical therapy treatments to enhance their motor skills is post-stroke patients. According to the data, stroke is the leading global cause of serious physical disability [15].

Doctors and therapists may benefit from the data regarding training outcomes provided by the remote monitoring of physiotherapy sessions in order to customize the exercises. This will aid patients in obtaining better rehabilitation outcomes in a shorter amount of time. Here, the objective of this study is to utilize wearable sensor networks, VR serious games, and IoT to monitor physical rehabilitation in order to increase patient involvement and track their progress. Thanks to serious games based on different VR settings, a patient with motor impairments can perform workouts in a very interesting and unobtrusive way while wearing a set of wearable technology. This helps the patient stay motivated during their rehabilitation process [3].

3.3 STEGANOGRAPHY-BASED MEDICAL PARADIGM FOR VIRTUAL REALITY'S SECURE MANAGEMENT OF MULTIMEDIA HEALTH INFORMATION

Steganography is the practice of concealing messages such that possible monitors are unaware that they are being conveyed. They are not aware that a secret communication is being conveyed, unlike with cryptography. In contrast to the former, which might make use of secret ink, the latter could contain a message like AHJKD [16]. This article recommends a steganography-based multimedia medical information service model as a means of safeguarding the integrity of the patient's healthcare data when utilizing specialist medical supplies, such as VR. The author suggested a model which attempts to prohibit the medical team from using VR to illegally access multimedia picture data obtained by specialized medical apparatus without the patient's consent.

Given that it combines both individual signatures and credentials in a hybrid cryptographic manner for digital medical care data, the proposed method has the properties that protect the person's confidentiality and privacy despite impairing the quality of the multimedia images they have taken using specialist medical equipment. In addition, because the person's signature data was encoded using steganography-based encryption techniques, data collected from medical imaging are viewed through VR and are not used without person's authorization [17]. It gathers the patient's medical information like his heart rate, blood pressure, body temperature, sleep check etc. so that the practitioner can safely transmit the patient's medical image data while effectively processing the user's ailment such as heart disease, diabetes, etc.

Figure 6.2 illustrates operational procedure for sharing user information with the clinical workforce. The operational procedures of the suggested paradigm can be generally categorized into three levels: wearables, heterogeneous networks, and feedback and analysis. Wearable device procedure depicts a stage in gathering patient's or user's data using cutting-edge medical technology such as smart watches, head-mounted displays (used for VR). In next phase, which is the heterogeneous network procedure, the user's medical imaging data procedure is transmitted through WLANs and cellular networks. The patient's medical imaging data is analyzed by approved persons/professionals during the analysis and feedback process. A steganography model is proposed for safeguarding IoMT-based medical data and information. Steganography is used to secure and protect medical information, as well as to conceal private information. The study's findings show that IoMT-based systems have a high level of data loss resistance as well as

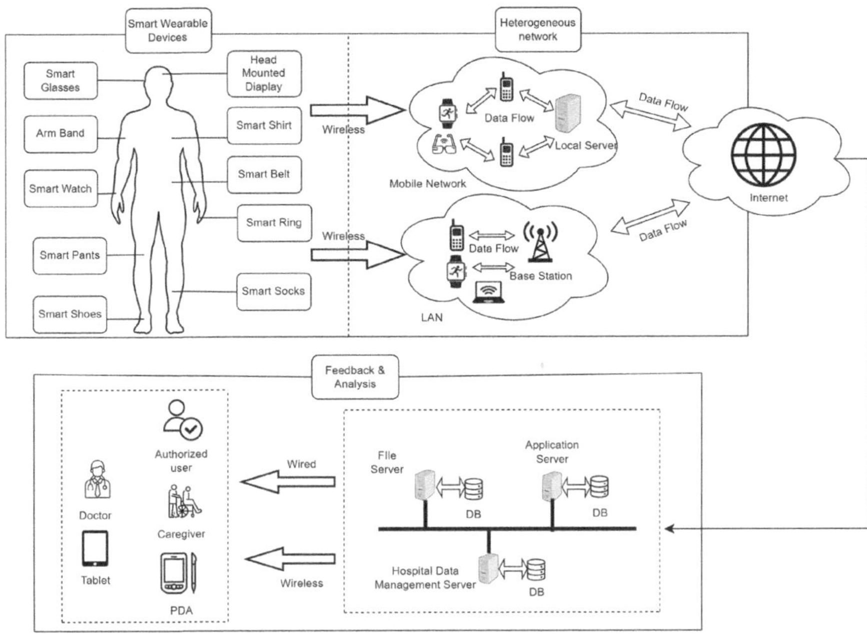

FIGURE 6.2   Transmission Process of Multimedia Information

a remarkable level of privacy and security protection. The performance measures are superior in terms of PSNR (66.45), RMES (0.98245), and MSE (0.8364) [18].

3.4   TREND OF METAVERSE AND AR, VR IN HEALTHCARE

Metaverse embraces integration as well as overlapping of the real and digital world, the merger of real and virtual economy or the amalgamation of real and virtual social lives or a combination of the real and virtual identities, or fusion of the virtual and physical assets. High-speed networks, cloud computing, IoT, AR/VR, edge computing, blockchain, AI, and other technologies are included. The adaptation of metaverse over current internet is due to the change in technology [19]. Therapy is one area where AR/VR has shown to be extremely useful. In aversion treatment, when patients encounter with situations that make them anxious in a secure, controlled environment under observation, psychiatrists and psychologists use it to customize surroundings for specific individuals [20].

The first Metaverse applications will be in patient care management, surgical simulations, diagnostic imaging modality, rehabilitation services, and healthcare management. With the aid of this technology, sufferers can better understand their diseases and available treatment options. AR/VR supports nursing staff at the time of care in a clinical setting. When AR is combined with radiology, doctors may clearly study internal anatomy by projecting medical images onto patients and arranging them with their bodies, even when they are moving. This includes

CT scan images [21]. Technology behemoths like Facebook, Microsoft, and others are currently heavily promoting Metaverse. People will unavoidably submit to every type of censorship, thus becoming targets of each and every form of commercial interests once the Metaverse is ready. According to research, Metaverse business model is slanted more in favour of platform owners, which weakens other rivals and frequently isn't good for the platform's long-term growth [22].

3.5 DENTAL RESEARCH IN MODERN WORLD

Due to the advancement of technology like AR/VR, IoT, AI, and the proliferation of mobile phones, telemedicine has increased [23]. There are currently a wide range of fascinating advances for both patients and healthcare professionals, as well as a fast growing number of uses for AR/VR technology in dental treatment [5]. Every imaginable sense, namely visual, auditory, and tactile, can be employed alone or in any combination, depending on the technique [24]. With the use of AR/VR technology, users may overlay virtually produced representations over recordings of patients moving naturally. Any 3D model may be enhanced to better reflect the unique patient situation in order to simulate various, plausible scenarios in advance without intrusive working procedures, for example, a prosthetic design for a prospective reconstruction. Such digital models are then examined in real-time, increasing efficiency in communication not only between dental professionals and the patient to increase treatment predictability and effectiveness but also with the sufferers to explain the complicated therapy stages [25]. The field of dentistry education is another interesting and promising one, transferring theoretical information and hands-on exercises to provide interactive training with all accessibility and impartial assessment [26]. Patients in rural locations can get dental care in an efficient manner. Early disease detection and monitoring provides the benefit of lowering patient risk while also lowering expenses. Among other research, the use of a smartphone camera for early diagnosis of dental caries, periodontitis [27], and oral cancer is being investigated [28]. In a setting like COVID-19, where there is a requirement to minimize interaction with people, it is anticipated to support a number of components and have an effect while offering the benefit of avoiding touch with the mask off [29].

A complete virtual environment can be used in postgraduate education [30] to learn difficult and sophisticated clinical protocols without endangering real patients, and professionals can continuously improve their skills while using AR/VR simulations. Soon, AR/VR will be able to completely transform dental education [31].

3.6 UTILIZATION OF AR EXERGAMING FOR THE ASSESSMENT OF PHYSICAL AND MENTAL ACTIVITY

A long-standing requirement in the healthcare and assisted living sectors is to encourage users' increased physical activity, which has been significantly decreased by today's sedentary lives [32]. Additionally, interventions and rewards for regularly adhering to a care plan are frequently needed. Today, AR technologies are widely used in the video game business, and typical gameplay situations encourage players to enhance their physical activity [33]. Exergames are a type of game that encourages players to engage in exercises and motions that they otherwise wouldn't [34]. The authors have created a prototype solution for serious exergame development that will not only support healthy lifestyle promotion but also assist medical specialists in evaluating user health conditions and in identifying hazards. To further guarantee simplicity, interoperability with other platforms, openness to integrate with other contemporary technologies, and inexpensive prices, the total system should also adopt a modular architecture and make use of commodity hardware. The suggested framework for creating AR games incorporates tools for sophisticated user interaction, tailored IoT technologies, and accurate evaluation of users' vital signs and activity.

The suggested framework for creating AR games includes tailored IoT technologies, instruments for sophisticated user interaction, and efficient evaluation of users' vital signs and activity. The prototype consists of three key components: (a) an AR-ready mobile framework built on [35]; (b) a program for IoT wearables that tracks user activity and biosignals; (c) a cloud platform with a web application endpoint that enables medical practitioners to remotely adjust the game's features and evaluate the outcomes. This method combines IoT technologies for biosignal and movement monitoring with AR development ideas for improved interactivity. Users and gamers can take advantage of AR's advanced interactivity features and track their health metrics while playing games (such as the amount of steps they took, their heart rate, and the tremor in their hand), and record the outcomes [36]. Additionally, they strive to consistently motivate and encourage elderly individuals to engage in exercises or motions that they otherwise wouldn't [37] and to adhere to a set schedule of tasks within the framework of their care plans. Indoor virtual reality exercise games exhibit promising outcomes in improving users' physical states while retaining high user satisfaction under COVID-19 distancing circumstances [38]. Patients with stroke have demonstrated improved balance using a telerehabilitation exergame platform that integrates mobile devices and remote sensors [39].

IoT, AR, cloud, and web technologies are all employed by this platform to suggest a prototype that, in addition to monitoring the user's current measures and providing the doctors with real-time health information, also gives them the ability to pre-define and control the game remotely. Furthermore, it has relatively minimal ownership costs because it can run on common and, in most cases, already owned devices and is hardware independent. In general, it can broaden the user's knowledge and provide an intriguing technique to enhance well-being in the overall ideas of quantified self-assisted life [35]. More sophisticated real-world interactions will be made possible through enhanced gameplay, and these interactions will be used to create more challenging game settings and challenges. The challenges will be improved in conjunction with healthcare professionals to better fit the user's treatment plans and rules for dynamic game parameter adjustments depending on the care plan and results monitoring will be put into place. Existing implementations of suggestions for applications utilizing quantified self will be included as part of this update [40]. Finally, to further improve user experience and increase gameplay excitement, multi-user activities will be supported both locally and remotely.

3.7 PAIN MANAGEMENT IN INPATIENTS USING VR

When the patient is in intense care, management of pain securely and effectively is a major concern. The majority of hospitalized patients experience pain, and one-quarter of that pain is severe [41]. VR headsets (also known as head-mounted displays) can help patients with psychiatric and psychological illnesses. VR helps in reducing anxiety and stress and, in addition to this, provides a fun environment for the patients to fix problems and experience pain [42]. Opioids are commonly used in pain management, which has a history of producing inconsistent and unsatisfactory results. According to data from the US Centers for Disease Control, even a single day of opioid medication can foretell a 6% chance of reliance one year later. Hence, there is a desperate call to implement proper pain management practices which should not only be safe and efficient but should also be drug free for such inpatients [43].

Under this investigation, authors have conducted a comparative efficacy study comparing "health and wellness" television programming with a scalable VR intervention in a varied population of patients who were admitted in hospital with pain. When compared to the control group watching "health and wellness" television channel in the room, the on-demand usage of VR in this trial was well handled and led to statistically massive improvements in pain management in a diverse group of hospitalized patients. These findings expand on past research and show that VR is a useful supplementary therapy to support conventional pain management techniques in patients who were admitted in the hospital [44]. The experiment specifically reduced examiner's communication and had not forced VR usage procedure after receiving the patient's initial instructions, collected the key outcome measure only from nonstudy nursing staff, and used a controlled intervention with possible therapeutic effects. Furthermore, the experiment included inpatients with every type of visceral and somatic pain, along with gastrointestinal, orthopedic, oncologic, neurological, and various types. It was challenging for any interface to provide persistent pain improvements throughout these heterogeneous, hospitalized patient population because a lot of the patients experienced complicated, biopsychosocial distress due to multi-factorial reasons and underwent multi-modal therapy.

Nevertheless, the VR intervention produced statistically significant gains from the very beginning as well as after using it for 48 and 72 hours. Patients were more satisfied with their VR experiences than they were with watching television, which is a step up from the current norm for in-room audiovisual interaction. Despite being statistically significant, the effect of VR had only a modest absolute impact on pain scores. Following the initial treatment, VR contributed to an incremental decrease of 1.18 point in pain versus that of a control group after multivariable correction; however, when examining the cumulative pain scores in the following 2 days, the incremental effect was just 0.59 points. According to Farrar and colleagues [45], these differences are less than 2 point cutoff for a minimum clinical relevant difference MCID on the Numeric Rating Scale. However, some researchers have found that MCID are closer to a 14% shift from the baseline (around 1.5 point on a scale of 0–10), which approximates the change seen in this research [46], [47].

It was noteworthy that just 120 patients signed up and followed the protocol despite 591 being evaluated for participation. Despite the fact that this study is a huge trial of randomized hospitalized patients for pain treatment using VR to our knowledge, it's crucial to highlight the decrease between the enrollment of patient's and completion of the study. The finding highlights the fact that many hospitalized patients were not eligible for or they were not interested in adopting emerging health techniques like virtual reality, and were happy with the earlier studies employing VR in hospitalized patients [48]. Many of those who were qualified to take part in the experiment declined to do so for a number of reasons [49].

Patients varied in their levels of skepticism, fear, vulnerability, concern over the equipment's potential psychological effects, and general unwillingness to be bothered. Although health technology holds out so much potential, we think it's critical for the ehealth society to acknowledge that aspirations might be dashed by clinical realities. It is not yet apparent how VR precisely reduces perception and experience of pain or to what extent different VR formats are useful [50]. In hypothesized processes, the benefit is frequently attributed to straightforward diversion. When the mind is engaged in an immersive task, it might be difficult to notice things outside the range of attention [51]. VR is supposed to produce an immersive distraction that prevents brain from processing pain by profusing visual, auditory, and proprioception senses [50].

4   A CASE STUDY: VR IN IOT-BASED ASSISTANCE MODEL FOR ALZHEIMER'S PATIENTS

Alzheimer's is a disease that affects the human brain. It badly affects people in their older ages. The illness grows with time and badly affects the daily routine works of the patients. Dementia, a term for memory loss and other cognitive impairments severe enough to interfere with daily life, is most frequently caused by Alzheimer's disease.

Brain consists of billions of neurons that further has specific task of thinking, learning, remembering, and many more activities. For smooth functioning of the brain, these neurons establish the communication among themselves. It behaves like the factories that receives the raw materials and consumes energy and produces some specific output functions. Scientists believe that Alzheimer's disease affects these neuron cells that can result in memory loss and can also affect other cognitive actions. These patients have common issues in that they even forget their basic daily life activities.

The case study has been performed in phases where the initial phase analyzes the behaviour of the patients and analyze the data received from the IoT sensors and detects the level of symptoms for the Alzheimer patients. According to patients' severity level, AR/VR-based assistance model is designed for the Alzheimer patients in the next phase. There are number of sensors that are embedded on the body of the patients to track their daily movement and other activities.

$$A(n) = a_1, a_2, a_3, ..., a_n \tag{1}$$

$$P(n) = p_1, p_2, p_3, ..., p_n \tag{2}$$

A_n represents a set of the sensors that are embedded on body of the Alzheimer patients. These sensors are like acceleration sensor, motion sensors, and other medical sensors. These sensors are called active sensors that continuously track the movement of the patients and periodically communicate the data to the cloud server that can be further processed and analyzed. There are other sets of sensors called passive sensors represented by P_n that can be used when required. These sensors are not embedded on the body of the patients and also they do not generate the data on a periodic basis. These are used in scenarios like smart homes or rooms where these patients are living under observations.

After receiving the data from the sensors, the data are analyzed and actions have been taken accordingly. The data analysis has been performed on cloud server and further action is decided based on the data received. The data received is from the periodic data and communicated from the active set of sensors.

Table 6.1 shows the criticality level of the data and also shows us what action needs to be performed at which level. When the decision system finds the data to be critical, it immediately triggers the actions that are needed to be performed, such as calling of an emergency service which has to be made. The emergency services include alerting the doctor, informing patient's family members, calling the local police and ambulance services or calling for immediate initial medical facilities available nearby.

The other two categories include severe level and mild level, where there are needs of assistance for the patients. The assistance could be made based on the VR-based applications. The application helps the patients in their Daily Life Activities (ADL) for severe level patients. The ADL activities include the basic activities like brushing, bathing, taking food, medicines, and walking etc. The assistance application-based model first triggers alarms and other signs that indicate the patients to perform the ADL activities and take the help of VR to feel like they are performing the ADL activities. VR heals the minds of patients and also helps them to perform their daily activities in a systematic manner. The above task could also be possible with the help of passive sensors only, but the VR adds extra benefits to it.

Social cognition can be considered as one of the major problems for the Alzheimer patients. As the patients are under continuous observation either in special care units or in their homes, their social interactions become very low and therefore VR emerges as a promising field for solving this problem. The VR plays

TABLE 6.1

Actions Performed for Alzheimer Patients

Data Category	Action to be Performed	Remarks
Critical level	Immediate action	Call emergency services
Severe level	VR-based assistance	Required ADL and social assistance
Mild level	VR-based assistance	Required social assistance

important role for their social interaction with their family and friends. There are various applications with which the patient can connect with his or her family and friends that can further give him or her feelings which are equal to physical interactions with them. The warmth of physical interactions actually did not happen, but VR's application will definitely improve the mental status of the patients.

5 CONCLUSION

The integration of IoT with the traditional healthcare system improves its service and its affordability to provide the healthcare services to the patients beyond the hospitals. The integration of AR/VR applications in fields of IoT-enabled healthcare makes its service more effective for the patients. Our study has reviewed the effects of AR/VR in healthcare fields like depression diagnostics and control, physical rehabilitation of stroke patients, dental treatment, pain management for the hospitalized patients, and assessment of mental health of patients. The study has presented a case study for detection, treatment, and guidance for Alzheimer patients based on their VR-based IoT-enabled environments. It shows that the field has lots of scope for further studies on AR/VR and in other healthcare fields also.

REFERENCES

[1] S. Latif, J. Qadir, S. Farooq, M. A. Imran, How 5g wireless (and concomitant technologies) will revolutionize healthcare? *Future Internet* 9 (4) (2017) 93.

[2] S. Dananjayan, G. M. Raj, 5g in healthcare: how fast will be the transformation? *Irish Journal of Medical Science* (1971-) 190 (2) (2021) 497–501.

[3] O. Postolache, D. J. Hemanth, R. Alexandre, D. Gupta, O. Geman, A. Khanna, Remote monitoring of physical rehabilitation of stroke patients using iot and virtual reality, *IEEE Journal on Selected Areas in Communications* 39 (2) (2020) 562–573.

[4] S. U. R. Singh, P. Sharma, P. Kukana, Study of revolutionizing healthcare with VR and AR technology (2016).

[5] T. Joda, M. M. Bornstein, R. E. Jung, M. Ferrari, T. Waltimo, N. U. Zitzmann, Recent trends and future direction of dental research in the digital era, *International Journal of Environmental Research and Public Health* 17 (6) (2020) 1987.

[6] G. Aloi, G. Caliciuri, G. Fortino, R. Gravina, P. Pace, W. Russo, C. Savaglio, A mobile multi-technology gateway to enable iot interoperability, in: *2016 IEEE First International Conference on Internet-of-things Design and Implementation (IoTDI)*, IEEE, 2016, pp. 259–264.

[7] M. Beri, B. Kumar, S. Tiwari, N. Sharma, H. Vashishtya, P. Chaudhary, Iot based health monitoring system built on esp32, in: *2022 2nd International Conference on Advance Com- puting and Innovative Technologies in Engineering (ICACITE)*, IEEE, 2022, pp. 454–458.

[8] F. G. Hamza-Lup, J. P. Rolland, C. Hughes, A distributed augmented reality system for medical training and simulation, *arXiv preprint arXiv:1811.12815* (2018).

[9] S. Srivastava, S. Prakash, An analysis of various iot security techniques: A review, in: *2020 8th International Conference on Reliability, Infocom Technologies and Optimization (Trends and Future Directions) (ICRITO)*, IEEE, 2020, pp. 355–362.

[10] G. E. Churcher, G. Bilchev, J. Foley, R. Gedge, T. Mizutani, Experiences applying sensor web enablement to a practical telecare application, in: *2008 3rd International Symposium on Wireless Pervasive Computing*, IEEE, 2008, pp. 138–142.

[11] S. Srivastava, S. V. Singh, R. B. Singh, H. K. Shukla, Digital transformation of healthcare: a blockchain study, *International Journal of Innovative Science, Engineering & Technology* 8 (5) (2021).

[12] P. Deepika Mathuvanthi, V. Suresh, C. Pradeep, Iot powered wearable to assist individuals facing depression symptoms, *International Research Journal of Engineering and Technology* 6 (2019) 1676–1681.

[13] P. K. Katkuri, A. Mantri, Study of behavioral changes and depression control mechanism using iot and vr, in: *Innovations in Computer Science and Engineering*, Springer, 2021, pp. 605–613.

[14] K. Lucki, M. Bach, M. Winfried Banzer, Rollator use and functional outcome of geriatric rehabilitation, *Journal of Rehabilitation Research and Development* 47 (2) (2010) 151.

[15] T. S. Jesus, I. L. Silva, Toward an evidence-based patient-provider communication in re- habilitation: linking communication elements to better rehabilitation outcomes, *Clinical Rehabilitation* 30 (4) (2016) 315–328.

[16] D. Kahn, The history of steganography, in: *International Workshop on Information Hiding*, Springer, 1996, pp. 1–5.

[17] M. Elhoseny, G. Ram´ırez-Gonz´alez, O. M. Abu-Elnasr, S. A. Shawkat, N. Arunkumar, A. Farouk, Secure medical data transmission model for iot-based healthcare systems, *IEEE Access* 6 (2018) 20596–20608.

[18] J. B. Awotunde, I. D. Oladipo, M. AbdulRaheem, G. B. Balogun, A. R. Tomori, An iomt-based steganography model for securing medical information, *International Journal of Healthcare Technology and Management* 19 (3–4) (2022) 218–236.

[19] K. Bhugaonkar, R. Bhugaonkar, N. Masne, The trend of metaverse and augmented & virtual reality extending to the healthcare system, *Cureus* 14 (9) (2022) e29071.

[20] B. Marr, The amazing possibilities of healthcare in the metaverse, *Internet Adresi* (2022). https://www.forbes.com/sites/bernardmarr/2022/02/23/the-amazing-possibilities-of-healthcare-in-the-metaverse.

[21] K. Ganapathy, Metaverse and healthcare: a clinician's perspective, *Apollo Medicine* 19 (4) (2022) 256–261.

[22] D. Chen, R. Zhang, Exploring research trends of emerging technologies in health metaverse: a bibliometric analysis, Available at SSRN 3998068 (2022).

[23] S.-Y. Park, Teledentistry and digital therapeutics (dtx) for dentistry, *Journal of Clinical Advances in Dentistry* 6 (1) (2022) 28–30.

[24] C. Pensieri, M. Pennacchini, Virtual reality in medicine, in: *Handbook on 3D3C Platforms*, Springer, 2016, pp. 353–401.

[25] T. Joda, G. O. Gallucci, The virtual patient in dental medicine, *Clinical Oral Implants Research* 26 (6) (2015) 725–726.

[26] S.-H. Lee, Research and development of haptic simulator for dental education using virtual reality and user motion, *International Journal of Advanced Culture Technology* 6 (4) (2018) 52–57.

[27] S.-J. Lee, I.-J. Kwon, Y.-D. Son, J.-H. Kim, M.-S. Lee, D. Kwon, E.-S. Song, B. Kim, J.-H. Lee, H.-K. Kim, Early detection of tongue cancer using a convolutional neural network and evaluation of the effectiveness of efficientnet (2022).

[28] J. Kü"hnisch, O. Meyer, M. Hesenius, R. Hickel, V. Gruhn, Caries detection on intraoral images using artificial intelligence, *Journal of Dental Research* 101 (2) (2022) 158–165.

[29] B. Askarian, F. Tabei, G. A. Tipton, J. W. Chong, Smartphone-based method for de- tecting periodontal disease, in: *2019 IEEE Healthcare Innovations and Point of Care Technologies, (HI-POCT)*, IEEE, 2019, pp. 53–55.

[30] S. Gargrish, Augmented reality and education: a comprehensive review and analysis of methodological considerations in empirical studies, *Journal of e-Learning and Knowledge Society* 19 (3) (2023) 99–109.

[31] A. Ayoub, Y. Pulijala, The application of virtual reality and augmented reality in oral & maxillofacial surgery, *BMC Oral Health* 19 (1) (2019) 1–8.

[32] P. Das, M. Zhu, L. McLaughlin, Z. Bilgrami, R. L. Milanaik, Augmented reality video games: new possibilities and implications for children and adolescents, *Multimodal Tech- nologies and Interaction* 1 (2) (2017) 8.

[33] T. Kari, J. Piippo, L. Frank, M. Makkonen, P. Moilanen, To gamify or not to gamify? gamification in exercise applications and its role in impacting exercise motivation (2016).

[34] J. Sween, S. F. Wallington, V. Sheppard, T. Taylor, A. A. Llanos, L. L. Adams-Campbell, The role of exergaming in improving physical activity: a review, *Journal of Physical Activity and Health* 11 (4) (2014) 864–870.

[35] D. Koulouris, A. Menychtas, I. Maglogiannis, On the development of augmented reality based exergames for assessing human activity and cognition on mobile devices, in: *The 14th PErvasive Technologies Related to Assistive Environments Conference, 2021*, pp. 521–526.

[36] D. Koulouris, A. Menychtas, I. Maglogiannis, An iot-enabled platform for the assessment of physical and mental activities utilizing augmented reality exergaming, *Sensors* 22 (9) (2022) 3181.

[37] E. Brox, L. F. Luque, G. J. Evertsen, J. E. G. Hern´andez, Exergames for elderly: social exergames to persuade seniors to increase physical activity, in: *2011 5th International Conference on Pervasive Computing Technologies for Healthcare (PervasiveHealth) and Workshops*, IEEE, 2011, pp. 546–549.

[38] P. Campo-Prieto, G. Rodr´ıguez-Fuentes, J. M. Cancela-Carral, Immersive virtual reality exergame promotes the practice of physical activity in older people: an opportunity during covid-19, *Multimodal Technologies and Interaction* 5 (9) (2021) 52.

[39] P. I. Burgos, O. Lara, A. Lavado, I. Rojas-Sepu´lveda, C. Delgado, E. Bravo, C. Kamisato, J. Torres, V. Castan˜eda, M. Cerda, Exergames and telerehabilitation on smartphones to improve balance in stroke patients, *Brain Sciences* 10 (11) (2020) 773.

[40] S. P. Erdeniz, A. Menychtas, I. Maglogiannis, A. Felfernig, T. N. T. Tran, Recommender systems for iot enabled quantified-self applications, *Evolving Systems* 11 (2) (2020) 291–304.

[41] M. Helfand, M. Freeman, Assessment and management of acute pain in adult medical inpatients: a systematic review, *Pain Medicine* 10 (7) (2009) 1183–1199.

[42] G. Singh, J. K. Sandhu, et al., Virtual and augmented reality technology for the treatment of mental health disorders: an overview, in: *2022 13th International Conference on Computing Communication and Networking Technologies (ICCCNT)*, IEEE, 2022, pp. 1–5.

[43] A. Shah, C. J. Hayes, B. C. Martin, Factors influencing long-term opioid use among opioid naive patients: an examination of initial prescription characteristics and pain etiologies, *The Journal of Pain* 18 (11) (2017) 1374–1383.

[44] B. Spiegel, G. Fuller, M. Lopez, T. Dupuy, B. Noah, A. Howard, M. Albert, V. Tashjian, R. Lam, J. Ahn, et al., Virtual reality for management of pain in hospitalized patients: a randomized comparative effectiveness trial, *PloS One* 14 (8) (2019) e0219115.

[45] J. T. Farrar, J. P. Young Jr, L. LaMoreaux, J. L. Werth, R. M. Poole, Clinical importance of changes in chronic pain intensity measured on an 11-point numerical pain rating scale, *Pain* 94 (2) (2001) 149–158.

[46] F. Salaffi, A. Stancati, C. A. Silvestri, A. Ciapetti, W. Grassi, Minimal clinically important changes in chronic musculoskeletal pain intensity measured on a numerical rating scale, *European Journal of Pain* 8 (4) (2004) 283–291.

[47] S. B. Bird, E. W. Dickson, Clinically significant changes in pain along the visual analog scale, *Annals of Emergency Medicine* 38 (6) (2001) 639–643.

[48] S. Mosadeghi, M. W. Reid, B. Martinez, B. T. Rosen, B. M. R. Spiegel, Feasibility of an immersive virtual reality intervention for hospitalized patients: an observational cohort study, *JMIR Mental Health* 3 (2) (2016) e5801.

[49] V. C. Tashjian, S. Mosadeghi, A. R. Howard, M. Lopez, T. Dupuy, M. Reid, B. Mar- tinez, S. Ahmed, F. Dailey, K. Robbins, et al., Virtual reality for management of pain in hospitalized patients: results of a controlled trial, *JMIR Mental Health* 4 (1) (2017) e7387.

[50] A. Li, Z. Montan̄o, V. J. Chen, J. I. Gold, Virtual reality and pain management: current trends and future directions. *Pain Management* 1 (2011) 147–157.

[51] K. McCaul, J. Malott, Distraction and coping with pain: Psychological Bulletin 95 (1984) 516–533, *Pain* 23 (3) (1985) 315.

7 Shooting Method for Solving Two-point Boundary Value Problems in ODEs Numerically and Applications to Medical Science

Jitender Singh

1 INTRODUCTION

For a positive integer $n > 1$ and real numbers a and b with $a < b$, let $X : [a,b] \to R^n$ be the $n \times 1$ column matrix function defined as follows:

$$X(z) = \left(X_1(z), X_2(z), \ldots, X_n(z) \right)',$$

where the prime denotes matrix transpose and $X_i : [a,b] \to R$, for each $1 \le i \le n$ is sufficiently smooth on the open interval (a,b). We consider the following first-order ordinary vector, differential equation

$$\frac{d}{dz} X(z) = f(z, X(z)), z \in [a,b]. \tag{1}$$

Throughout, the map $f : [a,b] \times R^n \to R^n$ is assumed to be sufficiently smooth and satisfies Lipschitz condition on the closed rectangle

$$R = [a,b] \times \bar{U} \subset [a,b] \times R^n$$

with a Lipschitz constant $K > 0$, that is,

DOI: 10.1201/9781003377818-7

$$\left\| f\left(z, X(z)\right) - f\left(z, Y(z)\right) \right\| \le K \left\| X(z) - Y(z) \right\|, \tag{2}$$

for all X, Y in $\bar{U}$ and $a \le z \le b$. For each $i = 1, \ldots, n$, let the coordinate functions $X_i(z)$ satisfy m initial conditions at $z = a$ and the remaining $(n-m)$ conditions at $z = b$, that is,

$$\left(X_1, X_2, \ldots, X_m \right)'(a) = \left(a_1, \ldots, a_m \right)' \in \mathbf{R}^m, \tag{3}$$

$$\left(X_{\sigma(1)}, \ldots, X_{\sigma(n-m)} \right)'(b) = \left(b_1, \ldots, b_{n-m} \right)' \in \mathbf{R}^{n-m} \tag{4}$$

where $\sigma : \{1, 2, \ldots, n\} \to \{1, 2, \ldots, n\}$ is a bijection.

The system $(1) - (4)$ defines a two-point BVP whose solution is not completely known at any of the two boundary points $z = a$ or b. Such BVPs are a common object of investigation in mathematical, physical, engineering, and medical and health care sciences. Most often, such BVPs do not possess a closed form solution although an approximate analytical solution may be found using topological methods such as the homotopy perturbation method. Consequently, one is forced to look for numerical solutions in order to unfold the inherent scientific information. In view of this, the differential equation in higher dimensions is converted to a nonlinear algebraic equation in higher dimensions by approximating $X(z)$ with a Galerkin type expansion in terms of a suitable orthogonal basis. Such basis functions should satisfy the boundary conditions of the BVP in hand. The nonlinear algebraic equation is then solved numerically for the unknown coefficients with the help of an iterative scheme such as Newton-Raphson or bisection.

An easy numerical procedure to solve two-point BVPs such as the one described in (1)–(4) is the shooting method. Due to generality and applicability of the shooting technique in solving many different types of BVPs in ODEs, different shooting methods have been developed in the literature, based on the type of the two-point BVP in hand [1–9].

Although the shooting technique is a direct numerical approach toward solving nonlinear BVPs, several difficulties arise during its implementation. For example, a reasonably good guess for the unknown initial conditions is desired to be made at one of the boundaries. Otherwise, the underlying Newton iterates may not converge. Also, the location of the root within the radius of convergence is not known in advance. This complexity increases with n and the use of shooting method may become impractical.

Ha [7] has discussed a shooting technique for nonlinear two-point BVPs and achieved rapid numerical convergence. Liu [10] has proposed Lie-group preserving schemes for integrating (1). Based on this, Liu [11] has developed a Lie-group shooting method for solving second-order nonlinear BVPs numerically.

Using a modification of Adomian decomposition, Wazwaz [6] has developed an efficient shooting technique to handle higher-order nonlinear two-point BVPs numerically.

In spite of plenty of available research on shooting techniques, their usage has been limited in the past. This serves as a motivation for the present chapter in order to highlight the power of the shooting techniques to efficiently solve higher-order two-point BVPs numerically. More precisely, we mainly describe the nonlinear shooting method of Singh [17] for higher-order two-point BVPs arising in physical situations.

The following well-known results for systems of ODEs can be found in Birkhöff and Rota [12]. The reader interested in implementing the shooting method can skip these results for the time being as well as the content of Section 3, and may jump to study the methodology explained in Section 4. The theory part can be studied later if needed.

Theorem 1.

If $X = A(z)$, $B(z)$ are any two solutions of (1) where $f(z, X(z))$ is continuous and satisfies Lipschitz condition of (2), then

$$\left\| A(a+h) - B(a+h) \right\| \le e^{K|h|} \left\| A(a) - B(a) \right\|, \ 0 < h < b - a. \tag{5}$$

Corollary 2.

Let $X(z,c)$ be a solution of (1) with $X(z,c) = c$, for some $c \in R^n$, and the hypotheses of Theorem 1 are satisfied. Let $X(z,c)$ exists on

$$\left\| c - c_0 \right\| \le k_1, |z - a| \le k_2,$$

for some $c_0 \in R^n$ and positive real numbers k_1, k_2. Then $X(z,c)$ is a continuous function of z and c. Further, if $c \to c_0$, then $X(z,c) \to X(z,c_0)$ uniformly on $|z - a| \le k_2$.

We recall that a smooth function $Y : R \to R^n$ is said to be an approximate solution of the differential equation $dX / dz = f(z, X(z)), X(0) = X_0$, with an error at most $\eta \ge 0$ if

$$\left\| Y(z) - X(z) \right\| < \eta \text{ for all } z \in [a,b],$$

with deviation at most $\epsilon \ge 0$ if $Y(z)$ is continuous and satisfies the differential inequality

$$dY / dz - f(z, X(z)) \le \epsilon.$$

Theorem 3.

(**Runge-Kutta Method**) *Let* $\mathcal{P} : a = z_0 < z_1 < \cdots < z_{s-1} < z_s = b$ *be a partition of the interval* $[a,b]$. *An approximate solution of the initial value problem*

$$\frac{dX(z)}{dz} = f(z, X(z)); X(a) = X_0, \ a \le z \le b,$$

is given by the following iterative scheme

$$X^0 = X_0; X^{i+1} = X^i + \frac{h}{6}(k_1 + 2k_2 + 2k_3 + k_4); i = 0,1,2,\ldots,$$

where $h = (b-a)/s$ *and*

$$k_1 = f(z_i, X^i),$$

$$k_2 = f(z_i + h/2, X^i + hk_1/2),$$

$$k_3 = f(z_i + h/2, X^i + hk_2/2),$$

$$k_4 = f(z_i + h, X^i + hk_3),$$

which is in an error $E = \mathcal{O}(h^5)$ *at each iterative step.*

The following well-known result is about the convergence of Newton iterates in higher dimensions (see for detail, Ortega [13], Tapia [14], Rall [15], and Gragg and Tapia [16]).

Theorem 4.

Let A *and* B *be Banach spaces. Let* U *be an open convex subset of* A. *Let* $F : U \rightarrow B$ *be such that map* F *is differentiable and satisfies*

$$\left\| \frac{dF}{dx} - \frac{dF}{dy} \right\| \le L \, \| x - y \|, \text{ for all } x, y, \in U. \tag{6}$$

For some $x_0 \in U$, *assume that* $F'(x_0)^{-1}$ *is defined on all of* B *and that* $h = L\beta\eta \le 1/2$ *for some positive real numbers* β *and* η, *where*

$$\left\| (dF \, / \, dx)(x_0)^{-1} \right\| \le \eta,$$

$$\left\| (dF \, / \, dx)(x_0)^{-1} F(x_0) \right\| \le \eta.$$

Define

$$t^* = \frac{1 - \sqrt{1 - 2h}}{\beta L}; t^{**} = \frac{1 + \sqrt{1 - 2h}}{\beta L}; S = \left\{ x \in U \mid \left\| x - x_0 \right\| \le t^* \right\}.$$

Then sequence of Newton iterates $\{x_k\}$, *where*

$$x_{k+1} = x_k - \left(\frac{dF}{dx}(x_k) \right)^{-1} F(x_k), k = 0, 1, 2 \ldots \tag{7}$$

is well defined in S *and converge to a solution* x^* *of* $F(x^*) = 0$ *which is unique in the set*

$$U \cap \{ x \mid \left\| x - x_0 \right\| < t^{**} \}.$$

Moreover if $h < 1 / 2$, *then the order of convergence is at least quadratic.*

The linear shooting method is described in Section 2. The technical detail about the nonlinear shooting technique is explained in Section 3. The numerical integration technique for the underlying BVP is then developed in Section 4 and is successfully implemented through examples in Section 5.

2 THE LINEAR SHOOTING METHOD

The linear shooting technique as we describe here converges rapidly for a wide class of linear BVPs in hand. The BVP (1)-(4) is called linear if the function $f(z, X(z))$ in (1) is of the form

$$A(z) X(z) + B(z),$$

where $A(z)$ is an $n \times n$ matrix function of z and $B(z) \in R^n$ is a column matrix function of z. Each of $A(z)$ and $B(z)$ is independent of $X(z)$. Consequently, the considered linear BVP can be described as follows:

$$\frac{d}{dz} X(z) = A(z) \cdot X(z) + B(z), z \in [a, b], \tag{8}$$

along with the boundary conditions given by (3)-(4). We follow the following steps of linear shooting technique. We construct the following set of linear IVPs

$$\frac{d}{dz}X(z) = A(z) \cdot X(z) + B(z), \tag{9a}$$

$$X(a) = \xi_0 + e_{m+i}, \tag{9b}$$

where

$$\xi_0 = (a_1, \ldots, a_m, 0, 0, \ldots, 0)' \in \mathbf{R}^n,$$

and $e_{m+i}, 1 \leq i \leq n-m$ is the element of the standard basis of $\mathbf{R}^n$ having its $(m+i)$-th entry 1 and each of the rest of the entries equal to zero. Using the theory of Wronskian, $(n-m)$ linearly independent solutions of (9) can be constructed, which remain linearly independent for all $z \in [a, b]$. Let $X^{(1)}, \ldots, X^{(n-m)}$ be those $n-m$ linearly independent solutions of (9), such that

$$X^{(i)}(z) = \left(X_1^{(i)}(z), \ldots, X_n^{(i)}(z) \right)',$$

$$X^{(i)}(a) = \xi_0 + e_{m+i}, 1 \leq i \leq n-m.$$

Then the solution of the BVP (8) can be expressed as a linear combination of the $n-m$ linearly independent column vectors $X^{(1)}, \ldots, X^{(n-m)}$, that is, there exist scalar $\alpha_1, \ldots, \alpha_{n-m}$ such that

$$X(z) = \alpha_1 X^{(1)}(z) + \cdots + \alpha_{n-m} X^{(n-m)}(z). \tag{10}$$

In order that the vector $X(z)$ in (10) satisfies the BVP (8), it must satisfy the remaining boundary condition at $z = b$. In view of this, we have

$$\alpha_1 X_{\sigma(i)}^{(i)}(b) + \cdots + \alpha_{n-m} X_{\sigma(i)}^{(i)}(b) = b_i, i = 1, \ldots, n-m \tag{11}$$

which defines a system of $n-m$ linear algebraic equations in $\alpha_1, \ldots, \alpha_{n-m}$ and hence can be solved using Gauss-elimination method. Thus, using the Runge-Kutta method, one can compute a numerical solution of (8) which satisfies the condition (11) at the second boundary. It is easy to implement the aforementioned procedure in MATLAB using the subroutine ode45 to solve the underlying $(n-m)$ IVPs at a discrete set of points in the interval $[a, b]$.

Linear BVPs arise frequently in hydrodynamic studies in fluid mechanics. In view of this, the linear shooting technique as explained here has been utilized in solving complex linear two-point BVPs in [18–21] arising from the Couette-Taylor instability and in [22] regarding the transient convection in ferrofluids.

3   THE NONLINEAR SHOOTING METHOD

Following Singh [17], let the $n - m$ tuple

$$c = (c_1, c_2, \ldots, c_{n-m})' \in R^{n-m}, n > m,$$

be independent of z such that the smooth vector function $X(z,c)$ satisfies (1)–(4), that is,

$$\frac{d}{dz} X(z,c) = f(z, X(z,c)); \tag{12a}$$

$$X(a,c) = X(a); X(b,c) = X(b). \tag{12b}$$

Assume that the functions $X(z,c)$ and f are defined on the closed rectangle R, where

$$R = [a,b] \times \bar{U} \subset [a,b] \times R^{n-m},$$

and are continuously differentiable in $R \setminus \partial R$ such that $\partial f / \partial X$ is nonsingular there. We observe that at point (z,c), and each $i = 1, 2, \ldots n - m$, we have

$$\frac{d}{dz}\left(\frac{\partial X}{\partial c_i}\right)(z,c) = \frac{\partial}{\partial c_i} \frac{dX}{dz}(z,c)$$

$$= \frac{\partial}{\partial c_i} f(z, X(z,c_i))$$

$$= \frac{\partial f}{\partial X}(z, X(z,c_i)) \frac{\partial X}{\partial c_i}(z,c) \tag{13}$$

If we let

$$X(a,c) = (a_1, \ldots, a_m, c_1, c_2, \ldots, c_{n-m})',$$

then we have

$$\frac{\partial X}{\partial c_i}(a,c) = e_{m+i}.$$

Consequently, for each component c_i of c, the derivative $\partial X / \partial c_i$ satisfies the following $(n-m)$ initial value problems (IVPs)

$$\frac{d}{dz}\left(\frac{\partial X}{\partial c}\right)(z,c) = \frac{\partial f}{\partial X}(z, X(z,c)) \cdot \left(\frac{\partial X}{\partial c}\right)(z,c), \tag{14a}$$

$$\left(\frac{\partial X}{\partial c}\right)(a,c) = [e_{m+1},\ldots,e_n]. \tag{14b}$$

In view of the aforementioned discussion, we have the following result.

Theorem 5

(Singh [17]). *The hypothesis of Theorem 4 is satisfied by the sequence of functions* $\left\{F\left(c^k\right)\right\}$ *defined as follows:*

$$F\left(c^k\right) = \tilde{X}\left(b,c^k\right) - \tilde{X}(b), k = 0,1,2,\ldots \tag{15}$$

on the closed rectangle $\bar{U} \subset \mathbf{R}^{n-m}$ *containing the point* c *in its interior, where*

$$\tilde{X}\left(z,c^k\right) = \left(X_{\sigma(1)}\left(z,c^k\right),\ldots,X_{\sigma(n-m)}\left(z,c^k\right)\right)' \text{ is in } [a,b]\times\bar{U}, \text{ such that}$$

$$\tilde{X}(b) = \left(b_1,b_2,\ldots,b_{(n-m)}\right)'.$$

The sequence $\left\{c^k\right\}$ *is defined recursively by the following:*

$$c^0 = c, c^{k+1} = c^k - \left(\frac{\partial F}{\partial x}\left(c^k\right)\right)^{-1} F\left(c^k\right), k = 1,2,\ldots \tag{16}$$

For proof of Theorem 5, the reader is referred to consult Singh [17]. The following corollary is immediate from Theorem 5.

Corollary 6

(Singh [17]). *The sequence* $\left\{c^k\right\}, k = 0,1,\ldots$ *as in (16) is well defined and lies in the set* $\{x \mid \|x-c\| < t^*\} \subset U_0$ *and converges to unique solution* c^* *of the equation*

$$F(x) = 0$$

on the set $U_0 \cap \{x \mid \|x-c\| < t^{**}\}$. *Further,* $\tilde{X}(z,c) \to \tilde{X}\left(z,c^*\right)$ *as* $c \to c^*$.

Remark.

The function defined by the sequence $\left\{F\left(c^k\right)\right\}$ as above, satisfies

$$\left\|F\left(c^{k+1}\right)-F\left(c^k\right)\right\| \le e^K \left\|\left(dF/dc\left(c^k\right)\right)^{-1} F\left(c^k\right)\right\|$$

and hence, is dominated by the sequence $\left\{c^k\right\}$. To see this, consider the partition

$$a = z_0 < z_1 < \cdots < z_{N-1} < z_N = b, z_i = a+i(b-a)/N; 1 \le i \le N, \text{ of } [a,b].$$

Since f satisfies Theorem 4 with Lipschitz constant K, we have the following or each fixed k and $a = z_{i-1}$, and any two solutions $X\left(z,c^{k+1}\right)$ and $X\left(z,c^k\right)$ of (12).

$$\left\|X\left(z_i,c^{k+1}\right)-X\left(z_i,c^k\right)\right\| \le e^{K(z_i-z_{i-1})}\left\|X\left(z_{i-1},c^{k+1}\right)-X\left(z_{i-1},c^k\right)\right\|$$

$\cdots$

$$\le e^{K(z_i-z_0)}\left\|X\left(z_0,c^{k+1}\right)-X\left(z_0,c^k\right)\right\|, \tag{17}$$

and correspondingly, the following is satisfied.

$$\left\|\tilde{X}\left(z_i,c^{k+1}\right)-\tilde{X}\left(z_i,c^k\right)\right\| \le e^{K(z_i-z_{i-1})}\left\|\tilde{X}\left(z_{i-1},c^{k+1}\right)-\tilde{X}\left(z_{i-1},c^k\right)\right\|$$

$\cdots$

$$\le e^{K(z_i-z_0)}\left\|\tilde{X}\left(z_0,c^{k+1}\right)-\tilde{X}\left(z_0,c^k\right)\right\|. \tag{18}$$

From (18) we obtain the desired assertion for $F\left(c^k\right), k = 0,1\ldots$ as follows:

$$\left\|F\left(c^{k+1}\right)-F\left(c^k\right)\right\| = \left\|\tilde{X}\left(1,c^{k+1}\right)-\tilde{X}\left(1,c^k\right)\right\|$$

$$\le e^K \left\|\tilde{X}\left(0,c^{k+1}\right)-\tilde{X}\left(0,c^k\right)\right\|$$

$$= e^K \left\|c^{k+1}-c^k\right\| = e^K \left\|\left(\partial F/\partial c\left(c^k\right)\right)^{-1} F\left(c^k\right)\right\|,$$

since the sequence $\left\{\partial F/\partial c\left(c^k\right)\right\}$ is constant. Also, $F\left(c^k\right) \to F\left(c^*\right) \to 0$ for $c^k \to c^*$.

4   THE NUMERICAL SCHEME FOR NONLINEAR SHOOTING METHOD

In this section, we develop a numerical scheme for applying the nonlinear shooting method described in Section 3. In view of Theorem 5, an arbitrary choice of the Lipschitz constant $\kappa > 0$ ensures at least quadratic convergence of the underlying Newton iterates. The underlying iterative scheme involves computation of an approximate numerical solution $X(z,c^*)$ of (1)-(4) which at $(k+1)$-th iteration involves simultaneous numerical integration of (12) from $z = a$ to $z = b$ to compute $F(c^k)$ followed by a numerical integration of IVPs defined by (14) for each c_i to numerically compute $\dfrac{\partial X}{\partial c}(b,c^k)$. The associated numerical integrations are to be performed on the interval $[a,b]$. In this view, we consider the following system of IVPs:

$$\frac{d}{dz}\begin{pmatrix} X \\ \dfrac{\partial X}{\partial c_i^k} \end{pmatrix}(z,c^k) = \begin{pmatrix} f\big(z, X(z,c^k)\big) \\ \dfrac{\partial f}{\partial X}\dfrac{\partial X}{\partial c_i^k}(z,c^k) \end{pmatrix}, \tag{19a}$$

$$\begin{pmatrix} X \\ \dfrac{\partial X}{\partial c_i^k} \end{pmatrix}(a,c^k) = \begin{pmatrix} \xi^k \\ e_{m+i} \end{pmatrix}, \tag{19b}$$

for each $i = 1,\ldots,n-m$, where

$$\xi^k = \big(a_1,\ldots,a_m,c_1^k,c_2^k,\ldots,c_{n-m}^k\big)'.$$

So, from (19), we have $(n-m)$ IVPs in ODEs, each of which is of order $2n$ and can be integrated numerically. We explain the procedure in the following steps.

Step 1. Using the fourth order Runge-Kutta method or the more efficient Runge-Kutta Fehlberg method, we solve the $(n-m)$ IVPs as in (19) for a finite set of points in the interval $[a,b]$, to obtain the solution at $z = b$, that is,

$$\begin{pmatrix} X \\ \dfrac{\partial X}{\partial c_i^k} \end{pmatrix}(b,c^k), \ i = 1,\ldots,\, n-m,$$

$$c^k = \left(c_1^k,\ldots,c_{n-m}^k\right), \ k = 0,1,2,\ldots,$$

with an appropriate step size h starting with an initial guess c^0 for $k = 0$.

Step 2. In the next step we extract the vector

$$\tilde{X}\left(b,c^k\right) = \left(X_{\sigma(1)}\left(b,c^k\right),\ldots,X_{\sigma(n-m)}\left(b,c^k\right)\right)'$$

and the Jacobian matrix $\dfrac{\partial \tilde{X}}{\partial c}\left(b,c^k\right)$ from the numerically computed solution in the preceding step so that we have

$$\frac{\partial \tilde{X}}{\partial c}\left(b,c^k\right) = \left(\frac{\partial \tilde{X}}{\partial c_1^{\,k}}\left(b,c^k\right), \frac{\partial \tilde{X}}{\partial c_2^{\,k}}\left(b,c^k\right), \cdots, \frac{\partial \tilde{X}}{\partial c_{n-m}^k}\left(b,c^k\right)\right). \tag{20}$$

Suppose the numerical solution is sorted within the specified tolerance (tol.), then this amounts to check if the following condition is satisfied

$$\tilde{X}\left(b,c^k\right) - \tilde{X}(b) < \text{tol.}, \tag{21}$$

so that at the k-th iteration, $\tilde{X}\left(z,c^k\right) \approx X(z)$ is the desired approximated solution within an error not exceeding tol. Otherwise, we go to the next step for implementing the next Newton's iteration.

Step 3. If $\tilde{X}\left(b,c^k\right) - \tilde{X}(b) \geq \text{tol.}$, then the $(k+1)$-th Newton iteration is performed to obtain c^{k+1} by solving the following system of $(n-m)$ linear algebraic equations in $c_1^{k+1},\ldots,c_{n-m}^{k+1}$ given by

$$\frac{\partial \tilde{X}}{\partial c}\left(b,c^k\right)c^{k+1} = \frac{\partial \tilde{X}}{\partial c}\left(b,c^k\right)c^k - \left\{\tilde{X}\left(b,c^k\right) - \tilde{X}(b)\right\}. \tag{22}$$

We use Gauss-elimination method in order to solve the linear system in (22) which is easy to implement in computer programs and is free from any type of numerical singularity.

With the computation of c^{k+1} using (22) one iteration of the shooting method is completed. The whole procedure is repeated through **steps 1–3** to obtain c^{k+2} till the numerically computed solution is within the specified tolerance, that is, it satisfies (21).

Nonlinear two-point boundary value problems (BVPs) arise in boundary layer flow over a stretching or shrinking sheet. Such situations commonly occur in industrial processes of making metallic sheets, manufacturing of chocolates in the food industry, magnetohydrodynamic drug targeting using Casson model in medical and health sciences. Most of the two-point BVPs arising in such applications can be solved numerically using the nonlinear shooting method as described before.

5　NUMERICAL EXAMPLES AND DISCUSSION

It is easy to write a program in MATLAB for simultaneously solving (20) and (22) recursively, till the scheme converges and meets the desired tolerance. The numerical codes for implementing the present numerical scheme can be easily written in MATLAB by following the excellent text of Mathews and Fink [23]. To justify applicability of the proposed numerical procedure of nonlinear shooting technique, we consider the following examples.

Example 1.

Consider the following second-order nonlinear BVP

$$\frac{d}{dz}\begin{pmatrix} X_1 \\ X_2 \end{pmatrix} = \begin{pmatrix} X_2 \\ 2X_1^3 - 6X_1 - 2z^3 \end{pmatrix},$$

$$X_1(1) = 2, X_1(2) = 5/2,$$

for $z \in [1,2]$. Here $n = 2, m = 1, c = c_1, a = 1, b = 2$, σ is the identity permutation of $\{1,2\}$ so that $\tilde{X}(z,c) = X_1(z,c)$, and

$$f(z, X(z)) = \begin{pmatrix} f_1 \\ f_2 \end{pmatrix}(z, X(z))$$

$$= \begin{pmatrix} X_2 \\ 2X_1^3 - 6X_1 - 2z^3 \end{pmatrix}.$$

We construct the approximate solution

$$X(z,c) = \left(X_1(z,c), X_2(z,c) \right)'$$

so that $X(z,c)$ and $\dfrac{\partial X}{\partial c}(z,c)$ satisfying the following system of equations

$$\frac{dX}{dz}(z,c) = f(z, X(z,c)); X(1,c) = \begin{pmatrix} 2 \\ c_1 \end{pmatrix},$$

$$\frac{d}{dz}\frac{\partial X}{\partial c_1}(z,c) = \begin{pmatrix} \dfrac{\partial f_1}{\partial X_1} & \dfrac{\partial f_1}{\partial X_2} \\[2ex] \dfrac{\partial f_2}{\partial X_1} & \dfrac{\partial f_1}{\partial X_1} \end{pmatrix}\frac{\partial X}{\partial c_1}(z,c)$$

$$= \begin{pmatrix} 0 & 1 \\ 6X_1^2 - 6 & 0 \end{pmatrix}\frac{\partial X}{\partial c_1}(z,c),$$

$$\frac{\partial X}{\partial c_1}(1,c) = \begin{pmatrix} 0 \\ 1 \end{pmatrix} = e_2.$$

In view of (19), we need to solve the following IVP numerically using Runge-Kutta method.

$$\frac{d}{dz}\begin{pmatrix} X_1 \\ X_2 \\ \dfrac{\partial X_1}{\partial c_1} \\ \dfrac{\partial X_2}{\partial c_1} \end{pmatrix} = \begin{pmatrix} X_2 \\ 2X_1^3 - 6X_1 - 2z^3 \\ \dfrac{\partial X_2}{\partial c_1} \\ 6\left(X_1^2 - 1\right)\dfrac{\partial X_1}{\partial c_1} \end{pmatrix}; \begin{pmatrix} X_1 \\ X_2 \\ \dfrac{\partial X_1}{\partial c_1} \\ \dfrac{\partial X_2}{\partial c_1} \end{pmatrix}(1,c) = \begin{pmatrix} 2 \\ c_1 \\ 0 \\ 1 \end{pmatrix}, \qquad (23)$$

where c_1 is the unknown constant, which is to be approximated, numerically. Now applying **steps 1–3** as explained in the preceding section, we compute the numerical solution of the given BVP. The exact solution is

$$X_1(z) = z + \frac{1}{z}, \ 1 \le z \le 2.$$

We choose a step size of $h = 0.02$ to numerically integrate the IVP (23) using Runge-Kutta method within a tolerance of 10^{-6}. To apply Runge-Kutta method, an initial guess for c_1^0 is needed, which can be specified as shown Table 7.1, where the convergence analysis of the solution is also shown for different initial guesses for c_1^0. Clearly, $c_1^0 = 0$ is appropriate corresponding to which the numerical convergence is achieved for first iteration within an error of the order of 10^{-8}. Larger the value of $|c_1^0|$, larger is the number of iterations required to have the numerical convergence within an error at most of the order of 10^{-8}.

The same example was considered by Ha [7] in which no numerical solution was found to exist with his numerical method for $c_1^0 \ge 1$. On the other hand, it is clear from Table 7.1 that the present numerical scheme converges

TABLE 7.1

Variation of k with c_1^0 for a Step Size of 0.02

c_1^0	k	c_1^k	$\left\| \tilde{X}\left(2,c^k\right) - \tilde{X}(2) \right\|$
-100	118	$-5.567960e-09$	$2.051692e-13$
-10	49	$-5.547987e-09$	$2.462031e-10$
-1.0	34	$-5.140315e-09$	$5.266837e-09$
0.0	01	$0.000000e-00$	$6.857203e-08$
0.1	05	$-5.554485e-09$	$1.661671e-10$
0.5	13	$-5.567931e-09$	$5.559997e-13$
1.0	32	$-4.726264e-09$	$1.036603e-08$
5.0	58	$-5.567060e-09$	$1.131273e-11$
10.0	62	$-4.687076e-09$	$1.084867e-08$
20.0	79	$-5.544791e-09$	$2.855325e-10$
50.0	98	$-5.276342e-09$	$3.591604e-09$

even for $c_1^0 \geq 1$. Moreover, for $c_1^0 = 0.6975$, the present numerical scheme converges in 20 iterations to the approximate numerical solution within an error of at most $3.483020e-07$, whereas Ha's paper mentions that his numerical method converged after 9982 iterations.

The system of ODEs in the above example is locally Lipschitz with the Lipschitz constant $\kappa \geq 40$ in the following set

$$R = \left\{ (X_1, X_2) \in \boldsymbol{R}^2 : |X_1 - 2| \leq 0.5 \right\}.$$

By Theorem 5, the present numerical scheme converges for every value of c_1^0 taken from the set R on the line $X_1 = 2$. However, for larger values of c_1^0, the rate of convergence may slow down as can be seen from Table 7.1. The numerically computed profiles of X_1 and X_2 with z are shown in Figure 7.1, where the solid lines denote the actual solution and the asterisks $*$ denote the numerically computed values. It is evident from the Figure 7.1 that the graph of numerically approximated solution using the present method is indistinguishable from that of the closed form solution.

In fact, the present numerical method will converge for all initial guesses in the BVPs originating from locally Lipschitz ODEs, where the Jacobian is computed only once for all iterations, thereby lowering the expenses of the numerical computations.

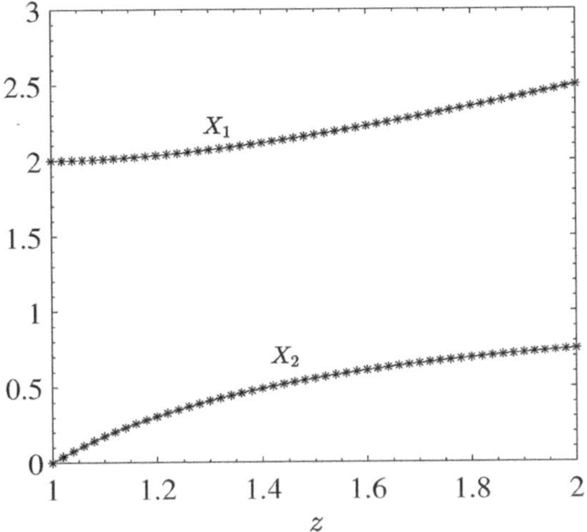

FIGURE 7.1   Numerically Computed Solutions (✳) vs the Closed form Solution (-) of the BVP Considered in *Example 1* (See Singh [17])

Example 2.

Consider the following fifth-order coupled nonlinear BVP arising in the boundary layer flow due to a stretching sheet under temperature variations.

$$f''' + ff'' - (f')^2 = 0; f(0) = 0, f'(0) = 1 = \theta(0), \qquad (24a)$$

$$\theta'' + \Pr \theta' f = 0; f'(5) = 0 = \theta(5). \qquad (24b)$$

If we let

$$f = X_1, \quad f' = X_2, f'' = X_3,$$

$$\theta = X_4 ; \theta' = X_5,$$

then

$$X(z) = (X_1, X_2, X_3, X_4, X_5)'$$

and the given nonlinear system (24) reduces to the following equivalent system

$$\frac{d}{dz}\begin{pmatrix} X_1 \\ X_2 \\ X_3 \\ X_4 \\ X_5 \end{pmatrix} = f(z, X(z)) = \begin{pmatrix} X_2 \\ X_3 \\ -X_1X_3 + (X_2)^2 \\ X_5 \\ -\Pr X_1 X_5 \end{pmatrix}, 0 \le z \le 5, \qquad (25a)$$

along with the following boundary conditions given by

$$X_1(0) = 0, X_2(0) = 1 = X_4(0); X_2(5) = 0 = X_4(5). \qquad (25b)$$

Here, $n = 5, m = 2, c = (c_1, c_2)', a = 0, b = 5$, and σ is the bijection with

$$\sigma(1) = 2, \sigma(2) = 4, \qquad (25c)$$

so that

$$\tilde{X}(z,c) = (X_2(z,c), X_4(z,c))'.$$

As before, let the approximate solution of (25) be

$$X(z,c) = (X_1(z,c), X_2(z,c), X_3(z,c), X_4(z,c), X_5(z,c))'$$

so that $X(z,c)$ and $\dfrac{\partial X}{\partial c}(z,c)$ satisfy the following IVP:

$$\frac{dX}{dz}(z,c) = f(z, X(z,c)), \qquad (26a)$$

$$\frac{d}{dz}\frac{\partial X}{\partial c_i}(z,c) = \begin{pmatrix} 0 & 1 & 0 & 0 & 0 \\ 0 & 0 & 1 & 0 & 0 \\ -X_3 & 2X_2 & -X_1 & 0 & 0 \\ 0 & 0 & 0 & 0 & 1 \\ -\mathrm{Pr}X_5 & 0 & 0 & 0 & -\mathrm{Pr}X_1 \end{pmatrix} \frac{\partial X}{\partial c_i}(z,c), \qquad (26b)$$

$$X(0,c) = \begin{pmatrix} 0 \\ 1 \\ c_1 \\ 1 \\ c_2 \end{pmatrix}; \frac{\partial X}{\partial c}(0,c) = \begin{pmatrix} 0 & 0 \\ 0 & 0 \\ 1 & 0 \\ 0 & 0 \\ 0 & 1 \end{pmatrix} = (e_3, e_5), \qquad (26c)$$

where c_1 and c_2 are the unknown missing boundary conditions to be approximated numerically using the shooting technique. So, we follow the **steps 1–3** of Sec. 4, to solve the IVPs defined by (26) numerically for a step size of 0.01 and a specified tolerance of 10^{-6}. The missing boundary conditions for each case Pr = 0.71, 1, 6 as obtained using the present numerical procedure are given in Table 7.2, where we find that for the nonlinear BVP (24), c_1 is independent of the parameter Pr while c_2 changes on changing Pr.

TABLE 7.2

Variation of the Number of Iterations k with Pr for the Convergence Within the Specified Tolerance

Pr	K	$c_1; c_2$	$\left\| \tilde{X}\left(5, c^k\right) - \tilde{X}(5) \right\|$
0.71	19	$-1.001396e + 00; -4.755625e - 01$	$8.784541e - 07$
1.0	16	$-1.001396e + 00; -5.872225e - 01$	$7.851039e - 07$
6.0	8	$-1.001396e + 00 ; -1.738095e + 00$	$2.235719e - 07$

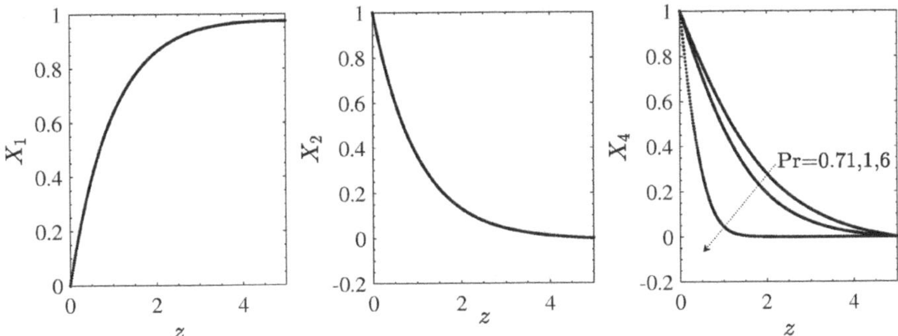

FIGURE 7.2   Plots of the Numerical Solution with z Using the Nonlinear Shooting Method for Various Values of Pr

The numerical scheme converges rapidly to the solution of the given BVP (24) within an error of the order of 10^{-7}. Figure 7.2 shows the numerically computed solution for the considered numerical values of the parameter Pr. The profiles for X_1 and X_2 are independent of Pr, while the profile for X_4 vary significantly on varying Pr. This can be understood physically since $X_4 = \theta$, the temperature of the boundary layer in the vicinity of the stretching sheet surface, which has to vary with changing Pr, the Prandtl number of the viscous fluid under consideration.

5.1   CASSON MODEL IN MEDICAL SCIENCES

In this section, we describe an application of the present numerical method to nonlinear problem arising in the magnetohydrodynamic Casson fluid flow in medical science. Casson fluid is a rheological plastic fluid that has an additional yield stress. The flow of a Casson fluid occurs when the shear stress exceeds the yield stress. The Casson model is intimately connected with modeling the flow of blood stream in medical science in hemodynamics. In view of this, the medicine mixed with magnetohydrodynamic (MHD) particles is injected into the blood stream near the location of the tumor. Simultaneously, the tumor site of the patient is also subjected to an externally applied magnetic field. The MHD particles behave like a heat source in the presence of magnetic field. As a result, cancer cells in the tissue located at the tumor site get destroyed. There is an analogy of hemodynamics with the flow of a Casson fluid over a stretching or shrinking sheet and can be understood as follows. In a cardiovascular system, the blood is a Casson fluid, where the blood flows over the inner wall of the blood vessels under an externally controlled magnetic field is modeled as a stretching sheet problem, where the inner wall of the blood vessel behaves like a stretching sheet [24], [25]. In [25], Singh et al. found that the wall shear stress at the inner wall of the blood vessels is likely to play a crucial role in the nonlinear dynamics of blood flow. The nonlinear system of ODEs describing the aforementioned blood flow along with suitable boundary conditions give rise to the following third-order nonlinear two-point BVP:

$$\left(1+\frac{1}{a}\right)f'''(\eta)+ff''(\eta)-f'^2-Mf'=0, \tag{27a}$$

$$f(0)=v_c, f'(0)-\left(d+\beta_1 f''(0)+\beta_2 f'''(0)\right)=0, \tag{27b}$$

$$\lim_{\eta\to\infty}f'(\eta)=0 \tag{27c}$$

where a is the Casson parameter, M is the dimensionless measure of the externally applied magnetic field, v_c, d, β_1, β_2, are the dimensionless forms of the initial flow velocity at the inner wall of the stretching sheet, the slip parameter, and the modified Navier's first and second-order slip parameters in modeling the flow. The nonlinear two-point BVP (27a)-(27c) can be easily handled using the present shooting method as in *Example 2*. It will be interesting to compare and combine the present technique with multimedia analysis of practical data and using intelligent systems [26–28].

Many other similar nonlinear high order BVPs can be handled efficiently with ease using the present numerical technique. Below, we provide some sample problems for the purpose; the first three problems have been taken from Vleggaar [29].

- $2f'''(\eta)+f(\eta)f''(\eta)=0;\quad f(0)=0, f'(0)=1=\theta(0),$

  $2\theta''(\eta)+\Pr\,\theta'(\eta)f(\eta)=0; f'(5)=0=\theta(5).$

- $\eta f'''+(f-1)(f''-f'/\eta)=0; f(1)=1/2, f'(1)=1=\theta(1),$

  $\theta''+\theta'(1+\Pr f)=0; f'(5)=0=\theta(5).$

- $\eta f''' + (f-1)(f'' - f'/\eta) - (f')^2 = 0; f(1) = 1/2, f'(1) = 1 = \theta(1),$

  $\theta'' + \theta'(1 + \Pr f)/\eta = 0; f'(5) = 0 = \theta(5).$

- Solve $y'' = 2yy', 0 \le t \le 1; y(0) = 0, y(1) = 2$ by taking initial guess $\alpha_0 = 0, 0.5, 1$. What do you observe?

- Solve the following BVP numerically

  $$y'' = 400y + 400\cos^2(\pi x) + 2\pi^2 \cos(2\pi x), y(0) = 0 = y(1).$$

6   CONCLUDING REMARKS

The linear shooting method is discussed in brief to solve linear two-point BVPs in ODEs. A good number of references are provided to encourage the reader about its usage.

The nonlinear shooting method for solving nonlinear higher-order BVPs is discussed in detail and the various steps involved in its implementation are described through concrete examples.

Based on the analysis, we have described a numerical scheme for obtaining numerical solutions of higher-order nonlinear two-point BVPs arising in different physical domains within the framework of ODEs. The numerical procedure is easy to implement in standard computer packages, such as MATLAB. The underlying numerical scheme is found to converge rapidly to a solution of the nonlinear BVP in hand. In view of the ease of applicability and high rate of convergence of the proposed linear and nonlinear shooting techniques, we recommend their use for handling a wide variety of linear and nonlinear BVPs, originating in diverse areas of science and technology. More importantly, the present numerical technique can be applied to the two-point BVPs arising in the modeling of blood flow dynamics in hemodynamics under magnetohydrodynamic and rheological conditions for treating tumor in patients.

REFERENCES

[1] H. B. Keller. "Numerical methods for two-point boundary value problems." *Soc. Indust. Appl. Math.*, Vol. **24**, pp. 161, 1976.

[2] A. Granas, R. B. Guenther, and J. W. Lee. "The shooting method for the numerical solution of a class of nonlinear boundary value problems." *SIAM J. Numer. Anal.*, Vol. **16**:5, pp. 828836, 1979.

[3] R. M. M. Mattheij and G. W. M. Staarink. "On optimal shooting intervals." *Math. of Comp.*, Vol. **42**:165, pp. 2540, 1984.

[4] J. Stoer and R. Bulirsch. Introduction to Numerical Analysis. Springer-Verlag, New York, 1993.

[5] M. E. Kramer and R. M. M. Mattheij. "Application of global methods in parallel shooting." *SIAM J. Numer. Anal.*, Vol. **30**:6, pp. 17231739, 1993.

[6] A. M. Wazwaz. "Approximate solutions to boundary value problems of higher order by modified decomposition method." *Comp. and Math. with Appl.*, Vol. **40**, pp. 67969, 2000.

[7] Sung N. Ha. "A nonlinear shooting method for two-point boundary value problems." *Comp. Math. Appl.*, Vol. **42**, pp. 1411–1420, 2001.

[8] A. M. Wazwaz. "A reliable algorithm for obtaining positive solutions for nonlinear boundary value problems." *Comp. and Math. with Appl.*, Vol. **41**, pp. 1237–1244, 2001.

[9] B. S. Attili and M. I. Syam. "Efficient shooting method for solving two-point boundary value problems." *Chaos, Solitons Fractals*, Vol. **35**, pp. 895–903, 2008.

[10] C. S. Liu. "Cone of non-linear dynamical system and group preserving schemes." *Int. Jour. Nonlinear Mech.*, Vol. **36**, pp. 1047–1068, 2001.

[11] C. S. Liu. "The Lie-group shooting method for boundary-layer problems with suction/injection/reverse flow conditions for power-law fluids." *Int. Jour. Nonlinear Mech.*, Vol. **46**, pp. 1001–1008, 2011.

[12] G. Birkhoff and G. C. Rota. *Ordinary differential equations*. John Wiley and Sons, New York, 1978.

[13] J. M. Ortega. "The Newton-Kantorovich theorem." *The Amer. Math. Monthly.*, Vol. **75**:6, pp. 658–660, 1968.

[14] R. A. Tapia. "The Kantorovich theorem for Newton's method." *The Amer. Math. Monthly.*, Vol. **78**:6, pp. 389–392, 1971.

[15] L. B. Rall. "A note on the convergence of Newton's method." *SIAM J. Numer. Anal.*, Vol. **11**:1, pp. 34–36, 1974.

[16] W. B. Gragg and R. A. Tapia. "Optimal error bounds for the Newton-Kantorovich theorem." *SIAM J. Numer. Anal.*, Vol. **11**:1, pp. 10–13, 1974.

[17] J. Singh. "A nonlinear shooting method and its application to nonlinear Rayleigh-Bénard convection." *ISRN Mathematical Physics.*, Vol. **2013**, Article ID 650208, 2013.

[18] J. Singh and R. Bajaj. "Couette flow in ferrofluids with magnetic field." *J. Magn. Magn. Mater.*, Vol. **294**, pp. 53–62, 2005.

[19] J. Singh and R. Bajaj. "Stability of non-axisymmetric ferrofluid flow in rotating cylinders with magnetic field." *Int. J. Math. Math. Sci.*, Vol. **23**, pp. 3727–3737, 2005.

[20] J. Singh and R. Bajaj. "Stability of ferrofluid flow in rotating porous cylinders with radial flow." *Magnetohydrodynamics*, Vol. **42**, pp. 46–56, 2006.

[21] J. Singh and R. Bajaj. "Non-axisymmetric modes of Couette-Taylor instability in ferrofluids with radial flow." *Magnetohydrodynamics*, Vol. **42**, pp. 57–68, 2006.

[22] J. Singh. "Energy relaxation for transient convection in ferrofluids." *Phys. Rev.* Vol. **82**, pp. 026311, 2010.

[23] J. H. Mathews and K. D. Fink, *Numerical Methods using MATLAB*, Pearson Prentice Hall, New Jersey USA, 2004.

[24] J. Singh, A. B. Vishalakshi, U. S. Mahabaleshwar and G. Bognar. "MHD Casson fluid flow with Navier's and second order slip due to a perforated stretching or shrinking sheet." *PLoS One.*, Vol. **17**:11, pp. e0276870, 2022.

[25] J. C. Misra, G. C. Shit and H. J. Rath. "Flow and heat transfer of a MHD viscoelastic fluid in a channel with stretching walls: some applications to haemodynamics." *Comput. Fluids*, Vol. **37**, pp. 1–11, 2008.

[26] N. Sharma, C. Chakraborty and R. Kumar. "Optimized multimedia data through computationally intelligent algorithms." *Multimedia Syst.*, Vol. **29**:5, pp. 1–17, 2022.

[27] N. M. Lutimath, H. V. Ramachndra, S. Raghav and N. Sharma. "Prediction of heart disease using genetic algorithms." *Proceedings of Second Doctoral Symposium on Computational Intelligence, Springer, Singapore*, pp. 49–58, 2022.

[28] N. M. Lutimath, N. Sharma and B. K. Byregowda. "Prediction of heart disease using random forest." *Emerging trends in Industry, 4.0 (ETI 4.0)*, IEEE, pp. 1–4, 2021.

[29] J. Vleggaar. "Laminar boundary-layer behaviour on continuous, accelerating surfaces." *Chem. Eng. Sci.*, Vol. **32**, pp. 15171525, 1977.

8 Key Management in Healthcare Using IoMT

Ramkrishna Mondal

1 INTRODUCTION

Technology plays a foremost protagonist in the growth and evolution of all sectors of our civilization and has become an inseparable part of daily life. Recent years have perceived technological development with a widespread range of applications in healthcare [1]. Information communication technology (ICT) and web services significantly impact the quality of services and people's lifestyles. Implementing ICT in the health sector is booming as one of the most rapidly growing areas in healthcare today. It has paved the road for a new area of research among doctors, scientists, and researchers trying to develop efficient and accurate technologies for dealing with health problems. In comparison, policymakers look at it from the viewpoint of providing affordable healthcare to everyone, imparting knowledge and creating interest among ordinary people. Appropriate use of ICT should be applied to achieve Global and National health, which can bridge the digital health revolution gap [2]. It became an active area of research and discussion only after 2000. A prime reason for digital health's growing popularity and awareness is the advancement in computer and communication technology, which has made healthcare information and services globally accessible at a meager cost. Different factors are driving toward better implementation and broader use of digital health services and technologies. It has several advantages, but the most important one is providing medical aid to one and all, irrespective of geographic restrictions, in a cost-effective manner, providing global expertise and holistic services in a time-bound manner. The role of satellite, Internet, and mobile communication plays a lot in the same [3]. Healthcare 4.0 is a word that developed later and came from Industry 4.0. The healthcare area is more digitalized than in earlier days. Recent changes in Healthcare 4.0 through the Internet of Things (IoT) and cloud computing to access healthcare operations remotely have made researchers famous from a smart city angle. Patients' sensitive and personal data lead to several challenges while protecting it from hackers. Therefore storing, accessing, and sharing patient medical information on the cloud needs security attention not to be compromised. Several cryptography algorithms have been designed to achieve secure medical data storage, sharing, and access in a cloud service provider.

DOI: 10.1201/9781003377818-8

However, such conventional solutions failed to reach the trade-off between the requirements of security solutions without a trusted third party and robust security. Blockchain-based security solutions also gained significant attention in the recent past due to their ability to provide strong protection for data storage and sharing with minimum computation efforts [4].

Internet of Medical Things (IoMT) can be considered as a subpart of IoT which comprises intelligent devices, such as wearables and medical or vital monitors, tailored toward monitoring people's health. Some of these wearables are intelligent devices that can monitor a user's physiological parameters such as oxygen saturation (pulse oximeter), blood glucose levels, heart rate, electrocardiogram (ECG) patterns, the electrical activity of cardiac pacemaker, etc., in real-time and transmit these data to the physician. It can be attached to the body, at home, community, clinic, or hospital setting. Numerous other devices include insulin pumps, cochlear implants, and pacemakers. These devices collect and transmit data via the Internet to healthcare providers. It enables healthcare providers to monitor a patient's health remotely. It also allows them to respond promptly to issues when they happen, rather than waiting for patients to visit the physician in person.

2   WHAT ARE IOT AND IOMT?

The Internet is used everywhere, in companies, organizations, governments, and many places. A prediction states that by 2020, machines using the Internet will increase to more than 50 billion [5]. IoT is defined as the connection of devices to the Internet, by which one can communicate with each other and sense the environment to collect and send data [6]. Common IoT applications are plenty, such as smart cities and industries, environmental monitoring, and health care [7]. IoT refers to various interconnected objects and devices that harvest information from the environment through sensors, and analyze it and act back on the physical world through actuators [8], [9]. In recent years, many applications affecting our daily lives have used IoT solutions. According to Gartner, by the end of 2020, we will have 5.8 billion IoT devices, increasing by 20% compared to last year [10].

The terms IoMT (Internet of Medical Things), IoHT (Internet of Health Things), and HIoT (Healthcare IoT) are now used interchangeably. While these technologies promise improved patient care, efficiency, and reduced costs, they also bring new risks, as many connected devices are unmanaged and unprotected. IoT systems have a complex architecture with various devices connected to provide a service to the end user [11]. Cyber-physical systems are central to any IoT architecture; they integrate human interference with computer-based structures and enable data-driven decision-making. IoT provides different real-time solutions to integrate high-sensitivity sensors into medical machines. The IoMT is an architecture of related software and hardware devices, which forms the medical IT systems by a network of connected nodes [12]. It can decrease needless hospital appointments and load on healthcare systems by connecting patients and doctors and making the transmission of medical data over a secure network. The market of IoMT consists of intelligent devices, such as wearables and medical/vital monitor devices used on the body, in a clinic, or hospital setting, in the home or the community, associated with real-time location, telehealth, and other services. Nearly 60% of international healthcare corporates have designed and applied Internet of Things technologies and expect an additional 28% to fully reply to their IoT topologies by 2020 [13]. Traditional medical systems are observing a rapid technological shift as the digital health revolution puts advanced connected healthcare devices in clients' hands and gives patients and doctors better access to healthcare services, even in remote locations [14]. As per Safeatlast [13], it is the expectation that the market of IoMT will be expanded from 32.4 billion USD (2015) to 156 billion USD% by 2020. The integrated technologies in IoMT systems may be classified into three main categories, namely, Local Patient Systems, End Medical Devices (i.e., Cloud-Enabled Solutions, Device Networks), and System of Control (i.e., Fireware, Controller, and Sensors). Different software developers, embedded systems, network operators, and semi-conductor companies are considered contributors to technology in IoMT ecosystem layers. Nowadays, North America's companies are leading the IoMT market. They provide insurance regulations and IoT medical devices. It is expected that the rise of IoT technology in the medical field will highly increase in the future. This increment is due to the medical knowledge awareness in American and European markets [15]. Philips contributed the highest with 129 patents, while both IBM and Fujifilm contributed the lowest with only 23 and 21, respectively. The patents related to healthcare technology from 1989 to 1999 were below 100 and after 1999 above 100 reaching a maximum in 2013 with more than 200 [16].

IoMT technology has provided many services, such as improving healthcare services, diseases management, data analysis, patient experience, and low-cost services. According to economic research [17], the market of IoT in the healthcare domain will rise to 120 billion $ by 2020. The vast, diverse diversity of IoT networks in healthcare faces many security risks in healthcare systems which have many reasons:

i. Medical technologies mainly exchange sensitive data about the diseased patient.
ii. Non-compatibility and complex issues of network connected many smart devices.
iii. Privacy and security issues; because of the critical data of physicians and patients.

In emergencies, medical staff rushes to use IoT solutions without considering security. Many security problems related to confidentiality and integrity appeared [18]. There is a rising security risk in the wireless sensor network (WSN) because all the data transmission in IoMT networks happens wirelessly. Security operations consume a colossal volume of computer resources, but there are limited resources available in wireless sensors [19]. The privacy and security issues in

IoMT became a crucial priority in healthcare due to the vital data of patients and doctors; any attack can represent a considerable risk and disastrous consequences such as loss of life, inappropriate treatment, or economic loss. It is highly mandatory to find all the possible threats to IoMT to support the decision-making process while analyzing and designing security solutions for the IoMT environment [20]. Still, IoMT faces serious threats related to security in general. Again, the IoMT system has different requirements for privacy and security because of the unique features of a healthcare environment [21].

Previous studies in the IoT field have mainly focused on Transmission Control Protocols (TCP)/IP layers. However, there needs to be more investigation of the threats in both physical and application layers. IoMT consists of multiple connected nodes. A set of connected IoT devices in the healthcare field shapes each node. It enhances the patient's treatment quality and the medical time responses [22]. Wireless communications, big data analytics, sensors, actuators, and cloud computing all drive IoT devices' integration in healthcare. The digital transformation in the medical industry has improved targeted and personalized medicine delivery by allowing continuous communication of healthcare information [23]. Medical systems usually collect and process critical and sensitive data about both patients' conditions to contribute to the decision-making process based on this information. Cyber attackers use the existing vulnerabilities in IoMT devices to gain access to the medical care network and get unauthorized contact with critical healthcare data; this is widely happening in countries in the Middle East and North Africa [24]. Continuous attacks on healthcare networks can represent a severe threat to patients' lives by misleading the decision-making process and thus negatively affecting the treatment process [25]. IoMT is a set of devices that uses the IoT for medical purposes, like monitoring and analyzing patient data [26]. This technology consists of Remote Patient Monitoring (RPM), along with the use of various devices e.g., the personal digital assistant (PDA) [26] available to the patient and intelligent medical devices. The technology reduces the costs related to medical examinations and gives medical professionals a better understanding of the patient's condition [27].

An application for the IoMTs was proposed in a study [28] that aimed to develop a platform that would record COVID-19 patients with mild symptoms who never needed to be hospitalized. This information helps to provide the appropriate health care and follow-up on their patient's condition at home. An exciting example of IoMT is based on wireless body area networks (WBANs), where sensors are implanted in the patient's body, and it senses the patient's biometrics and sends them wirelessly to the medical professional [29]. With the fast growth of the number of IoMT users, there have been fears of illegally exploiting these technologies. A report mentioned that for every 1,000 connected devices, around 164 attacks are threatening the sector [30]. Also, the health sector is the third industry targeted by attackers and poses a genuine concern [31]. Unfortunately, there still needs to be more research regarding how safe the IoMTs are, which is a serious concern as patients' data exposed to these attacks may violate their privacy – an attack or threat in their lives with a Denial of Service (DoS) attack. The attack may disrupt the patient's service, which affects the patient's rapid response and causes delays when one attempts to help [32]. Also, IoMT devices are vulnerable to zombies that carry out severe attacks on healthcare infrastructure [33]. Many documents emphasize how secure IoMTs are with regard to the security requirements, the attacks that the IoMTs are exposed to, and the proposed solutions to avoid or limit these attacks.

3   BACKGROUND OF IOMT

The invention of IoMT has enhanced RPM, reducing unnecessary hospital visits and the burden on healthcare systems by connecting patients to their physicians and allowing the transfer of health data over a secure network. Healthcare professionals (HCPs) can monitor patients' key biometrics in real-time, access healthcare data in remote locations, and keep track of any potential issues that might occur, thus helping to prevent any future complications. IoMT has the potential to give more accurate diagnoses, fewer mistakes, and lower costs of care, allowing patients to send health information data to doctors. Due to global pandemic, COVID-19, it is necessary to reduce in-person medical visits to prevent the spread, where IoMT has enhanced RPM, which helps monitor patients' vital signs, such as heart activities and glucose levels – the doctors can then be automatically alerted when necessary. IoMT can also help trigger emergency responses and keep chronic diseases in check. Those living in remote areas can share activity tracker information with a remote health provider using intelligent devices and get a medically informed recommendation. IoMT has revolutionized the operations of the health sector. A report from Forbes [34] states, "The IoMT is poised to transform how we keep people safe and healthy, especially as the demand for solutions to lower healthcare costs increases in the coming years"; and it can monitor, inform, and notify caregivers and provide healthcare providers with specific data to help identify issues for an earlier invention before they become critical [34]. IoMT helps insurance companies to view patient data more quickly and makes the processing of claims faster and more accurate. All stakeholders, including the pharmaceuticals and insurance companies, greatly benefit from IoMT due to the improved quality of patient care.

According to Kamalanthan et al. [35], IoMTs are divided into four categories:

i. *Wearable devices*: Smartwatches, temperature and pressure sensors, heart monitoring and muscle activity sensors, and glucose and biochemical sensors
ii. *Implantable devices*: Swallowable camera capsules for visualization of the gastrointestinal tract, embedded cardiac pacemakers, and implantable cardioverter-defibrillators (ICD)
iii. *Ambient devices*: Motion sensors, door sensors, and vibration sensors
iv. *Stationary devices*: Imaging devices like CT (Computerized Tomography) scans and surgical devices

3.1 Types of IoMT

IoMT systems provide the necessary assistance for various medical conditions based on devices they are divided in to two categories. The devices are implantable devices for specific conditions, e.g., pacemakers for heart conditions. Contrarily, the assisting devices are primarily wearables for an improved experience, e.g., smartwatches.

3.1.1 Implantable Medical Devices (IMDs)

A device implanted to replace, support, and enhance a biological structure is an IMD. e.g., a pacemaker for promoting the heart to beat at a regular rate [36] Recently, wireless IMDs are also available to solve problems with wired IMDs, e.g., infection and cable breakage [37]. IMDs primarily have small and long-life batteries. It consumes low power and less space, and small batteries that last long are essential to staying inside the human body for a long time, at least to last 5–15 years [38].

3.1.2 Internet of Wearable Devices (IoWDs)

A person wears a device to monitor their biometrics, e.g., heart rate, smart watches, fall detection bands, electrocardiograms (ECG), and blood pressure monitors [39]. These are currently widely used for non-critical patient monitoring [40]. The devices have sensor accuracy and battery life limitations and not likely to replace IMDs in critical conditions [41].

3.2 IoMT Systems Architecture

IoMT architecture helps better to understand the composition of different layers in the system. Several layers are proposed in different papers with different terminologies for these layers. There is no general agreement about the architecture of IoMT that the researchers agree with. Some researchers propose three layers, while some support the four-layer architecture and some five-layer [42] as depicted in Figure 8.1. The intelligent applications of IoMT interconnected devices give society personal and economic benefits.

3.2.1 Three-Layer IoMT Systems

They consist of basic Application, Network, and Perception layers.

1. Application Layer: The topmost layer of the IoMT architecture is the application layer. This layer provides personalized-based services according to user-relevant needs [43]. Its primary responsibility is to link the significant gap between the users and applications. Similar to a browser on a computer implementing application layer protocols like HTTP, HTTPS, FTP, and SMTP, there are also application layer protocols specified in the context of IoMT. However, HTTP is unsuitable in resource-constrained environments like IoMT because it is heavyweight and thus incurs a significant parsing overhead [44]. Some of the popular IoMT application layer protocols include Message Queuing Telemetry Transport (MQTT),

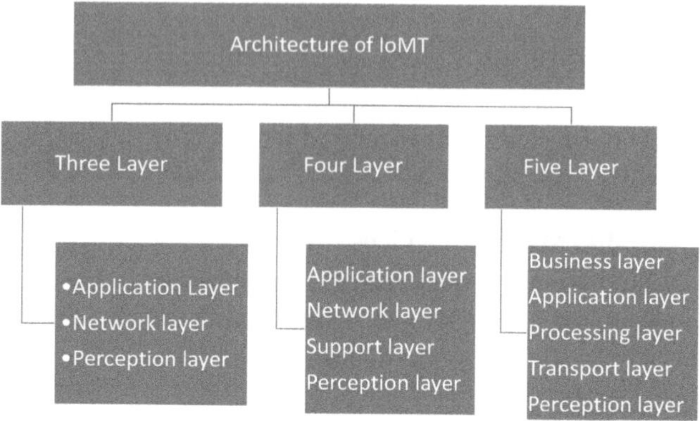

FIGURE 8.1 The Layered Architecture of IoMT (Three, Four, and Five Layers)

Secure Message Queue Telemetry Transport (SMQTT), Constrained Application Protocol (CoAP), Extensible Messaging and Presence Protocol (XMPP), Representational State Transfer Hypertext Transfer Protocol (RESTful HTTP), Simple Object Access Protocol (SOAP), and Websocket. All the user requests are fulfilled here; this layer is known as the cloud layer. The primary concern of this layer is data privacy, as heterogeneous devices communicate with different IoMT standards and different devices exchange a large number of data transactions and need to be secured [45]. Some data privacy techniques are also applied, which include Transport Layer Security (TLS), Domain Name System (DNS), and Secure Sockets Layer (SSL) [46]. Some of the protocols that provide data confidentiality, authenticity, and integrity are CoAP, XMPP, Data Distribution Service (DDS), and web socket [47].

2. Network Layer: The IoMT Network layer handles packets from source nodes to destination and network addressing. It transmits and processes the data collected by all devices and also connects these to other smart objects, servers, and network devices. The medium for the transmission can be wireless or wire-based. The technologies used in this layer for IoMT are Ethernet, wireless, 3G, local area network (LAN), Bluetooth, RFID, and NFC. Table 8.1 shows networking technologies used in IoMT. Ethernet connects stationary or fixed IoMT devices. IoMT uses WiFi systems for connecting the gateway to the end user, as IoMT devices can be stationary due to their continuous need for a reliable power source [48]. Many IoMT devices with low power during their connection with end users and other nodes use radio spectrums like 3G, LTE, and Bluetooth. For example, some medical devices in hospitals and clinics connect to other devices through WiFi or low-powered wireless personal area network (6LoWPAN) [49]. Wearables widely use Bluetooth for short-range communications. The Bluetooth Low-Energy

(BLE) standard was designed to meet the needs of low-power IoMT devices. It transfers only tiny portions of data and does not work for large files. ZigBee is a low-power wireless network carrying small data packages over short distances. The extraordinary thing about ZigBee is that it can handle up to 65,000 nodes [50]. It works effectively for IoMT devices due to its low-power capabilities.

3. Perception Layer: The primary responsibility of this layer is data collection (i.e., heart rate, temperature, and pressure), after which it is transferred to the network layer. The physical layer consists of sensors for sensing and gathering environmental information. The lowest layer is the perception layer of the conventional architecture of IoMT which, feels some parameters, identifies other smart objects in the environment and transforms them into electrical signals.

3.2.2   Four-Layer IoMT Systems

Current IoMT systems are mostly of four layers [51]. Current advances in IMDs, IoWDs, and IMDs mostly share the same architecture, given that IMDs can communicate with the gateways, as exemplified by Medtronic pacemaker [52]. The layers are as follows, -

1. *Sensor Layer/Perception layer:* This layer consists of small implanted or worn sensors that collect the patient's biometrics. The data are transmitted to the second layer over wireless protocols such as WiFi, Bluetooth, or the MedRadio frequency spectrum reserved for IMDs [53].
2. *Gateway Layer/Support layer:* Due to the processing and storage limitations of IoMT sensors, the data are transferred without processing to the second layer, i.e., the gateway layer. The devices in this layer can be the patient's smartphone or a dedicated access point (AP), which are generally more potent than sensors. In addition, they send the sensor data to the cloud over the Internet.
3. *Cloud Layer/Network Layer:* The cloud layer gets the data from the gateway for storage, analysis, and secure access. The analysis may include data processing to find any changes in the patient's health and presenting them to the physicians or patients for further action. The key generation server (KS) generates IDs and keys for various system nodes. The access to the sensors can be remotely managed and controlled from this layer.
4. *Visualization/Action Layer/Application layer:* In this layer, the data are presented to the physicians and the patients to track their health. This layer also includes the actions recommended by the physician based on the patient's health conditions. Examples of actions include prescribing or adjusting the dosage for various medicines

3.2.3   Five-Layer IoMT Systems

Because of the criticality of the healthcare field, it has become vital to manage many IoMT devices to provide reliability, and the need arises for flexible design

TABLE 8.1

Description of Perception Layer Devices in the Internet of Medical Things

IoMT Device	Function
Locator	Tracing the patients' location
Temperatures Measurement	They are providing results about body temperatures
Blood Pressure	We are monitoring the patients' pressure
Biometric Sensor	Uniquely identify the patients' identity
Heart Monitoring	Using both electrocardiographs (ECGs) for monitoring the heartbeats
Respiratory Rate	We are monitoring the breathing rate
Activity Monitoring	We are using gyroscope sensors for detecting patients' activities like (eating, sitting, or sleeping)
Electronic Cardiogram	Assess the main functions of the heart to ensure safety
Pulse Oximeters	It measures both pulse and oxygen rate
Biochemical Sensors	It detects biochemistry and harmful mixtures in the air

architecture. As presented by Singh et al [54], the top five IoT layers describe each layer, illustrating its primary functionality and for every function in the IoT layer, there is a security threat [55].

1. **Perception Layer:** This layer has primary responsibility in data collection (i.e., heart rate, pressure, and temperature) using sensors in the physical layer. After that, the collected data is transferred to the network layer [56]. Description of different devices is shown in Table 8.1.

Those devices will be classified into five categories as follows:

    i. Implantable Devices: These types of objects intended to be inside the patient's body for medical purposes, devices such as (Embedded Cardiac and Swallowable Camera Capsule) [57].

    ii. Tampering Devices: Sensors are the hardware that can be manipulated or tampered with physically by attackers; they can affect their functionality by stopping those sensors or modifying their configurations. Any medical equipment with a USB port can be damaged if the attacker plugs in an external device to destroy its functionality or uses vulnerabilities to control the equipment through malware [58].

    iii. Sensor Tracking: Health monitoring equipment has GPS sensors to share patients' locations in emergencies. If the equipment is not secured, attackers may spoof the data of GPS to track the patients' location [59]. Similarly, any sensor that uses fall detection or remote monitoring has its exploitations for revealing the patients' sensitive data [60].

    iv. Stationary Devices: This class contains immobile intelligent objects that do not always accompany the user. Devices may be, (a) Surgical Objects: Used tools by medical staff while performing surgeries and original transplants, [61] (b) Imagining Objects: Creating a visual simulation of the patient's interior body (i.e., MRI and X-rays) for medical analysis studies [62], and (c) Wearable Devices: The patient and the doctors use wearable objects to enable continuous monitoring and provide accurate results [63].

v. Ambient Devices: These objects aim to gather data about the patients' surrounding area for monitoring activity forms such as breathing, sleeping, eating, and walking and providing warnings to medical staff when suspicious activities are detected; below are some examples for ambient sensors:
- Pressure Sensors: Managing fluid and air rate in the room.
- Temperatures Measurement: Providing results about body temperatures.
- Doors Sensors: Sensing the door condition (open-close) to help states with Alzheimer's.
- Motion Sensors: Movement detections in small rooms.
- Daylight Sensors: Automatically adjust lighting power inside the room for natural light.
- Vibration Sensors: Analyzing the body activities during staying in bed.

2. **Transport/Network Layer:** This layer handles packets from senders to destinations and network addressing. The devices used in this layer for IoMT are as follows:
- *WiFi:* IoMT uses WiFi systems for connecting the gateway to the end user. IoMT devices can be stationary due to their continuous need for a reliable power source [64].
- *Radio Communication:* Many IoT devices with low power – during their connection with end-users and other nodes –– use radio spectrums like 3G, LTE, and Bluetooth. As an example, the IoT devices in hospitals and clinics connect other devices through WiFi or low-powered wireless personal area network (6LoWPAN) [65].

3. **Processing/Middleware Layer**: This layer is responsible for gathering and classifying the data from the devices in the perception layer, achieving service discovery, and controlling the device's access. Cloud technology became commonly used in IoMT environments (hospitals, clinics, healthcare centers, and sanatoriums) [66].
- **Cross-Site Request Forgery:** It is considered the most common attack in RESTful-based IoT architecture; the CSRF manipulates the user's application; this is done by making modifications by using the vulnerability in the web interface; without proper configurations of the web interface in the IoT layer can become defenseless to the CSRF attacks [67].
- **Session Hijacking:** This type of attack is common in RESTful-based IoT networks due to the mechanism that some IoT devices use to initiate the session connection to the web interface layer [68].
- **Cross-site Scripting (XSS)**: The XSS can inject side scripts to evade access controls through the IoT web devices' web pages; this is mainly done to exploit RESTful IoT systems [69].

4. **Application Layer:** This layer represents the interface where the users interact with the surrounding IoT devices over the Middleware-layer for managing, controlling, and interacting [70]. Due to a large amount of data, the healthcare industry tended to move to cloud platforms for scalability, integrity, and cost affordance [71]. Consequently, the potential attack risks increased to influence the healthcare field through different sophisticated attacks negatively [72]. The potential threats on this layer can be presented as follows:

   - SQL injection: SQL injection threat occurs when the attacker attempts to use the vulnerability in the backend of the software database; this is done through inserting a malformed SQL statement. As an operative, it has the capability to effectively launch an SQL injection attack which has the capability to steal patients' information or modify sensitive data, which may cause severe consequences in the healthcare environment overall [73].
   - Account Hijacking: Various IoT devices interact, whether with non-encrypted or weak encrypted channels at the network layer; the attacker can execute account hijacking by interrupting the packets during the authentication process of the end user. Old operating systems suffer from primitive vulnerabilities, the central aspect of such an attack [74].
   - Ransomware: Ransomware encrypts critical information and asks for enormous data decryption payments. Attackers can encrypt critical information, such as patient and physician data, mainly used to exchange the decryption key for money [75].
   - Brute Force: This approach depends on guessing passwords by trying all the possible characters, alphabets, and numbers. Brute-force attacks are dangerous, as limited protection exists to prevent such threats in IoMT devices. This is accredited to the sensors' derivative computation energy [76].
   - **Business Layer:** Primarily handle the business logic for the medical provider and support the business lifecycle (i.e., managing, observing, and adjusting) business procedures. It is also responsible for gathering information from the IoMT environment. Cyber-attacks impact on this layer is very high due to medical data sensitivity [77]. Those attacks can be the leading cause of information disclosure and deception; as information disclosure or fraud [78]. Illegal access to credential data can cause a considerable violation of the confidentiality of the IoMT network. The attacker can use any vulnerability to gain access to create, modify, or even delete data related to the patient's system in the healthcare domain, which can cause severe damage [79]. Infected data can disturb data integrity and lead to disastrous penalties. Threats such as Sinkholes and men in the middle can lead to data deception. About 56% of medical institutions do not provide a proactive approach to face such a threat.

TABLE 8.2

Comparison of Different Communication Technologies in IoMT

Technologies	Standard	Frequency	Range (m)	Data Rates
Zigbee	IEEE 802.15.4	2.4Hz	10–100	250kbps
Bluetooth	IEEE 802.15.1	2.4Hz	50–150	1 Mbps
Li-Fi	IEEE 802.15.7	>1 MHz	<10	1 Gbps
Wi-Fi	IEEE 802.11	2.4GHz & 5GHz	50	600 Mbps Max
LTE	3GPP	depends on number of bands	depends on bands	Uplink – 75Mbps Downlink-300Mbps
LTE-A	3GPP	depends on number of bands	depends on bands	Uplink-1.5 Gbps Downlink-3Gbps
5G	5G NR	depends on number of bands	depends on bands	50Mbps to > Gbps

4 IOMT COMMUNICATION TECHNOLOGIES

The most common types of networks for IoMT applications technologies are
Personal Area Networks (PANs), LANs, and Wide Area Networks (WANs). Each
network type involves many wireless technologies, as shown in Table 8.2. In the
following, we provide details of the architectures of the IoMT communication
environment. So many communication technologies are well known, such as
WiFi, ZigBee, Bluetooth, Li-Fi, and LTE, but there are also several emerging
networking options. The choice of one or a combination of communication technologies in IoMT is determined by the application and factors such as range, data
requirements, security, power demands, and device battery life.

5 SECURITY RISKS, PRIVACY, AND TRUST ISSUES IN IOMT ENVIRONMENT

Security is defined as a process by which unauthorized access to the system state is
prevented, and thus privacy is not compromised. Security requirements consist of
standard security requirements ensuring the security of patients' information and
system. It enables the users to protect and prevent IoMT-based healthcare systems
against known threats and attacks. IoMT devices produce a large volume of increasingly diverse real-time data, which is highly sensitive. Destroying the security of
the medical network or system could be disastrous. Also, the patient's privacy information exists at all stages of data collection, transmission, cloud storage, and data
republication. In the Information Technology (IT) field, three security features are
considered regarding security requirements. Confidentiality, integrity, and availability (CIA) are regarded as the prime objectives and are referred to as the CIA triad
[80]. In addition, other requirements to meet the specific needs of the IoMT environment are Data Confidentiality, Data Integrity, Data Availability, Authentication,
Information Privacy, Data Freshness, Scalability, Access Control, Mobility Support,
End-to-End Security, Auditing, Non-repudiation, Accountability, etc.

In the past decades, healthcare has witnessed a swift transformation from a traditional specialist/ hospital-centric approach to a patient-centric approach, particularly in the smart healthcare system (SHS). The IoMT performs a crucial role in the development of SHS by enabling patients' treatment compliance and behavioral change. It also provides a safe data transmission environment for interchanging medical data among diverse medical sectors. The concern for IoMT security, privacy, and trust occurs rapidly. Security, privacy, and faith have recently received more attention among the research community. Data storage and transmission are secured to ensure integrity, validity, and authenticity in data security. It also assures that only authorized users can be viewed and modified. Privacy-preserving (PP) is another critical objective to be considered while designing an SHS. However, achieving patient privacy is a challenge because an attacker can recognize a patient's health state based on the attended doctor's identity. In IoMT-enabled SHS, various symmetric and asymmetric encryption methods are used to achieve privacy. Recently, the literature has reported that there are better solutions to apply complex machine learning (ML) algorithms on resource-constrained devices such as IoMT. Machine-learning algorithm is tested to provide a secure mechanism for an authenticated user [81]. However, it can be resolved by deploying simple PP methods on IoMT devices and utilizing the benefits of the cloud for complex ML algorithms. Many works are reported in the literature based on cloud-related securing solutions for IoMT in SHS. Security of IoMT in any SHS plays a significant role compared to typical IoT-based infrastructures. Recently, extensive research has been done for securing IoMT-enabled competent healthcare [82].

The attack classification in the IoMT environment relies on its damaging level after successfully making the attack. As a result, the consequences of various cyber-attacks in the medical field demonstrate a strong need to develop proactive approaches for securing the IoMT environment. The layers of the IoMT system, the protocol stack, security issues, and vulnerabilities of various underlying techniques are varying. (Table 8.3) The cyber-attack threat in the healthcare industry may lead to:

- **Life Risk:** Any attack that occurs on devices connected directly to the patient may affect their functionality and the patient put the patient's life in danger [83].
- **Data Exposure:** When an attacker exploits a medical device or software, it may lead to patient data exposure, violating the typical roles of data privacy in the medical field [84].
- **Reputation Loss:** The occurred damages because of an attack, whether in device or software, may lead to brand value loss because of losing integrity and violating standard medical privacy rules [85].
- **Financial Loss:** The resultant damages by attacks on IoMT networks need to make damage control followed by a recovery plan. This process leads to an extra budget that negatively affects the healthcare organization's finances [86].

TABLE 8.3

Description of Attacks Threats for Each Layer in IoMT Environment

Layer	Attack Type	Risk Level
Perception layer	Side Channel	High
	Sensor Tracking	High
	Tag Cloning	Low
Network layer	Sinkhole	High
	Rogue Access	Low
	Denial of Service	High
	Man-in-the-middle	High
Middleware layer	XSS	Medium
	Session Hijacking	High
	CSRF	High
Application layer	SQL Injection	Medium
	Brute Force	High
	Account Hijacking	High
	Ransomware	High
Business layer	Disruption	High
	Information Disclosure	High

6 IOMT SYSTEMS SECURITY TECHNIQUES

There are several different techniques to secure IoMT systems. These techniques can be divided into three main categories: symmetric, asymmetric, and keyless, as shown in Figure 8.2. Symmetric and asymmetric techniques rely on cryptographic algorithms, while keyless plans are noncryptographic. One-factor authentication uses only one authentication technique to protect the system. In contrast, two-factor authentication adds a second authentication technique (factor), such as biometrics, to protect the system if one of the two factors is compromised.

6.1 SYMMETRIC-KEY ALGORITHMS

As shown in Figures 8.2 and 8.3, symmetric cryptography includes any cryptographic algorithm based on a secret/shared key between two or more nodes wanting to communicate. The key is to be generated and distributed before using asymmetric cryptography stage. These algorithms can be used for IoMT systems to allow hierarchical access to the patient's data and initiate secure connections without prior setup. Further, they can also be used in two-factor authentication, where they act as the first factor while other techniques, such as facial recognition and pattern-based, act as the second factor.

6.1.1 Hierarchical Access

This technique allows hierarchical access control to patients' data stored in the cloud layer. One approach utilizes a hierarchical role-based model and provides

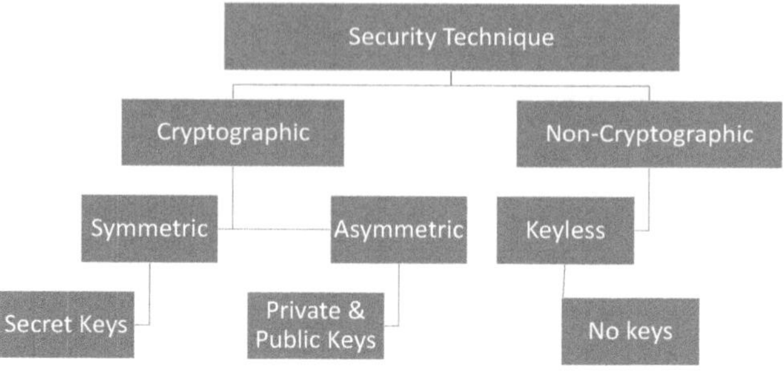

FIGURE 8.2   Security Techniques

authorization based on the user's role [87]. For example, all authenticated nurses can administer medicines, but prescribing a new medication requires a person authenticated as a doctor. Belkhouja *et al.* [87] have used the Chinese remainder theorem (CRT) to support this hierarchal access where the user with a higher privilege can access any patient's data. In contrast, the user with a lower privilege can access part of the data related to their roles.

6.1.2   Wireless Signal Characteristics

This technique utilizes wireless signal characteristics to secure IoMT systems by generating keys without prior connections. Radio signal strength (RSS) is one of these characteristics, and it measures the received signal power, which varies based on the medium it passes through. IMDs can be excellent candidates for this technique since the RSS value variation inside the human body differs from outside [88]. This key can secure the communication between a headless cardiac pacemaker and a subcutaneous (under-the-skin) implant without prior knowledge of the keys.

6.1.3   CHF with XOR

CHF is a one-way mathematical function that converts an arbitrary size data to a fixed size. Exclusive-OR (XOR) can be used to check if one of its operands is different. In a medical setting, initial parameters (i.e., a sensor ID and a shared key) can be XORed together and then hashed. Then, these hashed parameters are shared from the KS to the sensor and gateway nodes.

Combining the CHF, a symmetric key, and the XOR operator can secure the IoMT systems' communications using new authenticated key agreement protocols, as illustrated by Alzahrani *et al.* [89] and Xu *et al.* [90]. This technique also supports unique identification parameters for the system's nodes.

6.1.4   Gait-Based Technique

This technique uses the human walking pattern to generate unique symmetric keys. They claim that their system can generate three times the number of bits per gait cycle than those caused by similar state-of-the-art techniques [91]. The gait cycle is one cycle of movement between two repetitive events while walking.

It outperforms finger-based systems by generating binary keys at different times, which provides randomness to the keys without direct user interaction with the system.

6.1.5 Facial Recognition

This technology is a one-way that IoMT systems can rely on authenticating users by scanning their faces. As a first factor, shared keys and facial recognition may use as the second factor in continuous role-based authentication [92]. It helps secure the connection between the sensor and the medical controller in the gateway layer based on each authorized user's privilege. Since this technique continuously scans the user's face while using the system, it can secure the system in a medical setting.

6.1.6 Pattern-Based Technique

This technique is similar to the facial recognition system but uses a pattern-based technique as a second factor [93]. This technique uses a tab pattern generated by the patient to control the sensor. After successfully passing the first factor with the medical controller in the gateway layer, the controller sends a random tab pattern as a second factor to the user before executing a sensitive command.

6.2 Asymmetric-Key Algorithms

Asymmetric cryptography includes cryptographic algorithms that use two keys, a public and a private, with one of them for encryption/validation and the other used for decryption/signature. Asymmetric cryptography is also known as public-key cryptography. The public key is known to everyone, and the private key is only known to its owner (Figure 8.3). Some of the known algorithms in this category include Rivest–Shamir–Adleman (RSA) and Elliptic-Curve Cryptography (ECC). ECC is the most common encryption technique for securing IoMT systems due to its lightweight characteristics. An ECC key with a size of 160 bits is as good as the 1024-bit RSA key and is 15 times faster.

This section discusses the integration of asymmetric cryptographic algorithms in IoMT systems. It includes asymmetric keys with CHF, homographic encryption (HE), or digital signatures. Also, similar to symmetric keys, asymmetric keys can use for two-factor authentication. They act as the first factor for authentication, with other techniques, such as smart cards, as a second factor. Smart cards are extensively used in hospitals nowadays.

6.2.1 CHF with ECC

CHF function and ECC keys can be a secure certificateless channel between patients and medical doctors. The idea of combining the ECC and the CHF is to allow a certain way for sharing keys between the KS (KGS) in the cloud layer and the nodes in the IoMT sensor and gateway layers, respectively. The ECC public key of the KGS and initial parameters, such as a node ID, are hashed together using CHF; then, they go to the nodes in the IoMT sensor and gateway layers. The nodes can generate their asymmetric keys with the help of the received hashed

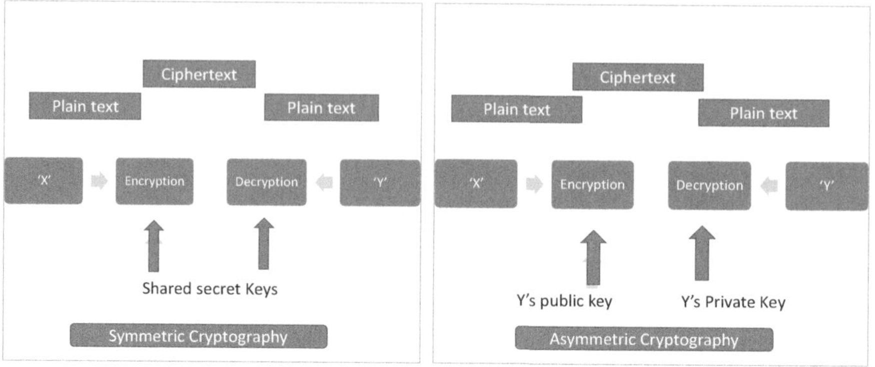

Symmetric and Asymmetric Cryptography

FIGURE 8.3   Symmetric and Asymmetric Cryptography

values. It can also overcome the overhead in certificate management for data storage and sharing in the cloud [94]. By dividing the patient's data into subsets and converting them using ECC keys and CHF, they can securely share among the system's entities. The average energy consumption in this technique is around 30% less than in similar fashions.

6.2.2 Homomorphic Encryption (HE)

HE is an encryption technique that preserves data confidentiality and allows limited mathematical operations on encrypted data. This technique protects the patient's data privacy and stores them as ciphertext in the cloud layer for mathematical operations, such as data integrity. However, this technique differs from other techniques since it allows only the patient to see their data, not the medical staff, except during emergencies. There are three different schemes for HE: partial HE (PHE), somewhat HE (SHE), and fully HE (FHE). PHE supports one mathematical operation an unlimited number of times, while SHE supports only a limited number of functions. FHE supports a total number of functions; therefore, it can be suitable for fast data aggregation without compromising data confidentiality. Hence, it is ideal for healthcare monitoring systems in hospitals. Optimal HE (OHE) is a modification of FHE. It differs from FHE in that it is based on the Step-size Firefly Optimization (SFFO) algorithm, in which the key with the maximum breaking time is selected [95]. This technique reduces the computation time and increases the breaking time by 2% to 8% compared to other HE and non-HE techniques.

6.2.3 Digital Signatures

Digital signature techniques can be used even in a small IoMT system. Generally, they can verify the data/command authenticity using the sender's (Alice) private and public keys for signature and verification, respectively. In IoMT systems, digital signatures can be integrated into the sensor's firmware with an add-on software shim, intercepting and validating the sensor's wireless communications. These techniques require storing a list of authorized users' (i.e., medical staffs') public keys in the sensor's firmware to validate them.

6.2.4 Smart Cards

This technique differs from the first three techniques since it relies on physical keys [96]. These keys utilize as a second factor, with the ECC keys as the first factor for authentication. In IoMT settings, the medical staff must first enter a key and use their smart cards to access the system. This technique helps the procedure be resistant to cyber-breaks if one of the factors is stolen or lost. This has made them quite common nowadays.

6.3 KEYLESS ALGORITHMS

The techniques in this category can be based on biometrics, token-based security, or proxy-based techniques. Cutting-edge technologies such as blockchain technology and AI also fall in this category since they can use for security without pre-shared keys.

6.3.1 Biometrics

The biometric sensors used to identify users' physical characteristics are the most common technique employed to provide security for IoMT systems since they are easy to use. Biometric factors include fingerprint and ECG-based sensors that are handy in emergencies. The fingerprint sensors are based on reading the fingerprint image, while the ECG-based sensors record the heartbeat activities to encrypt the data. Fingerprint sensors reduce the messages' size during transmission and the computational overhead compared to the ECG-based techniques [97]. The performance of the fingerprint sensors is based on the extraction algorithm used. Popular algorithms used in these sensors are Delaunay Triangulation-based feature representation, Pair-polar coordinate-based feature representation, and Minutia Cylinder-Code-based feature representation. According to Zheng *et al.*, Delaunay performs better and is less complicated than the other techniques.

6.3.2 Token-Based Security

User authentication can be possible using software or hardware tokens. For instance, the x-auth-token field in the hypertext transfer protocol (HTTP) header can use as a software token embedded in the user's web browsers [98]. Cloud data analytics companies use these tokens, e.g., IoT Ubidots, to secure the connection between the cloud layer and the nodes in the IoMT sensor and gateway layers. Likewise, RFID can use as a hardware token for secure logistic management of sensors in a hospital information system (HIS).

6.3.3 Proxy-Based and Light-Based Systems

Proxy-based systems are middleware devices that control the communication between the sensors and any device communicating with them, such as medical controllers. Besides, they can provide full-duplex secure communications between these devices, where they can simultaneously communicate. Middleware devices can be a set of microprocessors inside a jacket or a belt to be worn by the patient [99]. Light-based communication technologies, such as Light-Fidelity (Li-Fi), can be used to secure the monitoring capabilities for HIS. Since Li-Fi does not use wireless communications, it has no interference with the hospital network, substantial free operation frequency, and short coverage range for enhanced security.

6.3.4　Blockchain Technology and AI

These are new techniques for use in IoMT systems due to their success in providing security in other fields, such as finance. The blockchain technology typically uses in IoMT systems as a security management sharing technique for the data between the patient and other parties such as doctors and insurance companies. On the other hand, AI systems can detect anomaly behaviors (leading to attacks) in network flows and patients' data. However, there are some challenges for these techniques to be adopted by IoMT systems. AI systems require a large amount of data; hence, they may need to be better at detecting rare attacks. Blockchain technology and AI use in IoMT systems, mainly in the cloud layer [100], [101].

7　IOMT SYSTEMS RISKS AND LIST OF ATTACKS

In this section, we explore possible attacks targeting such systems, including physical and network attacks. Table 8.4 summarizes the security requirements for IoMT systems, possible attacks, and countermeasures. The countermeasures for 11 out of the 14 attacks on keyless methods, and more than half of all countermeasures rely on two-factor authentication methods.

7.1　PHYSICAL ATTACKS

These attacks target the physical components (e.g., sensors, physical keys) of the IoMT systems to extract patient data or security keys. They require some component of the IoMT systems to be physically accessible to the attacker. These attacks can be summarized as follows:

7.1.1　Physical Security Token Loss

It includes any attack where the attacker steals an authorized user's physical security token, such as a smart card, to access the system. The violated security requirements are authentication, authorization, anonymity, and forward secrecy. Kumari *et al.* showed that integrating asymmetric keys, such as ECC, with smart cards can mitigate such attacks since stealing the intelligent card is insufficient to hijack the system [96]

7.1.2　Impersonation/Presentation

In this attack, the attacker impersonates an authorized user's identity, e.g., by replicating the fingerprint or face print. It can target any node in the IoMT system.

The attack violates authentication, authorization, anonymity, and forward secrecy security requirements. It can avoid using symmetric/asymmetric techniques, such as CHF, or keyless techniques, such as biometrics [97].

7.1.3 Tampering

Any modification to the IoMT systems' data at the collection, transit, or storage stage is considered a tampering attack. It may include attaching external devices to alter the data and attack sensors during emergencies. It violates data confidentiality and integrity and can be mitigated by combining symmetric keys with facial recognition or using keyless methods [97]. Such an attack intends to tamper with the reliability of the sent messages' data to achieve their own goals, which could lead to doctors making wrong decisions that can potentially harm patients [102].

7.1.4 Side Channel

These attacks occur during the communications among devices in the IoMT system. They are due to leaked information about cryptographic operations in communications. Maji *et al.* suggest that the datagram transport layer security (DTLS) protocol can be used to avoid them. Blockchain technology and AI can act as other detection and mitigation strategies.

7.1.5 Radio Frequency (RF) Jamming/Desynchronization

RF Jamming attacks target the system's availability, which is dangerous for critical systems such as IoMT systems. Blockchain technology and AI can reduce the effects of such intrusions by finding alternative routes or terminating the channel connection with the attacker [103]. The attacker disables the ability of patients and hospitals to communicate with each other. Wireless networks are usually the target [104]. Continuous packets are sent from DoS attacks, disrupting all communications on every channel with any form of security. These jamming attacks either operate selectively or non-selectively [105]. However, by shifting the frequency and moving between frequencies, the effects of this attack can be minimized, as mentioned [106].

7.2 NETWORK ATTACKS

Other attacks may target the communication between different layers of the IoMT system, such as Bluetooth or Internet links. These attacks usually aim to steal or fabricate patients' data or block the connections between the IoMT systems' layers.

7.2.1 DoS/DDoS

These attacks load the system's communication links with many undesirable connections making it unavailable for regular contacts. They may also cause network fragmentation. Thus, a fragmentation attack is a particular type of DDoS. Blockchain technology and AI can reduce the effects of such intrusions by finding alternative routes or terminating the channel connection with the attacker [103], similar to those mentioned in the RF jamming attacks.

7.2.2 Sniffing

A sniffing attack passively intercepts the data transmitted between two nodes, violating patient data confidentiality. Any encryption algorithm, i.e., symmetric, asymmetric, or keyless, can mitigate these attacks [107].

7.2.3 Man-In-The-Middle

MITM attack is an eavesdropping attack. After a successful sniffing attack, the attacker can alter the intercepted data before sending them to the original destination. For example, the attacker can change the patient's biometric data transmitted from any two layers in the IoMT system (i.e., from the sensor layer to the gateway layer). It can do using unmanned aerial vehicles (UAV), resulting in a drone-in-the-middle (DitM) attack, as discussed by Sethuraman *et al.* [107] This attack violates authorization in addition to data confidentiality requirements and can mitigate using encryption or two-factor authentication techniques.

7.2.4 Relay

After a successful sniffing attack, the attacker can relay the intercepted data to a third node without altering them and for instance, sending the patient's data after blocking them (i.e., from the sensor layer) to the attacker's computer before sending them to the intended layer (i.e., gateway layer). This attack can mitigate using asymmetric keys, such as hierarchal access, supporting secure session keys [103].

7.2.5 Replay

After a successful sniffing attack, the attacker can resend the intercepted data later to the original destination without altering them. By repeating this process, this attack may also result in a DoS/DDoS attack. It can mitigate using a timestamp, which is part of some symmetric, asymmetric, and keyless techniques [96]. This can cause physical damage to the medical systems. System connections are initially recorded and replayed later in the receiving device. The hacker would have the ability to leak, steal, disclose private patient information, access specific medical systems without authorization, and obtain a high privilege within them [108].

7.2.6 Clock Synchronization

This attack targets the clock synchronization protocol, which is necessary for real-time systems like IoMT systems. The attacker successfully initiating this attack can make relay, replay, and MITM attacks not easily detectable. This attack can mitigate using two-factor techniques like ECC with smart cards [96].

7.2.7 Parallel Session

These attacks break one-way authentication protocols that use asymmetric keys. The effects of attacks are authentication and authorization violations, which can avoid using two-factor techniques, such as ECC with smart cards [96].

7.2.8   Brute Force

The attacker in this type of attack tries many credentials until successful. One way is the so-called dictionary attack, which relies on known passwords or words in dictionaries. These attacks can also perform in the offline phase after capturing the encrypted data decrypted with powerful machines. Their short, simple, or factory-set default passwords can guess using a simple python script, making them easier to find online; therefore, IoMT systems can be affected. These attacks have violated authentication and authorization security requirements as the parallel session attacks but can be alleviated using keyless methods, such as biometrics. This attack includes most targeted devices and is not limited to remote medical sensors of patients [109].

7.2.9   Stepping Stone

Instead of relying on one computer/host to attack the IoMT system, a chain of hosts can attack the system. Sethuraman *et al.* perform this attack using a series of UAVs to extend the communication link between the UAVs and the attacker's computer. Hence, the attacker can launch an attack in restricted areas (i.e., in a hospital) that are not directly accessible by the attacker [107]. This attack violates the authentication and authorization security requirements, but it can avoid using keyless methods, such as AI.

7.2.10   Eavesdropping Attacks

Such attacks depend on the gathering of sensitive data. They exist in two forms: active and passive eavesdropping. Passive eavesdropping scans wireless access points to determine which medical device connects them. In contrast, the opponent monitors the data sent and received during transmission in passive eavesdropping. Then, they use this data to gather information more efficiently and faster [110].

7.2.11   Data-Interception Attack

During the execution of a man-in-the-middle attack, the opponent can intercept the data and forward it at another time. It permits third parties to eavesdrop on Address Resolution Protocols (ARP) so that handshakes are successfully captured. It uses it to enter a system and medical records without authorization and obtain encryption keys if it catches it [111].

7.2.12   Malicious Data injection

In this attack, a legal entity is created that can grant authentication into the system. This attack causes severe effects on the IoMT systems, leading to the end of patients' lives by creating messages containing false information and sending it to the doctors and the hospital's databases. In addition, the attacker blocks the correct and accurate message sent by a legitimate user and then injects the wrong message within the system [112]. The wrong script system presents a false update, as a hacker mimics a legitimate backup server. As a result, it can access the IoMT devices without authorization and provides a tailgate [113].

7.2.13   Flooding Attacks

These attacks attempt to overburden the medical system and deplete its resources by flooding and injecting methods using fraudulent information and fake request [114]. ICMP Flooding Attacks is a flood of Internet Control Message Protocols (ICMP) or Ping a DoS, which uses an ICMP echo request or a ping to attack medical devices [115]. In SYN Flood Attack or "half-open" attack a hacker would usually use this attack on IoMT connections that utilize a device with a higher capacity due to TCPs for communication (i.e., a web server/email) [116].

7.2.14   The Black-Nurse Attack

ICMP attacks target CPUs and firewalls with a DoS attack that prevents medical staff and patients from transporting Internet traffic within the LAN [117].

7.2.15   Dictionary Attacks

This attack occurs when accessing medical systems without authorization when the security measures are not stringent enough for the IoT device. These attacks rely on a group of dictionary words to guess passwords. This attack comprehensively covers time and resources, ranging from minutes and hours to even days [118]. In this attack, they rely on a group of numbers known as the Personal Identification Number (PIN).

7.2.16   Birthday Attacks

Often users rely on weak hashes, as two passwords may contain the same hash. The hacker exploits this weakness and accesses the medical systems without authorization [119]. The best solution to protect the systems from such attacks is to use secure hash algorithm mechanisms.

7.2.17   Worms

It is the most dangerous and destructive form of malware present within things [120]. They can self-reproduce without human intervention via a connected device and take advantage of its vulnerabilities. It affects all devices and data security services (confidentiality, safety, and availability), which leads to data loss and even sometimes affects patients' health and even is the reason for the loss of human lives. They are programmed to affect specific industrial control systems [121]. Recently, one of the articles introduced a few "dubbed" malicious Internet worms targeting a network [122]. A worm can be executed and utilized to attack an IoMTs device to collect and steal information to destroy a specific device.

8   THE FRAMEWORK OF SECURITY OF IOMT

As the previous section shows, only some techniques can provide a secure environment for IoMT systems. Hence, we propose a framework capable of protecting IoMT systems from the 14 attacks mentioned in the previous section. The framework also fulfills all the security requirements required by IoMT systems. The framework has three parts based on the IoMT security model stages.

TABLE 8.4

List of Common Attacks and Countermeasures

Attacks	Security	Countermeasures
Physical security token loss	• Authentication	• Asymmetric (two factor)
Impersonation	• Authorization	• Asymmetric
	• Anonymity	• Keyless
	• Forward secrecy	
Tampering	• Data confidentiality	• Symmetric (two factor)
	• Data Integrity	• Keyless
Side channel		• Keyless
RF Jamming	• Availability	
DoS/DDoS		
Sniffing	• Data Confidentiality	• Symmetric/asymmetric
MITM	• Data confidentiality	(two factor)
	• Authorization	• Keyless
Relay	• Authorization	
Replay		
Clock synchronization	• Secure key exchange	• Asymmetric (two factor)
Parallel session	• Authentication	
Brute force	• Authorization	• Keyless
Stepping stone		

8.1 SECURING DATA COLLECTION

The first step in securing IoMT systems is to ensure how other systems interact with them, which protects the patient's data collection stage. Two-way factor authentication techniques are good options to provide such security and resistance to some of the attacks mentioned. If one of the two factors is compromised, the other can still provide essential overall security. ECC keys commonly use as first-factor authentication techniques due to their lightweight keys and reliable protection [94], [123], [124].

8.2 SECURING DATA IN TRANSIT

To enhance the IoMT systems' security when connected to other devices over the network, we advise utilizing some security protocols, such as CoAP. The rest of the layers can be linked using Secure HTTP (HTTPS) or TLS version 1.3 [125]. Thus, it is convenient for use in IoMT systems. To reduce the certificate management overhead in the cloud layer, certificateless cryptography, an ID-Based Cryptography (IBC) branch, can be used [126], [127]. The protection from these attacks provides the system with confidentiality, integrity, non-repudiation, authentication, and secure key exchange.

8.3 Securing Data in Storage

Some of the attacks in IoMT systems target the availability and integrity of the system, such as DoS/DDoS, RF jamming, and stepping-stone attacks. These attacks can be detected using AI techniques. AI techniques used to build detection models with mitigation techniques imposed on these models. For example, Deep Neural Networks (DNN) can be used to build intrusion detection models. Once this model detects suspicious activity, termination of the compromised connection imposes to mitigate the attack. Adopting these intrusion detection models in the cloud layer can warn the system administrator when such attacks occur, which can verify early signs (if they exist) from the EC nodes in the gateway layer.

9 ADVANTAGES AND DISADVANTAGES OF IOMT IN HEALTHCARE

There are enormous advantages of IoMT in healthcare but there are limitations too [128]. Below Table 8.5 shows both advantages and disadvantages of IoMT in healthcare.

10 CONCLUSION AND FUTURE TRENDS

Due to the demand for using IoMT sensors to reduce healthcare spending and provide better care for patients, securing these devices has become extremely important. However, IoMT sensors tend to have constrained resources, and some require external devices to connect them. The key management is

---

TABLE 8.5

Advantages and Limitations of IoMT

Advantages	Limitations/Challenges
• Real-time interventions in emergency	• Security of IoT data- hacking and unauthorized use of IoT
• Cost reduction	
• Reduced morbidity and financial burden due to less follow-up	• Lack of standards and communication protocols
• Optimal utilization of resources and infrastructure	• Errors in patient data handling
	• Data integration
• Reduced response time in case of a medical emergency	• Need for medical expertise
	• Managing device diversity and interoperability
• Standardization/compatibility and uniformity of data available	
	• Scale- Data volume and performance
• Capability to sense and communicate health-related information to a remote location	• Physician compliance
	• Data overload in healthcare facility
	• Mobile hesitation
	• Security policy compliance

modular, composed of a platform key management layer, which establishes ad hoc, point-to-point secure channels between devices in the IoMT system, and of a data key management layer, which provisions keys for end-to-end encryption of patient data, with the help of the platform key management's point-to-point security. The platform key management enables point-to-point secure communications channels between devices of the IoMT monitoring platform and is a prerequisite for data key management. The function of the platform key management proposes data security, but its capabilities are much more diverse. Furthermore, the ability to develop a distributed platform key management domain further improves scalability and resiliency against attackers. Data key management introduces a significant paradigm shift, giving the patient complete control over the data protection keys to a patient, significantly reducing the degree to which a patient needs to trust the healthcare provider. At the same time, the design is remarkably scalable; it can thus serve a practically unlimited number of sensors from a total number of healthcare providers. On the other side, the tree-based key derivation facilitates data access to be highly efficient at configurable scales. Finally, the complete solution and each of its parts easily generalize to other IoT applications [129].

IoMT technology has brought about a drastic enhancement in RPM. It can connect entire networks of medical devices worldwide. However, the increasing rate of intrusions in the healthcare network has badly affected the security and privacy of patients and the healthcare sector. Also, their resource constraints, e.g., limited battery power and limited processing power, have reduced the efficiency of some security mechanisms like cryptography. In conjunction with IoMT devices, ML can help build more efficient intrusion detection system (IDS) for medical organizations to support thousands of patients and manage sizable amounts of data. Characteristics of ML techniques make it possible to design IDS with high detection rates and low false favorable rates while the system adapts quickly to changing malicious behaviors. It shows that K Nearest Neighbors (KNN) is the best model for healthcare monitoring systems as it gives the lowest execution time and generates an accuracy rate of 97.67%. The ideal IDS should be based mainly on eight parameters: Accuracy, Execution time, Area under the ROC (AUC) score, Precision, Recall, F1 score, True Positive, and False Positive. These gives solution when applied it in the IoMT system, which is under MITM and DoS attacks, and are successfully detected. Results show that all ML methods performed significantly better with combined features than using only one of the two features. Future work is on to develop IDS using Fuzzy Logic, one of the most powerful tools for reasoning under uncertainty for intrusion analysis. With Fuzzy Logic, it intends to effectively identify the intrusion activities in the network since it could give a reasonable conclusion in cases where situations do not explicitly define in the rule-based knowledge representation. Furthermore, a more robust and secure solution is arrived by integrating the various newer developmental techniques. Wearable IoMT devices can collect patients' data for condition monitoring and alerts, while implanted devices can inject medicine remotely. Data security and computation overhead remain the two main issues of the IoMT cloud-based system. Traditionally, network security involves encryption, authentication, and authorization. However, these approaches may not be feasible for IoMT devices with severe power constraints. Considering the importance of security and privacy parameters in IoMT, various literature was explored and the factors analyzed that could negatively impact security and privacy. Accordingly, IoMT security challenges have identified numerous challenges addressed with cryptographic techniques, algorithms, and approaches proposed by various recent researchers with the rise in the usage of IoMT devices, to identify new threats and patterns that arise, both technical and behavioral. Insufficient power in IMDs led to the operation of these devices without proper security defenses. Moreover, new factors have emerged, such as "the fear of not knowing how IoMT devices work", making these devices more vulnerable to security threats. Additionally, the author suggested improvements to enhance the security of future Medical Body Area Network (MBAN) applications based on IEEE standards.

REFERENCES

[1] Pradhan, Bikash, Deepti Bharti, Sumit Chakravarty, Sirsendu S. Ray, Vera V. Voinova, Anton P. Bonartsev, and Kunal Pal, "Internet of things and robotics in transforming current-day healthcare services," *Journal of Healthcare Engineering,* vol. 2021, p. 1–15; Article ID 9999504. http:doi.org/10.1155/2021/9999504, 2021.

[2] C. (. Chakraborty, Digital Health Transformation with Blockchain and Artificial Intelligence (1st ed.)., CRC Press. https://doi.org/10.1201/9781003247128, 2022.

[3] M. P. A. A. N. A. Shilpa Srivastava, "The technological growth in eHealth services," *Computational and Mathematical Methods in Medicine*, vol. 2015, p. 18 Article ID 894171. https://doi.org/10.1155/2015/894171, 2015.

[4] H. R. A. J. A. e. a. Mahajan, "Integration of healthcare 4.0 and blockchain into secure cloud-based electronic health records systems," *Applied Nanoscience*, 2022. https://doi.org/10.1007/s13204-021-02164-0.

[5] H. R. A. M. H. Ghorbani, "Security challenges in the Internet of things: a survey," In *2017 IEEE Conference on Wireless Sensors (ICWiSe),* pp. 1–6; IEEE, 2017, November.

[6] K. B. A. M. K. J. P. P. R. R. P. P. &. G. D. Fizza, "QoE in IoT: A vision, survey, and future directions," *Discover the Internet of Things* vol. 1, no. 1, pp. 1–14., 2021.

[7] U. S. S. A. T. C. &. S. M. A. Shanthamallu, "A brief survey of machine learning methods and their sensor and IoT applications," In *2017 8th International Conference on Information, Intelligence, Systems & Application (IISA)*, August 2017.

[8] R. B. S. M. a. M. P. J Gubbi, "Internet of things (IoT): A vision, architectural elements, and future direction," *Future Generation Computation Systems*, vol. 29, no. 7, pp. 1645–1660, 2013. https://doi.org/10.1016/j.future.2013.01.010.

[9] I. e. a. Essop, "Generating datasets for anomaly-based' intrusion detection systems in IoT and industrial IoT networks," *Sensors*, vol. 21, no. 4, p. 1528, 2021.

[10] Gartner, "Gartner says 5.8 billion enterprise and automotive IoT endpoints will be in use in 2020," 2019. https://www.gartner.com/en/newsroom/pressreleases/2019-08-29-gartner-says-5-8-billion-enterpriseand-automotive-io.

[11] A. M. A. S. Y. M. M. M. M. M. Gul S, "A survey on the overview of internet of things (IoT)," *International Journal of Recent Trends in Engineering and Research*, vol. 4, no. 3, pp. 251–257, 2018.

[12] F. e. a. Alsubaei, "IoMT-SAF: Internet of medical things security assessment framework," *Internet of Things*, vol. 8, p. 100123, 2019.

[13] Y. Perwej, K. Haq, F. Parwej, M. Mumdouh, M. Hassan, The internet of things (IoT) and its application domains. *International Journal of Computer Applications*, vol. 975, no. 8887, p. 182, 2019 Apr.

[14] S. Gritzalis, "Enhancing privacy and data protection in electronic medical environments," *Journal of Medical Systems*, vol. 28, no. 6, pp. 535–547, 2004.

[15] B. M. R. a. P. S. Vinoth, "Internet of Medical Things (IoMT) using hybrid security and near field communication (NFC) technology," *International Journal of Computer Applications*, vol. 174, no. 7, pp. 37–40, 2017.

[16] N. Internetmedicine.com., "Top 40 medical device companies | Internetmedicine. Com," *Internetmedicine.com*, p. 2019. Web, 14 August 2019.

[17] A. e. a. Mavrogiorgou, "Internet of medical things (IoMT): Acquiring and transforming data into HL7 FHIR through 5G network slicing," *Emerging Science Journal*, vol. 3, no. 2 Web, p. 64, 2019.

[18] S. R. e. a. Moosavi, "Performance analysis of end-to-end security schemes in healthcare IoT," *Procedia Computer Science*, vol. 130, pp. 432–439, 2018.

[19] A. M. H. N. T. a. N. E. M. K. A Mawgoud, *Security Threats of Social Internet of Things in The Higher Education Environment*, Cham: Springer, 2019.

[20] D. a. C. S. Kavitha, "Security threat management by software obfuscation for privacy in Internet of medical thing (Iomt) application," *Journal of Computational and Theoretical Nanoscience* vol. 14, no. 7, pp. 3100–3114, 2017.

[21] S. H. a. P. N. CR Varun, "Survey on energy efficient routing issues in IOMT," *International Journal of Scientific Research in Computer Science, Engineering and Information Technology*, pp. 112–117, 2019.

[22] W. A. S. a. M. B. Osei-Bonsu, "The current ethical and regulatory status of the internet of medical things (Iomt) and the need of a new IoMT law," *The Journal of Healthcare Ethics & Administration*, vol. 4, no. 2, pp. 32–38, 2018.

[23] S. a. V. S. Smagulov, "Challenges of digital transformation in healthcare," *Intellectual Archive*, vol 8, no. 1 (SI), 2019. doi:10.32370/ia_2019_01_si_5.

[24] A. e. a. A Mawgoud, "Cyber security risks in MENA region: Threats, challenges and countermeasures," In *International Conference On Advanced Intelligent Systems and Informatics*, Cham, 2019.

[25] A. a. A. A. Gupta, "Ethical Hacking and Hacking Attacks," *International Journal of Engineering and Computer Science*, vol. 6, no. 6, pp. 2319–7242, 2017.

[26] M. D. S. K. &. M. R. Ahmed G, "An efficient routing protocol for the Internet of medical things focusing on hot spot node problems," *International Journal of Distributed Sensor Networks*, vol. 17, no. 2, p. 1550147721991706, 2021.

[27] P. T. O. K. K. A. E. &. R. D. Harvey, "Security and privacy of medical internet of things devices for smart homes," In *2020 7th International Conference on Internet of Things: Systems, Management and Security (IOTS)*, 2020, December.

[28] G. M. S. C. C. C. Yang T, "Combining point-of-care diagnostics and internet of medical things (IoMT) to combat the COVID-19 pandemic," *Diagnostics (Basel)*, vol. 10, no. 4, p. 224, 2020. doi:10.3390/diagnostics10040224.

[29] M. &. C. S. Kumar, "A lightweight cloud-assisted identity-based anonymous authentication and critical agreement body area network," *IEEE Systems Journal*, vol. 15, no. 2, pp. 2779–2786, 2020.

[30] FDA, "Design considerations and premarket submission recommendations for interoperable medical devices," Food and Drug Administration; HHS, September 2017.

[31] K. K. V. V. T. U. N. S. &. T. C. Karmakar, "Towards a security enhanced virtualised etwork infrastructure for internet of medical things (IoMT)," In *2020 6th IEEE Conference on Network Softwarization (NetSoft)*, 2020, June.

[32] Y. L. F. W. &. L. B. Sun, "Security and privacy for the Internet of medical things enabled healthcare systems: A survey," *IEEE Access*, vol. 7, pp. 183339–183355, 2019.

[33] K. Angrishi, "Turning Internet of things (IoT) into the Internet of vulnerabilities (iov): IoT botnets," *arXiv preprint arXiv:1702.03681*, 2017.

[34] N. Sharma, C. Chakraborty, & R. Kumar, Optimized multimedia data through computationally intelligent algorithms. *Multimedia Systems*, vol. 29, no. 5, pp. 2961–2977, 2023.

[35] S. S. K. A. a. V. R. K Kandasamy, "IoT cyber risk: A holistic analysis of cyber risk assessment frameworks, risk vectors, and risk ranking process," *Eurasip Journal on Information Security*, vol. 2020, no. 1, p. 8, December 2020.

[36] M. Beri, B. Kumar, S. Tiwari, N. Sharma, H. Vashishtya, & P. Chaudhary (2022, April). "IoT based health monitoring system built on ESP32," In *2022 2nd International Conference on Advance Computing and Innovative Technologies in Engineering (ICACITE)* (pp. 454–458). IEEE.

[37] J. E. F. a. A. D. Redish, "Wireless communication with implanted medical devices using the conductive properties of the body," *Expert Review of Medical Devices*, vol. 8, no. 4, pp. 427–433, 2011.

[38] N. Sharma, M. Soni, S. Kumar, R. Kumar, N. Deb, & A. Shrivastava. "Supervised machine learning method for ontology-based financial decisions in the stock market," *ACM Transactions on Asian and Low-Resource Language Information Processing*, vol. 22, no. 5, pp. 1–24.

[39] A. Phaneuf., "Latest trends in medical monitoring devices and wearable health technology," November 2021. [Online]. Available: https://www.businessinsider.com/wearable-technologyhealthcare-medical-devices.

[40] D. Srivastava, N. Sharma, D. Sinwar, J. H. Yousif, & H. P. Gupta (Eds.). (2023). *Intelligent Internet of Things for Smart Healthcare Systems*. Boca Raton: CRC Press.

[41] V. M. a. A. U. A Kos, "Challenges in wireless communication for connected sensors and wearable devices used in sport biofeedback applications," *Future Generation Computer Systems*, vol. 92, pp. 582–592, 2019.

[42] K. S. Z. R. &. K. S. Khan R, "Future internet: The internet of things architecture, possible applications and key challenges," In *10th International Conference on Frontiers of Information Technology*, 2012.

[43] J. W. C. Z. a. J. L. H Suo, "Security in the internet of things: A review," In *Proceedings -2012 International Conference on Computer Science and Electronics Engineering, ICCSEE 2012*, vol. 3, no. March, 2012.

[44] IOT, "Application layer protocols for IOT: IOT Part 11," April 2021. [Online]. Available: https://www.engineersgarage.com/tutorials/applicationlayer-protocols-for-iot-iot-part-11/85.

[45] A. K. J. P. a. M. R. S Rizvi, "Securing the Internet of Things (IoT): A security taxonomy for IoT," In *Proceedings -17th IEEE International Conference on Trust, Security and Privacy in Computing and Communications and 12th IEEE Internatiol Conference on Big Data Science and Engineering,* Institute of Electrical and Electronics Engineers Inc, September 2018.

[46] B. S. K. a. T. Gnanasekaran, "A systematic study of security issues in Internet-of-Things (IoT)," In *Proceedings of the International Conference on IoT in Social, Mobile, Analytics and Cloud, I-SMAC 2017,* Institute of Electrical and Electronics Engineers Inc., October 2017.

[47] D. J. a. N. K. SN Swamy, "Security threats in the application layer in IOT applications," In *Proceedings of the International Conference on IoT in Social, Mobile, Analytics and Cloud, I-SMAC 2017,* Institute of Electrical and Electronics Engineers Inc., October 2017.

[48] H. V. a. A. C. SR Pokhrel, "Adaptive admission control for IoT applications in home WiFi networks," *IEEE Transactions on Mobile Computing*, vol. 19, no. 12, pp. 2731–2742, December 2020.

[49] S. S. J. P. S. P. S. Hwang, "A survey of the self-adaptive IoT systems and a compare and analyze of IoT using self-adaptive concept," *KIPS Transactions on Computer and Communication Systems [Internet]*, vol. 5, no. 1, pp. 17–26, 2016 January 31.

[50] AltexSoft, "Internet of Things (IoT) architecture: Key layers and components |AltexSoft," April 2021. [Online]. Available: https://www.altexsoft.com/blog/iot-architecture-layers-components/.

[51] H. J. a. J. Ibarra, "Digital forensic investigation for the Internet of medical things (IoMT)," *Journal of Forensic Legal & Investigative Sciences*, vol. 5, no. 29, 2019.

[52] Medtronic, "Pacing systems - Azure | Medtronic," November 2020. [Online]. Available: https://europe.medtronic.com/xden/healthcare-professionals/products/cardiacrhythm/pacemakers/azure.html.

[53] F. C. Commission(FCC), "Medical device radiocommunications service (MedRadio)," 2020. [Online]. Available: https://www.fcc.gov/medicaldevice-radiocommunications-service-medradio.

[54] A. D. K. a. J. H. Singh, "IoT based information and communication system for enhancing underground mines safety and productivity: Genesis, taxonomy and open issues," *Ad Hoc Networks*, vol. 78, pp. 115–129, 2018.

[55] T. a. E.-u. H. Aziz, "Security challenges facing IoT layers and its protective measures," *International Journal of Computer Applications*, vol. 179, no. 27, pp. 31–35, 2018.

[56] H. F. a. M. A. A Azza, "IOT perception layer security and privacy," *International Journal of Computer Applications*, vol. 182, no. 49, pp. 25–28, 2019.

[57] Y.-S. a. S.-S. S. Jeong, "An IoT healthcare service model of a vehicle using implantable devices," *Cluster Computing*, vol. 21, no. 1, pp. 1059–1068, 2016.

[58] J. a. R. S. Liebowitz, "Biological warfare: Tampering with implantable medical devices," *IT Professional*, vol. 17, no. 5, pp. 70–72, 2015.

[59] Y.-S. Jeong, "An efficient IoT healthcare service management model of location tracking sensor," *Journal of Digital Convergence*, vol. 14, no. 3, pp. 261–267, 2016.

[60] P. P. D. D. a. D. D. Ray, "A systematic review and implementation of IoT- based pervasive sensor-enabled tracking system for dementia patients," *Journal of Medical Systems*, vol. 43, no. 9, pp. 1–21, 2019.

[61] D. B. J. a. W. J. K. Dziak, "Wirelessly interfacing objects and subjects of healthcare system – IoT approach," *Elektronika ir Elektrotechnika*, vol. 22, no. 3, pp. 66–73, 2016.

[62] A. J. A. M. a. N. C. Mazayev, "Interoperability in IoT through the semantic profiling of objects," *IEEE Access*, vol. 6, pp. 19379–19385, 2018.

[63] L. a. R. M. Celic, "Seamless connectivity architecture and methods for IoT and wearable devices," *Automatika*, vol. 61, no. 1, pp. 21–34, 2019.

[64] S. R. H. L. V. a. A. L. C. Pokhrel, "Adaptive admission control for IoT applications in home Wifi networks," *IEEE Transactions on Mobile Computing*, vol. 19, no. 12, pp. 2731–2742, 2019.

[65] S. e. a. Hwang, "A survey of the self-adaptive IoT systems and a compare and analyze of IoT using self-adaptive concept," *KIPS Transactions on Computer and Communication Systems*, vol. 5, no. 1, pp. 17–26, 2016.

[66] G. e. a. Bouloukakis, "Automated synthesis of mediators for middleware-layer protocol interoperability in The IoT," *Future Generation Computer Systems*, vol. 101, pp. 1271–1294, 2019.

[67] E. e. a. Semastin, "Preventive measures for cross site request forgery attacks on web-based applications," *International Journal of Engineering & Technology*, vol. 7, no. 4, 15, p. 130, 2018.

[68] M. S. e. a. Hossain, "Survey of the protection mechanisms to the SSL-based session hijacking attacks," *Network Protocols and Algorithms*, vol. 10, no. 1, p. 83, 2018.

[69] P. a. R. T. Tripathi, "Cross site scripting (XSS) and SQL-injection attack detection in web application," *Proceedings of International Conference on Sustainable Computing in Science, Technology and Management (SUSCOM)*, Amity University Rajasthan, Jaipur - India, February 26-28, 2019, Available at, 2019. https://ssrn.com/abstract=3356292 or http://dx.doi.org/10.2139/ssrn.3356292

[70] X. a. N. A. Sun, "Dynamic resource caching in the IoT application layer for smart cities," *IEEE Internet of Things Journal*, vol. 5, no. 2, pp. 606–613, 2018.

[71] S. a. R. M. Mendhurwar, "Integration of social and IoT technologies: Architectural framework for digital transformation and cyber security challenges," *Enterprise Information Systems*, vol. 15, no. 4, pp. 1–20, 2021 Apr 21.

[72] V. Dyagilev, "Target attacks on IoT and network security vulnerabilities increase," *LastMile*, vol. 6, pp. 72–73, 2018.

[73] Y. a. J. H. P. Bansal, "Multi-hashing for protecting web applications from SQL injection attacks," *International Journal of Computer and Communication Engineering*, vol. 4, no. 3, pp. 187–195, 2015.

[74] V. a. A. K. Dutt, "Cyber security: Testing the effects of attack strategy, similarity, and experience on cyber attack detection," *International Journal of Trust Management in Computing and Communications*, vol. 1, no. 3/4, p. 261, 2013.

[75] D. K. Mishra, "Cyber security guidelines for healthcare providers threats and defense from ransomware," *International Journal of Engineering Research and V6.12*, vol. 6, p. 12, 2017.

[76] D. e. a. Stiawan, "Investigating brute force attack patterns in IoT network," *Journal of Electrical and Computer Engineering*, vol. 2019, pp. 1–13, 2019.

[77] L. I. a. K. Lee, "The Internet of things (IoT): Applications, investments, and challenges for enterprises," *Business Horizons*, vol. 58, no. 4, pp. 431–440, 2015.

[78] J. e. a. Feng, "Securing traffic-related messages exchange against inside-and-outside collusive attack in vehicular networks," *IEEE Internet of Things Journal*, vol. 6, no. 6, pp. 9979–9992, 2019.

[79] N. A. e. a. Kamalanathan, "Improving the patient discharge planning process through knowledge management by using the internet of things," *Advances in Internet of Things*, vol. 3, no. 2, pp. 16–26, 2013.

[80] CIA, "A survey on CIA triad for cloud storage services," April 2021. [Online]. Available: https://www.researchgate.net/publication/311951056_A_survey_on_CIA_triad_for_cloud_storage_services.

[81] D. M. E.-D. M. M. H. a. N. E. Hussein, "A blockchain technology evolution between business process management (BPM) And internet-of-things (IoT)," *International Journal of Advanced Computer Science and Applications*, vol. 9, no. 8, pp. 442–450, 2018.

[82] A. B. a. V. V. Thavavel Vaiyapuri, "Security, privacy and trust in IoMT enabled smart healthcare system: A systematic review of current and future trends," *International Journal of Advanced Computer Science and Applications(IJACSA)*, vol. 12, no. 2, pp. 731–737, 2021.

[83] Y. a. P. B. Fathy, "Quality-based and energy-efficient data communication for the internet of things networks," *IEEE Internet of Things Journal*, vol. 6, no. 6, pp. 10318–10331, 2019.

[84] H. A. a. M. M. H. El Zouka, "Secure IoT communications for smart healthcare monitoring system," *Internet of Things*, vol. 1, no. 13, p. 100036, 2019 Aug 28.

[85] R. Kunnavil, "Healthcare data utilization for the betterment of Mankind - an overview of big data concept in healthcare," *International Journal of Healthcare Education & Medical Informatics*, vol. 5, no. 2, pp. 14–17, 2018.

[86] V. a. K. A. Dutt, "Cyber security: Testing the effects of attack strategy, similarity, and experience on cyber-attack detection," *International Journal of Trust Management in Computing and Communications*, vol. 1, no. 3/4, p. 261, 2013.

[87] S. S. a. M. H. T Belkhouja, "Role-based hierarchical medical data encryption for implantable medical devices," In *2019 IEEE Global Communications Conference (GLOBECOM), 9–13 December 2019*, 2019.

[88] K. K. S. P.-S. C. G.-P. S. C.-P. a. N. C. MF Awan, "RSS-based secret key generation in wireless in-body networks," In *2019 13th International Symposium on Medical Information and Communication Technology (ISMICT)*, 2019.

[89] A. I. A. A. a. K. A. BA Alzahrani, "A provably secure and lightweight patient-healthcare authentication protocol in wireless body area networks," *Wireless Personal Communications*, vol. 117, no. 1, pp. 47–69, 2021 Mar.

[90] C. X. W. L. J. X. a. H. C. Z Xu, "A lightweight mutual authentication and key agreement scheme for medical internet of things" *IEEE Access*, vol. 7, pp. 53922–53931, 2019.

[91] Y. S. a. B. Lo, "An artificial neural network framework for gait-based biometrics," *IEEE Journal of Biomedical and Health Informatics*, vol. 23, no. 3, pp. 987–998, 2019.

[92] B. D. a. D. C. VH Tutari, "A continuous role-based authentication scheme and data transmission protocol for implantable medical devices," In *2019 Second International Conference on Advanced Computational and Communication Paradigms (ICACCP) 25–28 February 2019*, 2019.

[93] e. a. S Maji, "A low-power dual-factor authentication unit for secure implantable devices," In *2020 IEEE Custom Integrated Circuits Conference (CICC)*, 2020.

[94] A. V. a. G. S. T Bhatia, "Towards a secure incremental proxy re-encryption for e-healthcare data sharing in mobile cloud computing," *Concurrency and Computation: Practice and Experience*, vol. 32, no. 5, pp. 1–16, 2020.

[95] G. Kalyani and S. Chaudhari, "An efficient approach for enhancing security in Internet of Things using the optimum authentication key," *International Journal of Computers and Applications*, vol. 42, no. 3, pp. 306–314, 2020.

[96] S. J. M. Y. A. V. K. M. A. Adesh Kumari, "ESEAP: ECC based secure and efficient mutual authentication protocol using smart card," *Journal of Information Security and Applications*, vol. 51, p. 102443. 2020.

[97] e. a. Zheng G, "Finger-to-heart (F2H): Authentication for wireless implantable medical devices," *IEEE Journal of Biomedical and Health Informatics,.,* vol. 23, no. 4, pp. 1546–1557, 2019.

[98] N. I. a. S. Hadj, "Smart ECG monitoring through IoT," In *Smart Medical Data Sensing and IoT Systems Design in Healthcare*, USA, IGI Global, 2020, pp. 224–246.

[99] S. Kulac, "A new externally worn proxy-based protector for non-secure wireless implantable medical devices: Security jacket," *IEEE Access*, vol. 7, pp. 55358–55366, 2019.

[100] A. G. T. S. D. U. a. R. J. AA Hady, "Intrusion detection system for healthcare systems using medical and network data: A comparison study," *IEEE Access*, vol. 8, pp. 106576–106584, 2020.

[101] T. S. M. Z. A. E. a. R. J. L Gupta, "Fault and performance management in multi-cloud virtual network services using AI: A tutorial and a case study," *Computer Networks*, vol. 165, Art no. 106950, 2019.

[102] P. N. a. M. K. R. Yao Liu, "False data injection attacks against state estimation in electric power grids," *ACM Transactions on Information and System Security (TISSEC)*, vol. 14, no. 1, p. 13, 2011.

[103] H. Z. D. G. W. L. R. Y. a. S. L. X Chen, "Merging RFID and blockchain technologies to accelerate big data medical research based on physiological signals," *Journal of Healthcare Engineering*, vol. 2020, pp. 1–17, 2020.

[104] A. P. a. L. Lazos, "Selective jamming attacks in wireless networks," In *2010 IEEE International Conference on Communications*, 2010.

[105] A. L. a. Q. Y. Kanika Grover, "Jamming and anti-jamming techniques in wireless networks: A survey," *International Journal of Ad Hoc and Ubiquitous Computing*, vol. 17, no. 4, pp. 197–215, 2014.

[106] Z. A. B. a. A.-R. Amoudi., "An analysis of clever grid attacks and countermeasures," *Journal of Communications*, vol. 8, no. 8, pp. 473–479, 2013.

[107] V. V. a. S. W. SC Sethuraman, "Cyber attacks on healthcare devices using unmanned aerial vehicles," *Journal of Medical Systems*, vol. 44, no. 1, pp. 1–10, 2019.

[108] J. P. H.-K. K. U. M. K. a. D. W. Junghyun Nam, "An offline dictionary attack on a simple threeparty key exchange protocol," *IEEE Communications Letters*, vol. 13, no. 3, pp. 205–207, 2009.

[109] P. K. a. H.-J. Lee, "Security issues in healthcare applications using wireless medical sensor networks: A survey," *Sensors*, vol. 12, no. 1, pp. 55–91, 2012.

[110] S. C. a. M. G. Daojing He, "Droneassisted public safety networks: the security aspect," *IEEE Communications Magazine*, vol. 55, no. 8, pp. 218–223, 2017.

[111] T. H. a. T.-H. L. Chun-Wei Yang, "Modification attack on qsdc with authentication and the improvement," *International Journal of Theoretical Physics*, vol. 52, no. 7, pp. 2230–2234, 2013.

[112] M. R. H. Mohsenian-Rad, "False data injection attacks with incomplete information against intelligent power grids," In *Global communications conference (GLOBECOM)*, Citeseer, 2012.

[113] B. E. H. M. a. A. N. Satish Vadlamani, "Jamming attacks on wireless networks: A taxonomic survey," *International Journal of Production Economics*, vol. 172, pp. 76–94, 2016.

[114] H. Harshita., "Detection and prevention of ICMP flood DDoS attack," *International Journal of New Technology and Research*, vol. 3, no. 3, 2017.

[115] T. S. a. A. R. Mitko Bogdanoski, "Analysis of the syn flood dos attack," *International Journal of Computer Network and Information Security (IJCNIS)*, vol. 5, no. 8, pp. 1–11, 2013.

[116] G. K. D. F. a. A. S. Yuquan Shan, "Preliminary study of fission defenses against low volume dos attacks on proxied multiserver systems," In *2017 12th International Conference on Malicious and Unwanted Software (MALWARE)*, 2017.

[117] G. M. a. C.-C. L. Chee-Wooi Ten, "Cy- cybersecurity for critical infrastructures: Attack and defense modeling," *IEEE Transactions on Systems, Man, and Cybernetics-Part A: Systems and Humans*, vol. 40, no. 4, pp. 853–865, 2010.

[118] M. B. a. T. Kohno., "Hash function balance and its impact on birthday attacks," In *International Conference on the Theory and Applications of Cryptographic Techniques*, 2004.

[119] D. A. Vidhate J, "Security attacks in IoT: A survey," In *2017 International Conference on I-SMAC (IoT in Social, Mobile, Analytics, and Cloud) (I-SMAC)*, 2017.

[120] L. O. M. a. E. C. W... Nicolas Falliere, "Stuxnet dossierWhite paper, Symantec Corp," *Security Response*, vol. 5, no. 6, p. 29, 2011.

[121] S. E. a. I. Profetis., "Hajime: Analysis of a decentralized internet worm for IoT devices," *Rapidity Networks*, vol. 16, p. 1–8, 2016 Oct 16.

[122] F. J. a. D. M. Evan Cooke, "The zombie roundup: Understanding, detecting, and disrupting botnets," *SRUTI*, vol. 5., p. 6, 2005.

[123] M. K. a. S. M. A. P Kasyoka, "Certificateless pairing-free authentication scheme for wireless body area network in healthcare management system," *Journal of Medical Engineering & Technology*, vol. 44, no. 1, pp. 12–19, 2020.

[124] S. J. M. A. V. K. a. M. A. A Kumari, "ESEAP: ECC based secure and efficient mutual authentication protocol using smart card," *Journal of Information Security and Applications*, vol. 51, pp. 1–12, 2020.

[125] S. a. C. W. JA Salowey, "TLS 1.3," November 2020 [Online]. Available: https://www.ietf.org/blog/tls13/.

[126] R. Kumar, N. Sharma, & S. Kumar (2022, April). Image Intelligence in Cyber Security using Sensing System towards the Future Generation Intelligence. In 2022 2nd International Conference on Advance Computing and Innovative Technologies in Engineering (ICACITE), April. IEEE, pp. 298–300, 2022.

[127] N. M. Lutimath, H. V. Ramachandra, S. Raghav, & N. Sharm. "Prediction of heart disease using genetic algorithm." In *Proceedings of Second Doctoral Symposium on Computational Intelligence: DoSCI 2021*. Springer Singapore, pp. 49–58, 2022.

[128] A. A. K. A. I. &. T. B. S. Mawgoud, "A secure authentication technique in internet of Medical Things through Machine Learning," *arXiv*. https://doi.org/10.6084/m9.figshare.13311479.v2, 2019.

[129] D. V. G. M. J. B. C. K.-F. a. J. R. M De Ree, "A key management framework to secure IoMT-enabled healthcare systems," In *IEEE 26th International Workshop on Computer Aided Modeling and Design of Communication Links and Networks (CAMAD)*, 2021.

9 Security Issues Related to COVID Data Using Artificial Intelligence (AI)

Ramkrishna Mondal

1 INTRODUCTION

The coronavirus outbreak has stirred the digital health revolution that has been building for the past decade. However, the full potential of the digital process can only be felt once the core structural reforms in healthcare do not take place, along with a significant boost in digital infrastructure. The way digital technologies have helped in the coming years, it has become imperative for the world to increasingly adopt and integrate digital innovations to make healthcare more accessible, interconnected, and affordable [1]. Healthcare savings could reach $150 billion by 2025 due to this technology, of which half are clinical savings and the other half are financial and operational costs [2]. Most healthcare systems will soon need to find an answer to a similar question [3]. The budget is far more complex in the US, with the US Government paying for approximately 50% of care [4]. Data that belong to healthcare systems are incomplete, imperfect, and underused, yet these data do exist, and healthcare systems probably have more data than any other stakeholder. Currently, as 80% of the data, i.e., 41 zettabytes (410 trillion GB) of digital information available, is unstructured, AI will be required to detect patterns and trends that our gray matter is unable to decipher [5]. Technology companies seek access to those data while promising to help the healthcare systems mitigate their three historical weaknesses: access to care, quality of care, and inefficiency. Three initiatives need prioritizing. First, massive public investment is necessary so that hospitals, which are the current healthcare data giants, are equipped to develop their algorithms. Several examples show that it is feasible [6]. Second, public hospitals or groups should be allowed to implement non-conventional business models complementary to their typical funding sources. And third, the global community needs to be realistic: public investment will only be able to fund the development of some of the algorithms required because several of them should be available per condition, and there are thousands of diseases [7].

DOI: 10.1201/9781003377818-9

Leading experts have repeatedly outlined the value asymmetry between current AI algorithms and data [8]. AI expects to affect global productivity, equality and inclusion, environmental outcomes, and several other areas in the short and long term [9], [10]. It also reported that AI's potential impacts indicate both positive and negative impacts on sustainable development [11], [12]. There needs to be more studies assessing the extent to which AI impacts sustainable development. In the 2030 Agenda for Sustainable Development Goals (SDGs), 17 (SDGs) and 169 targets were internationally agreed upon [13]. It is a critical research gap, as AI may or may not influence the ability to meet all SDGs.

1.1 AI AND SOCIETAL CONSEQUENCES

Sixty-seven targets (82%) within the society group could benefit from AI-based technologies. Diversity is one of the primary values of subsidiary innovation and resilience, which will become essential in a society exposed to changes associated with AI development. These lead to a very high energy requirement and carbon footprint, and green growth of Information Communication and Technology (ICT) is therefore essential [14], [15]. Societal resilience is also promoted by decentralization, i.e., by implementing AI technologies adapted to different regions' cultural backgrounds and particular needs.

1.2 AI AND ECONOMIC OUTCOMES

Technological advantages provided by AI may also positively impact the achievement of several SDGs within the economy. It identified benefits from AI on 42 targets (70%) from these SDGs. In contrast, negative impacts are reported in 20 marks (33%), as shown in Figure 9.1. Although Acemoglu and Restrepo say a net positive impact of AI-enabled technologies associated with increased productivity, the literature also reflects potential adverse effects that are mainly related to increased inequalities [16–18] Though the linkages in economy are primarily positive, trade-offs cannot be neglected. For instance, AI can negatively affect social media usage by showing users content suited to their preconceived ideas. This may lead to political polarization and affect social cohesion in the context of SDG 10 on inequality reduction [19]. AI has the potential to identify sources of inequality and conflict [20], and therewith can reduce inequalities, by using simulations to assess how virtual societies may respond to changes. The work by Dalenberg [20] highlights the need to modify the data preparation process and explicitly adopt the AI for selection processes to avoid biases.

1.3 AI AND ENVIRONMENTAL CONSEQUENCES

It identified 25 targets (93%) for which AI could act as an enabler. Benefits from AI could be derived from analyzing interconnected databases to develop joint actions to preserve the environment. Furthermore, AI will help low-carbon energy systems with renewable energy and energy efficiency, all of which are needed to address climate change. Another example is target 15.3 for combating desertification and restoring degraded land and soil [21]. According to Mohamadi et al. [22], neural networks can be used to improve vegetation cover types based on satellite images. Furthermore, though there are many examples of AI to improve biodiversity monitoring and conservation [23] increased access to AI-related information about ecosystems may drive the overexploitation of resources.

1.4 TOWARD SUSTAINABLE AI

Worldwide the growing economic reputation of AI may increase inequalities due to the maldistribution of educational and computing resources. One area where this conflict is fundamental is healthcare: Panch et al. argue that although the enormous personal healthcare data could lead to the development of potent tools for diagnosis and treatment, the numerous problems with data ownership and privacy call for careful policy intervention [24]. Figure 9.1 shows a schematic representation of these dynamics, emphasizing the role of technology. The first step is to make adequate policy and legislation to help direct the vast potential of AI toward the maximum benefit for individuals and the environment. This is required to achieve the SDGs.

The above schematic representation (Figure 9.1) showing the identified agents and their roles in the revolution of AI. Technology affects individuals through technical results, which change how people interact with environment. In contrast, individuals would interact with technology through new needs to be satisfied. Also, technology developers affect the government through lobbying and influencing decision-makers. Governments touch individuals through policy and legislation, and individuals require new legislation consistent with the changing

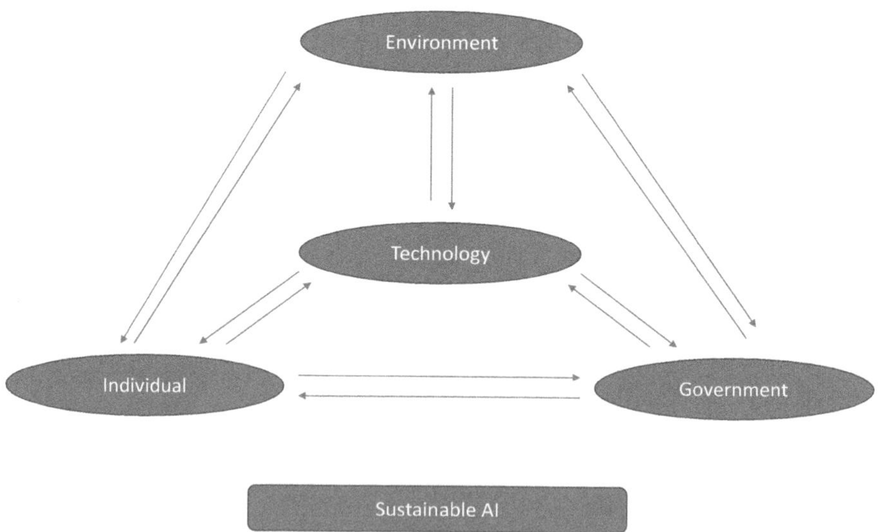

FIGURE 9.1 Interaction of AI, Environment, Economy and Society

circumstances of the governments. The environment intermingles with technology by the resources for technological development, and is affected by the environmental impact. Moreover, the environment is affected negatively or positively by the needs, impacts, along with choices of individuals and governments, which in turn require environmental resources. Finally, AI applications with positive societal welfare implications may not always benefit each individual separately, and this dilemma of collective vs. individual benefit is relevant in the scope of AI applications but is different from one that the application of AI itself should be solved [25]. AI is also called the new electricity, as the invention of electricity transformed how we live; AI is poised to change our world. Research says that global AI healthcare spending will equal $36.1 billion by 2025. In 2017, China announced its goal of becoming a global AI leader by 2030. In 2019, the US issued an order directing all to implement strategic objectives aimed at accelerating AI research and development [26]. Moreover, it is essential to mention that higher awareness from society on digitalization and Industry 4.0 technologies through improved education and development of "digital" professionals will be of great importance. Future research will cover the technologies mentioned above related to digitalization in medicine and healthcare, including virtual experiments, biological additive manufacturing, the development of cybersecurity, and pandemic predictive extensive data analysis [27].

2 AI AND HEALTHCARE

2.1 What Is AI?

The terminology "Artificial Intelligence" was first coined by McCarthy in 1956. As per John McCarthy [28], AI is the science and engineering of producing intelligent machines which do similar works by computers to understand human intelligence but not confine themselves to biologically observable methods [5]. AI is the evolution of computers that can complete tasks that typically require human intelligence, such as perception, speech recognition, decision-making, and language translation [29]. Machine learning (ML) is a subset of AI defined as enabling computing advances through testing and adaptation scenarios and by using trends and patterns for improved decision-making [7]. ML models have been shown to augment the decision-making capacity of clinicians in neurosurgical applications. Viewing ML in a human and machine context rather than a human-machine setting is essential [30]. Deep learning (DL) is a subclass of ML, having networks capable of learning in an unsupervised manner, from unstructured or unlabeled data. Natural Language Processing (NLP) is the capacity of a computer program to comprehend spoken human language. Fuzzy Logic (FL) is a multivalued logic like human thinking and interpretation. This can combine human heuristics (a problem-solving technique) that finds rapid computer-assisted decision-making. FL can quantify all these multiple variables. The National Aeronautics and Space Administration's (NASA) innovative project used FL to identify gray and white matter and normal tissue and tumor cells in real time [31].

2.2 AI AND HEALTHCARE INTERRELATIONSHIP

AI will expectantly place back the "humanity" aspects in healthcare through letting clinicians to focus on patient rather getting drowned in voluminous data [32]. In a thought-provoking article, "Surgery, Virtual Reality, and the Future", Vosburgh emphasized that AI should ideally address the problems surgeons have, not what engineers think they have [33]. It is an irony that the AI application in neurosciences assumes a better understanding of the intellectual functioning of the biological brain [34]. AI aims to mimic human cognitive functions. NLP procedures target turning texts into machine-readable structured data, which ML can then analyze [35]. Amalgamation of clinicians and data scientists, supported by the growing strength of clinical informatics, are beginning to yield positive results. Like other disruptive technologies in the past, its potential for causing a considerable impact should not be underestimated [36]. AI is the foundation of PM, which will eventually be a part of neurological management. PM assumes the handiness of gigantic computing power and algorithms, which can learn by themselves at an unprecedented rate [37]. DeepMind Technologies Ltd, a subsidiary of the Google, uses AI with data-driven tools and methods and ML to progress healthcare. Microsoft, International Business Machines (IBM) Corporation, and Apple are capitalizing heavily in health-related AI [38]. The Gartner hype cycle for evolving technologies labels the different phases of innovations. The phases are trigger, peak of inflated expectations, trough of disillusionment, and scope of enlightenment and a plateau of productivity [39]. AI is conventionally defined as a computer system's problem-solving, reasoning, and learning ability [40]. There is potential for AI systems to work more efficiently, with increased reliability, and for longer hours, than paid human workers. Experts in the field have described the scope of AI to address longstanding deficiencies in healthcare and improve patient care [41]. AI also has the potential to enhance medical devices, especially by working synergistically with robotic technologies in improving the rate and scope of their iterative improvements. Potential uses of AI are well described in the literature, some proven, and some which are speculative. Thus far, studies have shown that AI can outperform human doctors in several specific tasks, affecting a range of fields such as dermatology, cardiology, and radiology [42], [43]. The DL capacity of AI would enable systems to detect characteristics and patterns unrecognizable to humans. It was evident with the Deep Patient initiative, in which a research group at Mount Sinai Hospital, New York, trained a program using the electronic health records of 700,000 patients and then used the program to predict disease in another sample of 76,214 patients [44]. This may initiate a recursive self-improvement cycle, whereby improvements also improve the improvement process [45]. It can be argued that the growing amount of speculation about "singularity" is premature and diverts our attention from more immediate social and ethical issues resulting from current-day machine intelligence [46]. AI is a broad term encompassing a range of technologies that aim to use human-like intelligence to solve problems [47]. These expert systems are now widely used by services such as the NHS 111 telephone triage service (currently being beta-tested as a mobile app in the UK [48]) and other commercial symptom-checking apps [49]. Another approach to AI is using ML techniques, including artificial neural networks (ANNs). Using an ANN approach, computer programs create decision-making networks of artificial "neurons" that operate similarly to biological nervous systems [50]. AI and ML differ in that AI is created through automated iterative improvements, while ML is created by human experts. AI maximizes the "area under the curve" (AUC) by graphing false negative rates against actual positive rates. The program will maximize the "area under the curve" (AUC) when the false negative rate is graphed against the actual positive rate [51]. The potential roles of AI techniques in healthcare delivery and medical research are becoming increasingly evident [52], [53]. Studies have highlighted the efficacy and potential of AI-enabled health applications. Role of AI in healthcare happens in the following areas:

2.2.1   Healthcare Administration

Healthcare delivery has become complex, with healthcare infrastructure in many countries being stretched to its capacity because of administrative burdens and resourcing constraints [54]. Health services can also use optimized ML algorithms to support clinic scheduling and patient prioritization, thus reducing waiting times and creating more efficient use of services [55].

2.2.2   Clinical Decision Support

Clinical decision support systems are computer programs that draw upon clinical data and knowledge to support decisions made by healthcare professionals [56]. ANNs can tolerate a certain amount of noise in the data, but sometimes this can impact the predictions [57].

2.2.3   Patient Monitoring

The adoption of electronic health records and the proliferation of smartphones and fitness monitoring devices have created unprecedented access to digital data and the potential to exploit AI techniques for monitoring patients. For example, in hospitals, waveform pattern learning can improve the monitoring and analysis of ECG, electroencephalographs, electromyographs, and Doppler ultrasounds. Such virtual health assistants have been found to increase medication compliance and reliable follow-up [58].

2.2.4   Healthcare Interventions

ML programs integrated with electronic health records can analyze individual patients' biometric and other medical data and recommend treatment plans based on current clinical guidelines. Recent computer vision has been used for several years for the automated analysis of 3D medical images [59]. Still, facial analysis is also now used to assess a patient's condition [60].

The "Turing test" was the intelligent behavior of a computer which has the ability to achieve human-level performance in cognition-related tasks [61]. AI in medicine can be dichotomized into virtual and physical [62]. Traditionally, we used statistical methods to establish these patterns and associations. An example of this approach is Google's artificial brain project launched in 2012, which trained itself to recognize cats based on 10 million YouTube videos, improving efficiency by reviewing more images. After three days of learning, it could predict a picture of a cat with 75% accuracy [63].

3 HISTORY OF AI

AI isn't a new technology. Instead, it began in 1956 at the Stanford University, where scientist John McCarthy devised the term during leading the Dartmouth Summer Research Project. Since then, the AI field has experienced many ups and downs [64]. Historically, we needed more computational power and support technologies to process vast amounts of data. In early 2011, the field started to see progress, with advances in computer processing capabilities and access to large data sets required to train AI systems. Also, in 2011, computer scientist Andrew N proved that computers could learn. Cognitive technology is used interchangeably with AI, such as the famous Watson computer that won Jeopardy! Challenge in 2011. One function of Watson is to rank evidence and provide patient-relevant, evidence-based treatment options. Vice President of IBM Analytics Steven Astorino describes cognitive computing as the "ability of computers to simulate human behavior of understanding, reasoning, and thought processing" [65].

ICT is a fundamental element of digitized organizations which can facilitate operational effectiveness and enhance competitive advantage [66]. In Fourth Industrial Revolution (4IR) era, advanced digital technologies and devices are extensively applied for innovation and value creation across industries [67]. Hospitals and healthcare providers, particularly in developed economies, are aggressively arraying digital technologies, such as AI, ML, intelligent sensors and robots, big data analytics, and the Internet of Things (IoT), for better quality of care and operational efficiency [68]. In a study by Aruba [69], a Hewlett-Packard Enterprise company, reported that worldwide, more than 60% of hospitals implemented IoT in their facilities. There are changing trends in ICT starting from data analysis to DL to Fuzzy set as shown in Figure 9.2 below.

It is apparent that AI has enormous and wide-reaching potential, from simple operational process innovation to the most sophisticated treatments of emergency patients [70]. Policies and ethical guidelines for healthcare services incorporating AI and its applications need to catch up to the speed of advances in AI [71]. Miyashita and Brady et al., argued that AI may not provide the same benefits in the medical field like general business, but the application of AI may improve patient outcomes, and is not intended to primarily improve healthcare services or significantly reduce costs soon [72].

4 REAL-WORLD AI APPLICATION CASES IN HEALTHCARE

According to the World Health Organization [73], 60% of factors related to health and quality of life relate to lifestyle factors, such as exercise, diet, sleep, stress

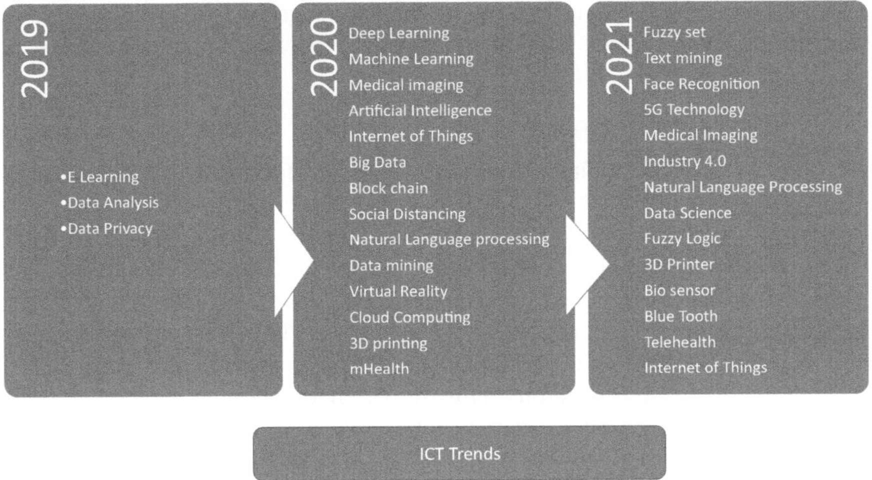

FIGURE 9.2   Recent ICT Trends (2019 to 2021)

reduction, substance and medication abuse, and/or recreation [74]. AI-aided technologies and applications can provide lifestyle interventions based on an individual's vital signs through digital devices. Within healthcare organizations, AI-based technologies are set to significantly transform healthcare systems operation, optimization, and interaction with patients, to provide care services to increase the overall efficiency of patient outcomes. Various applications are as follows:

4.1   CLINICAL APPLICATION

4.1.1   Disease Prediction and Diagnosis

Despite the increasing application of AI in healthcare, the research mainly concentrates around cancer, nervous system, and cardiovascular diseases, because they are the leading causes of disability and mortality. However, infectious and chronic diseases (e.g., type 2 diabetes inflammatory bowel disease, difficile infection) have also been getting considerable attention [75]. In another study on 1,634 images of cancerous and healthy lung tissue, the algorithm identified healthy cases and distinguished, as accurately as three pathologists, between two common types of lung cancer [76]. In the United States, more than 6% of adult populations are affected by depression. Predicting major depressive disorder was 74% accurate by image heatmap pattern recognition [77]. In a 260 patient cohort study, Abedi V. et al [78] found that the model can better diagnose acute cerebral ischemia than trained emergency medical respondents. Although noisy data and experimental limitations reduce the clinical utility of the models, DL methods can address these limitations by reducing the dimensionality of the data through layered auto-encoding analyses. Examples include: analysis of more than 1,400 images from 308 histopathology regions of skin to detect basal cell carcinoma and differentiate malignant from benign lesions, achieving a diagnostic accuracy of >90% compared with experts; or examination of more than 41,000 digital screening breast mammographic for identifying dense or non-dense breast tissue, where the interpreting radiologist accepted 94% of the 10,763 DL assessments [79].

4.1.2 Diagnostic Assistance

AI is predictable to facilitate the diagnosis of patients with specific diseases. Taylor [80] reported that "60% of all medical errors are for diagnostics errors and an estimated 40,000 to 80,000 deaths each year in U.S. hospitals". The Mayo Clinic, a premier healthcare organization in the US, noted for its innovation in patient care and health technology, employed AI for cervical cancer screening to identify precancerous changes in a woman's cervix. The AI-based solution uses an algorithm employing over 60,000 cervical images from the National Cancer Institute to identify precancerous signs. Researchers reported that the algorithm functions at a much higher accuracy rate (91%) than a trained human expert (69%) and can reduce diagnostic time also [81]. In addition to radiology, the use of ML algorithms in medical image analysis has been expanded widely to most medical departments that use images for fields such as pathology, dermatology, cardiology, gastroenterology, and ophthalmology.

4.1.3 Treatment Effectiveness and Outcome Prediction

Treatment effectiveness and outcome prediction are also essential areas with potential clinical implications in disease management strategies and personalized care plans. A decade ago, only molecular and clinical information was exploited to predict cancer outcomes. Electronic health records (EHRs) are practical tools for documenting and sharing healthcare information. Integrating machine learning-based modeling explicitly designed for administrative datasets can facilitate the detection of potential complications to improve healthcare resource utilization and outcomes at a personalized level [82].

One of the goals of Precision Medicine (PM) in cancer is the accurate prediction of optimal drug therapies from the genomic data of individual patient tumors. For example, Costello J. C. et al. [83] analyzed 44 drug sensitivity prediction algorithms on 53 breast cancer cell lines with available genomic information to fulfill dose-response growth inhibition values for each cell line exposed to 28 therapeutic compounds.

4.2 TRANSLATION APPLICATION

4.2.1 Drug Discovery and Repurposing

About 25% of all discovered drugs resulted from a chance when different domains were brought together accidentally [84]. Targeted drug discovery is preferred in pharmaceuticals due to the explicit mechanism, higher success rate, and lower cost when compared to traditional blind screening. ML is now utilized in the drug discovery process due to the following: (1) high costs of drug development; (2) increasing availability of three-dimensional structural information that can guide the characterization of drug targets, and (3) extremely low success rates in clinical trials. Despite these novel approaches in drug discovery, there are important challenges, including data access and the fact that in general, different data sets are stored in a variety of repositories. Another example includes the use of NLP for identification of hidden or novel associations that might be important in the detection of potential drug adverse effects based on scientific publications [85].

4.2.2 Clinical Trial and in Silico Clinical Trials

Clinical trial design has its roots in classical experimental design. However, the clinical investigators are not able to control various sources of variability. Ethical issues are paramount in clinical research. Subject enrollment can become lengthy and costly [86]. In a study, placebo-controlled Phase III clinical trial study was designed where investigators used virtual treatments on synthetic Crohn's disease patients. Results showed a positive correlation between the initial disease activity score and the drop in the disease activity score but with different medications efficacy [87].

4.3 PUBLIC HEALTH & ADMINISTRATION RELEVANCE

4.3.1 Epidemic Outbreak Prediction

The infectious disease distribution pattern between population groups with known probabilities are based on prior knowledge of ecological and biological features of the environment. Early epidemic prediction (such as peak and duration of infection) is possible if model parameters are partially known [88]. In another study, Kesorn K. et al. [89] predicted the morbidity rate of dengue hemorrhagic fever in central Thailand by estimating the infection rate in the female Aedes aegypti larvae mosquitoes and achieved a prediction accuracy of >95% and 88% in the training and test set, respectively.

4.3.2 Precision Health

Genetic and biomedical studies have continued investigation efforts to reveal connections between genes and human traits or diseases. Many studies rely on large-scale sensitive genotype or phenotype data and sharing across institutions is paramount for the success of such studies [90].

4.3.3 Nursing and Managerial Assistance

Healthcare staff is often flooded with much paperwork in the care process. AI can reduce such works of the staff. In addition, AI has been identified as a potentially effective tool for conversing with patients and family members in hospitals [91]. An AI-assisted system of the University of Pittsburgh Medical Center can also listen and learn from conversations between doctors and patients in hospital rooms. The Johns Hopkins University Hospital, Baltimore, Maryland, in May 2016, announced collaboration with GE healthcare partners to use predictive analytics based on AI technologies to support a more efficient operational flow [92].

TABLE 9.1

Current Application of AI in Healthcare

Technology	Application Areas
Robotics	Medical device, Health IT
Digital secretary	Medical device, Health IT
Machine Learning	Diagnostic medical image, Health IT
Image processing	Diagnostic medical image, Health IT
Natural Language Processing	Medical device, Health IT
Voice recognition	Medical device, Health IT
Statistical analysis	Medicine, Health IT
Big Data analysis	Medicine, Health IT
Predictive modeling	Medicine, Health IT

4.3.4 Smart IoT Devices, Signal, and In Vitro Diagnostic Analysis

Various technology giants such as IBM, Google, Apple, and Samsung are competing to develop and commercialize devices and services that can assist in improving the user health by acquiring health information from daily life using a combination of IoT technologies and wearable devices. In a recent review, Torkamani et al., examine the core disciplines that enable high-definition medicine given our recent technological advances and high-resolution data [93].

4.3.5 AI Using Electronic Medical Records (EMRs)

Various attempts are being made to develop AI systems using EMRs. EMR firms in the United States, like as Allscripts, are actively adopting deep learning (DL) techniques based on artificial neural networks (ANN) to handle complicated non-linear correlations in medical data [94,95]. As DL algorithms are based on ANN resembling the network of neurons in the human brain and can learn very complex non-linear relationships, they are being actively used in the tasks dealing with medical data [95]. There are many such examples in recent years. Accordingly, several studies on the use of AI-based technologies in health care are currently being conducted (Table 9.1).

AI technology holds both great promises to transform mental healthcare and potential pitfalls. However, caution is necessary in order to avoid over-interpreting preliminary results, and more work is required to bridge the gap between AI in mental health research and clinical care [96].

5 ROLE OF AI DURING COVID ERA

AI is one of such technology which can easily track the spread of this virus, identifies the high-risk patients, and is useful in controlling this infection in real time. It can also predict mortality risk by adequately analyzing the previous data of the patients. AI can help us to fight this virus by population screening, medical help, notification, and suggestions about the infection control [97]. The physician is not only focused on the treatment of the patient but also the control of disease with the AI application. Major symptoms and test analysis are done with the help of AI with the highest of accuracy. Main applications of AI in COVID-19 pandemic are as follows:

5.1 EARLY DETECTION AND DIAGNOSIS OF THE INFECTION

AI can quickly analyze irregular symptoms and other "red flags" and thus alarm the patients and the healthcare authorities [98]. It helps to provide faster decision-making, which is cost-effective. AI is helpful in the diagnosis of infected cases with the help of medical imaging technologies.

5.2 MONITORING THE TREATMENT

AI can build an intelligent platform for automatic monitoring and prediction of the spread of this virus. A neural network can also be developed to extract this disease's visual features, which would help in proper monitoring and treatment of the affected individuals [99]. It has the capability of providing day-to-day updates of the patients and to provide solutions to be followed in COVID-19 pandemic.

5.3 CONTACT TRACING OF THE INDIVIDUALS

AI can help analyze the level of infection by this virus identifying the clusters and "hot spots" and can successfully do the contact tracing of the individuals and also to monitor them. It can predict the future course of this disease and likely reappearance.

5.4 PROJECTION OF CASES AND MORTALITY

This technology can track and forecast the nature of the virus from the available data, social media, and media platforms, about the risks of the infection and its likely spread. Further, it can predict the number of positive cases and death in any region.

5.5 DEVELOPMENT OF DRUGS AND VACCINES

AI is used for drug research by analyzing the available data on COVID-19. It is helpful for drug delivery design and development. This technology is used to speed up drug testing in real time. In contrast, standard testing takes plenty of time and hence helps to accelerate this process significantly, which may not be possible by a human. It has become a powerful tool for diagnostic test designs and vaccination development [100].

5.6 REDUCING THE WORKLOAD OF HEALTHCARE WORKERS

Healthcare professionals have a very high workload due to a sudden and massive increase in the number of patients during the COVID-19 pandemic. Here,

AI is used to reduce the workload of healthcare workers [101]. It helps in early diagnosis and providing treatment at an early stage using digital approaches and decision science, offering the best training to students and doctors regarding this new disease [102].

5.7 PREVENTION OF THE DISEASE

With the help of real-time data analysis, AI can provide updated information, which is helpful in the prevention of this disease. It can be used to predict the probable sites of infection, the influx of the virus, the need for beds, and healthcare professionals during this crisis. AI is helpful for future virus and disease prevention, with the help of previous mentored data over data prevalent at different times. It identifies traits, causes, and reasons for the spread of infection.

AI is not only helpful in the treatment of COVID-19-infected patients but also for their proper health monitoring. The post-COVID era shall continue to tickle our minds in seeking new solutions to newer problems. Developing disease surveillance AI-based platforms that can monitor and track the rising number of disease cases would be needed to predict pandemics [103]. Such platforms would perform real-time surveillance of population demographics. It performs tasks requiring thinking, learning, problem-solving, and decision-making. Smartphone applications and wearable devices generate continuous data that can be useful for COVID-19. Contact tracing using smartphone data can help identify these individuals and may limit the spread of COVID-19 by breaking the chain of transmission.

The 21st century witnessed pandemics of infectious diseases such as Ebola, SARS, Middle East respiratory syndrome, and Zika virus. An early diagnosis is critical to preventing, controlling, and managing any pandemic. Rapid diagnosis of COVID-19 positive cases is based on nucleic acid tests such as the reverse transcriptase real-time polymerase chain reaction (RT-PCR), which is regarded as the standard gold test for diagnosis [104]. As the pandemic evolves and variants of SARS-CoV-2 emerge, it becomes necessary to rapidly screen positive cases to prevent further spread. This has implications, especially during a pandemic when resources are scarce and time is premium [105]. The COVID-19 Severity Score combines multiplex biomarker measurements and risk factors to predict mortality in a statistical learning algorithm [106]. An ML system to analyze images of patients' white blood cells for signs of an activated immune response against sepsis may be helpful [107]. AI and its role in vaccine development analysis of the SARS-CoV-2 genome sequences and bioinformatics have accelerated the development of vaccines for this novel virus [108]. The next challenge has been met when AI has impacted the distribution of vaccine doses globally. Data may be used for predictive modeling and help the decision-makers by providing vital information for planning cost-effective global distribution and vaccine access. AI is applied in the medical field during the coronavirus disease 2019. Still, as a two-sided coin, AI has its limitations, such as accuracy, privacy, and reliability. Another primary concern regarding the AI models is privacy-related risks. In the future, AI will likely play a significant role in training, teaching, patient care, and research [109]. The coronavirus disease 2019 (COVID-19) is a significant worldwide threat. The latest advancements in computational techniques based on AI, ML, and Big Data can help detect, monitor, and forecast the severity of the COVID-19 pandemic. AI also provides a solution for contact tracing, prediction, and drug development, thus reducing the workload of the medical industry [110]. We eventually used an interpretive structural model (ISM) to build a framework of interrelationships among the identified factors, which will help healthcare stakeholders to realize the requirements for the successful implementation of AI [111].

Major disease areas where AI tools are used are cancer, neurology, and cardiology. One study reviewed the AI applications in stroke in more detail in areas of early detection and diagnosis, treatment, outcome prediction, and prognosis evaluation [35].

In the past, practical medical information could only be reached using textbooks, journals formatting the guidelines, and expert opinions, including master-apprentice relationships. In addition, physicians gain experience by directing patient treatments and observing the outcomes. Digesting this extensive knowledge and experience is a significant limitation of targeted patient care. AI has already come forward to assist by blending a large amount of patient data to promote and elaborate the effectiveness of physicians [112]. If we ask real questions, AI has the potential to reveal the remarkable information hidden in big data, which may have a role in clinical decisions [113]. Baxt et al. have proved the predictive superiority of ANN in patients with suspected myocardial ischemia admitted to the emergency department with chest pain [114]. The algorithms in ML offer performance improvement by automatizing model-forming for constituting patterns or decision support using the examined data [115]. There are four types of ML methods; the most popular ones are supervised and unsupervised learning methods, and the others are semi-supervised and reinforcement learning methods. DL is the recently developed field of ML, and consists fundamentally of neural networks with several layers of hidden neurons [115]. A new statistical DL-based pattern recognition method for left ventricle endocardium tracking has demonstrated superiority compared to current state-of-the-art endocardium tracking methods in ultrasound data [116]. Convolutional neural network (CNN), a featured subtype of ANN, is also derived from DL with hidden multilayers to evaluate the data. CNN has been tested and shown to help calculate coronary artery calcium in cardiac CT angiography using a supervised type of ML [117].

6 GLOBALIZING AI FOR IMPROVED CLINICAL PRACTICE

AI technologies are facilitating the work of modern healthcare organizations to leverage the power of big data in clinical practice [35]. AI-based systems improve clinical decision-making using multiple layers of information and pre-specified algorithms [118]. In addition, recent AI technologies like ML can learn from existing data and perform predictive operations resulting in a robust performance in clinical settings [118]. Such innovations will likely serve the healthcare industry by minimizing human error, savings costs, and maximizing informed decision-making [118]. However, critical challenges may affect the applications of AI in clinical settings, which include the effects on patient-provider communication, safety and efficacy of health services, and humane aspects of caregiving [35]. These issues suggest carefully analyzing different ethical aspects before adopting AI in clinical practice. Several agencies have started developing guidelines and regulatory frameworks for using AI in clinical practice, which has presented its "Ethics guidelines for trustworthy AI", which proposed that the development of AI should be lawful, ethical, and robust [119]). Moreover, using AI to integrate genomic, epigenetic, and behavioral data can better inform personalized diagnosis and treatment across populations [118]. AI can also analyze a population's economic, political, and technological challenges and inform clinical decision-making accordingly, which can help achieve equality and sustainability in global health systems [35]. Recent initiatives taken by the World Health Organization (WHO) and the International Telecommunication Union (ITU) for benchmarking AI in healthcare show promise to improve AI-driven processes and outcomes [120]. Globally, health systems face multiple challenges: an increase in the burden of illness, multimorbidity, and disability driven by aging and epidemiological transition, greater demand for health services, higher societal expectations, and increasing health expenditures [121]. A further challenge relates to inefficiency, with poor productivity [122]. These health system challenges exist against a background of fiscal conservatism, with misplaced economic austerity policies that constrain investment in health systems. A fundamental transformation of health systems is critical to overcoming these challenges and achieving universal health coverage (UHC) by 2030. ML, the most tangible manifestation of AI – and the newest growth area in digital technology – holds the promise of achieving more with less and could be the catalyst for such a transformation [123]. But the nature and extent of this promise have not been systematically assessed. To date, the impact of digital technology on health systems has been equivocal [124]. Is AI the ingredient for such a transformation to have the same fate as earlier attempts at introducing digital technology? AI's broad definition arguably has some crossover with existing statistical techniques [125]. The recent explosion in progress in this field is attributable to a subset of AI – ML and one family of techniques DL where computers are programmed to learn associations based on large quantities of raw data, DL systems have been applied extensively and set new benchmarks in areas of the economy where high-quality digital data are plentiful. There is a strong economic incentive to automate prediction tasks [126]. In these cases, DL algorithms have been able to uncover associations of predictive value, typically for a single use case, with large amounts of data and human expertise to curate the data and tune the algorithms involved [127]. Policymakers modify health system functions of organization and governance, financing, and resource management to achieve health system outputs (health care services and public health) and system goals [128]. ML can improve hypothesis generation and hypothesis testing tasks within a health system by revealing previously hidden trends in data. Therefore, while ML models are more challenging to interpret, they can incorporate many more variables, are generalizable across a much broader array of data types, and produce results in more complex situations [129]. These methods have been deployed in the research context to screen, diagnose, and predict future events. These deployments are in disparate areas, typically in hospital than community settings, and in most cases, based on data from single centers, with implications for reproducibility and generalizability [130]. This, in turn, allows savings to be invested in existing non-automatable tasks and in creating new non-automatable studies, some of which involve directly working on the automating technology [131]. Most interestingly, there are a number of publications in this area in the last 20 years, from 1999 to 2018. The growth of interest is noticeable from below 25 in 1999 to more than 250 in 2018, especially during the previous five years, and continued growth in the future can be forecast [131].

7   ETHICAL ISSUES IN AI

Most studies comparing the efficiency of AI vs. clinicians have unreliable designs and the validation of the algorithms developed in samples from sources other than the one used to train algorithms [132]. Continuous reevaluation and calibration after adopting algorithms suspected of overfitting should be necessary to adapt the software to the fluctuation of patient demographics [24]. Ongoing monitoring and privacy violations can increase the stigma around chronically ill or more disadvantaged citizens [133]. Universities have created new curricula, including doctor engineering, to answer the need to educate future medical leaders about the challenges of AI in medicine [134]. Ambient clinical intelligence (ACI) is a digital environment around physician and patient, which are sensitive, adaptive, and responsive [135]. It can, for instance, analyze the interview and automatically fill in patients' EHRs. Many projects are underway to develop an ACI, and much needed to solve modern problems in the physician workforce. While scientific progress should remain rigorous and transparent in developing new solutions to improve current healthcare, health policies should be focused on tackling the ethical and financial issues associated with this cornerstone of the evolution of medicine [136]. WHO recognizes and agrees that AI holds great promise for public health and medical practice. The World Health Organization (WHO) has endorsed a set of fundamental ethical principles for the use of AI in health:

1. Protecting human autonomy:
2. They promoted human well-being, safety, and the public interest, not harm.
3. They ensure transparency, explain ability, and intelligibility.
4. Fostering responsibility and accountability.
5. Ensuring inclusiveness and equity.
6. Promoting AI that is responsive and sustainable.

Finally, the report discusses practical know-how for implementing of the WHO guidance for the stakeholders. The considerations are intended only as a starting point for context-specific discussions and decisions by diverse stakeholders [137]. In the US, health information privacy and confidentiality are discussed in Health Insurance Portability and Accountability Act (HIPAA). A case study says that a technology company, Google DeepMind, does not have a direct patient care service and thus has held data on millions of patients since November 2015 without consent [138]. The problem is complicated, and the reasoning in an AI application is difficult and often too complex to understand [139]. Another aspect that the financial motivators for the sole purpose of coding a higher level of care must be tempered and significantly impact the funding a healthcare organization provides [140]. Hoyle and Shepherd [141] argued that Health Information Management (HIM) professionals are positioned as advocates for the ethical use of technology and data and they must urge healthcare organizations to consider the ethical frameworks and practice guides deemed appropriate for health information technologies. These activities will support the HIM professionals in a healthcare organization to "provide the clinical truth in their coding and resist the perverse incentives" [141]. AI in healthcare has enormous promise to evolute healthcare, but it has ethical issues which must be addressed. For achieving full potential of AI in healthcare, four major ethical issues need to be considered: (i) informed consent, (ii) safety and transparency, (iii) algorithmic fairness and biases, and (iv) data privacy [142]. The danger is unknown, and using machines will severely limit the ability to assign blame and take ownership of the decision-making. Modern computing approaches can hide the thinking behind an Artificial Intelligent System (AIS) output, making meaningful scrutiny impossible [143]. However, an easy, essential component of figuring out the protection of any healthcare software relies upon the capacity to check out the software and recognize how the software would fail. AI can go from being extremely intelligent to extremely naive in an instant. All AI systems will have limits, even if AI bias is managed. The human decision-maker must be aware of the system's limitations, and the system must be designed to fit the demands of the human decision-maker. Furthermore, people may accept decision support system results without questioning their limits. This failure will be repeated in other areas, such as criminal justice, where judges have modified their decisions based on risk assessments later which have been revealed to be inaccurate [144]. Unlike doctors, technologists are not obligated by law to be accountable for their actions; instead, ethical principles of practice are applied in this sector. Instead of asking if they were aware of the hazards and poor decision-making, they should be asked if they could grasp and recognize those risks [145]. Evidence suggests that AI models can embed and deploy human and social biases at scale. There are no guidelines or standards to report and compare these models, but future work should involve this to guide researchers and clinicians [146]. AI will be increasingly used in healthcare and hence needs to be morally accountable. Not using AI is also possibly unscientific and unethical [147]. The focus of AI should be on making or using hi-tech machines and ensuring that it remains person-centric and humanity grounded. That is why AI technology is transdisciplinary; it requires contributions from all sectors, including medical sciences, social sciences, law, economics, and humanities, besides technological advances [148]. The term "responsible AI" is also often interchangeably used with ethics. However, these two are different concepts, even if being tightly knitted. Responsibility is the practical aspect of ethics. Following are the ways to maintain ethics in designing AI-based healthcare systems [148].

1. Ethics in design, which refers to the dogmatic and technical methods that consider the cultural aspect during the creation of AI systems.
2. Ethics in the application is more about the behavioral ethics of developing and adopting AI systems in health care.
3. Ethics for diverse stakeholders may refer to the rules and governing requirements that safeguard the veracity of all players as they develop and implement AI systems.

Understanding these ethical constructs may inform how complex AI systems can effectively serve the population's health needs, contingent upon the actions of individual and collective human intelligence in social contexts. The "Ethical AI Toolkit", invented by Smart Dubai Office, admonishes individuals and organizations affording AI services [148]. The World Intellectual Property Organization too is in the lead as it released a major report on AI. The WHO is trying to create a focus group for AI by collaborating with the ITU and International Labour Organization [149]. These kinds of efforts can lay down powerful platforms in shaping standards and benchmarks to guide national policymakers [149]. In such a scenario, the increasing trend of using newer technologies such as AI may further increase health disparities in digitalization [150].

8 MERIT AND DEMERITS OF AI

The healthcare sector is considered one of the world's largest and fast-growing industries. Innovations and novel approaches have always remained the prime aims of bringing massive development. The condition has been steadily revolutionizing with recent advancements in ML. AI lies in the computer science department, which stresses the creation of an intelligent machine that works and reacts just like human beings. Every coin has two sides. Similarly, AI can also be considered a boon and a bane, depending on how one uses it. In this section, we will discuss both AI's merits and demerits [151].

8.1 AI A BOON

AI's first and foremost advantage is that the chances of error are almost negligible. Committing mistakes is very much typical among humans. However, machines with algorithms and decisions considering previous data seldom commit mistakes. Business organizations greatly benefit from this and are using it in all their domains due to its ability to solve complicated problems using calculations, which minimizes errors. Organizations are using digital assistants to interact with their users, which save their time, and the demand of the users' businesses also gets fulfilled.

8.2 AI A BANE

High cost, Unemployment, Lacks creativity, AI in the wrong hands, Proper operating skills, No enhancement with experience.

The only methods to curb the limitations are, creating awareness. The proper usage of AI and its reach to all the masses can be achieved by creating awareness among the people about its importance and benefits. Along with it, we need to create a proper firewall to prevent hacking of the system. Hacking and gaining access to the system can prove to be harmful. So, good firewalls and hi-tech cyber security should be developed to protect the system's safety [152]. The tech giants, policymakers, and department experts must be consulted before designing an AI for a product or facility [153]. AI is a platform that has allowed us to explore new horizons and improve and widen our thinking. Even though these demerits are hindering the usage and productivity of AI, realizing the value of AI, steps are being taken to reduce or prevent such problems and use it to its full potential. AI may not solve the problem of the transmission of infectious diseases. However, AI is a tool for an early warning system which can give a timely heads-up to health professionals and potentially save thousands of lives if the disruptive power of AI is used in a good way [154].

9 CHALLENGES OF AI APPLICATIONS IN HEALTHCARE

The challenges are incredibly daunting in healthcare because human lives are at stake. Some challenges that need to be addressed with wisdom are as follows.

9.1 ACCOUNTABILITY OF THE SYSTEM USE

Dr. Stephen Hawking had observed that with the rapid growth of AI, the world is fast approaching to a point where the human power will be out of control. Lupton [155] stressed that moral and ethical behavior patterns are required to be developed for AI in a positive way for society.

9.2 AI DIVIDE

One characteristic that distinguishes healthcare from other service industries is that patients trust medical staff unconditionally [156]. Suppose an AI-based technology/system assumes the role of a doctor. However, even people with experience in digital technologies and AI would need help in trusting an AI system.

9.3 CYBERSECURITY FOR PRIVACY AND SECURITY

Disease-related data are challenging to share and regulate diverse databases which contain personal information. It is necessary to have some rules and regulations that AI technology should observe, such as ethics, laws, and personal values which regulate their behavior in society.

9.4 MANAGERIAL CONTROL LOSS

In the healthcare sector, patients are getting treated by doctors and nurses. However, good health is the amalgamation of healthy living habits, good diet, regular exercise, and daily well-beings, in addition to quality medical services. A related concern is that AI could make healthcare providers complacent and less likely to check results and challenge errors [157].

9.5 JOB LOSS AND THE PAIN OF TRANSFORMATION

Amazon announced that by 2025, it would re-educate its 100,000 employees through training programs on new technologies by 2025 to prepare for more highly skilled jobs in the AI era. Jeff Wilke, Amazon's worldwide consumer CEO, stated, "technology changes work, and employee have the opportunity to take advantage of those changes". As discussed earlier, radiology is a medical specialty that may disappear because AI can analyze diagnostic medical images more accurately than humans. However, it is argued that AI will permit radiologists to deliver more focused diagnostic services to patients [158]. Though, due to AI-related technologies some jobs will be lost, but at the same time many new jobs will be created to support implementing AI-based systems and devices. This could be problematic if the technology fails and staffs can only recognize errors or carry out necessary tasks with computing assistance [157]. However, there are also concerns that technology-fueled increases in productivity will make specific healthcare jobs redundant [159].

9.6 ETHICAL CONSIDERATIONS

Concerns have been raised that datasets used to train AI systems have inherent biases and are often not representative of the wider population [157]. The difficulties in validating the outputs of AI systems have raised concerns about accountability, transparency, and human control. At a practical level, both patients and healthcare providers will need to be able to trust AI systems if they are to be implemented successfully in healthcare.

9.7 REGULATORY COMPLIANCE

As the use of AI in the clinical space increases and evolves, legal and regulatory risk will increase, particularly since traditional regulatory principles still need to be attuned to AI. This implies a regulatory framework that supports technological innovations but safeguards the leakage of sensitive information to unauthorized third parties and protects the patient's right to privacy.

9.8 PROVIDER–PATIENT RELATIONSHIP

A well-functioning provider–patient relationship is still the essence of healthcare. The success of providing care depends on collaboration, empathy, and shared decision-making. Empathy skills of healthcare providers have been shown to influence patient outcomes positively [160]. AI can assist in improving efficiency and quality but is limited by its inability to possess some human characteristics, such as compassion, empathy, and the human touch.

AI has a huge potential to alleviate some of healthcare providers' challenges. Optimizing the benefits of AI will require a balanced approach that enhances accountability and transparency while facilitating innovation, fostering responsible access to data to develop computing abilities further, and building trust between providers, patients, researchers, and innovators. Looking into the future – taking cues from the history of automation – AI is unlikely to displace humans but will redefine their roles and establish itself as an indispensable cognitive assistant [161]. In summary, this colossal joint effort based on a new collective intelligence will exponentially improve the quality of medical research, resulting in a radical change for the better in the healthcare model [162]. As much healthcare data is siloed and unstructured, one challenge is the need for more mature data to serve as a foundation for AI strategies [7]. The ethical challenges presented by data science have also been an area of debate. These challenges can be mapped within the conceptual space and described by three branches of research: the ethics of data and privacy, the ethics and morality of algorithms, and the ethics and values of practices [163]. The most important issue when developing ML in a clinical setting is the issue of trust when both clinicians and patients accept the recommendations provided by the system [164]. Furthermore, missing data is not random. Missingness can be due to incompleteness, inconsistency, or inaccuracy [165]. Other limitations are the lack of interoperability across technology platforms over time and the massive expansion of structured and unstructured data elements. NLP can process and contextualize different medical words and expressions [166].

However, clinical medicine has always required doctors to handle vast amounts of data, from history and physical exams to laboratory and imaging studies and new genetic data. The ability to manage this complexity has always set good doctors apart [7]. The full maturity of many AI applications is yet to be realized. Even within current medical regulations, lines of responsibility are sometimes clear when medical errors occur. It needs to be clarified where responsibilities should lie when AI agents increasingly support or even autonomously deliver healthcare services [167]. Governments across the world have increasingly adopted favorable positions in adoption of AI and some governments have actively involved themselves in the application of AI in healthcare, while others have supported private developers in the development of relevant AI applications [35]. As successes of AI in medicine become more evident [168] governments and funders may be required to formulate strategies outlining how AI gets applied in healthcare delivery and how this process will be funded. An increasingly recognized issue is the potential for bias by the AI program toward specific population sub-groups if inappropriate sampling and training of the algorithms have occurred [169]. Clinicians have traditionally been slow adopters of new technology, relying on tried and trusted methods to deliver clinical care

[170]. Also important is the availability of a user-friendly interface and integration with existing health information technology systems [171], [172]. Finally, the authors discuss an overview of the need to implement transdisciplinary solutions that can be used to mitigate this bias [173]. Available literature indicates that AI-based systems used in healthcare have flaws that adversely affect its ability to perform at an expected level [174]. Under these circumstances, the bias in a discussion can be conceived as an outcome of the methods and their associated selection processes used for experimentation. On this matter, Gurupur et al. [175] have explained how methods used for analysis can affect the accuracy of the outcome. In their experiment, the investigators have emphasized computationally more powerful techniques that consume more computational power for analyzing healthcare data. It is worth noting that the analysis accuracy is also dependent on the input data used for this purpose. Henriksen and Kaplan [176] emphasize how hindsight bias affects the healthcare delivery system. Additionally, they also identify outcome bias being correlated with the influence of outcome knowledge acquired by the investigator/s. Hindsight bias is an important concept that cannot be obviated in a discussion involving AI-based healthcare systems. For instance, a transdisciplinary perspective advocates healthcare outcomes or health status improvement as a joint function of both micro-level and macro-level predictors [177].

10   IMPLICATIONS OF AI APPLICATIONS IN HEALTHCARE

Therefore, while the digital or AI divide is narrowing, and consumer behavior has been changing across industries, it is required to do more and more research, and increase the actual use of AI in the healthcare industry. Researchers suggest several approaches to best manage AI applications in healthcare.

a. First, it is the need of the hour to establish a legal outline for information access and sharing for AI applications. Real-time data acquisition and sharing are required to enhance AI performance in healthcare. Johnson et al. [178] suggested that healthcare organizations prioritize data quality improvement efforts for validity and assess whether reported values should be trusted. The qualitative collection of accurate and realistic data is vital because disease patterns vary depending on individual characteristics.

b. Second, social consensus must be reached regarding the critical sides of AI, including data sharing, confidentiality, and liability.

c. Third, applications of AI-based systems need collaboration of specialists in multidisciplinary areas for care service. Therefore, a collaborative environment must be developed in the development–application–analysis phases of AI application.

d. Fourth, instead of focusing solely on the job-destroying possibilities of AI, efforts should be made to best utilize the surplus workforce in new areas of value creation. Radiologists have an important role in bridging the gap between medical research and information and communication technology, and efforts should be made to increase their value in hospitals [158].

e. Lastly, information protection systems should be further strengthened to avoid the patient data leakage through cyberattacks or operational errors in healthcare institutions. The assurance of security will help promote the agreement of patients to use their medical data for public purposes.

11 FUTURE TRENDS OF AI IN HEALTHCARE

Challenges will ultimately be overcome, but they will take much longer than they will take for the technologies to mature. AI systems will not replace human clinicians, and over time, human clinicians may move toward a job designed based on empathy, persuasion, and big-picture integration. Although there are instances where AI can perform better than humans, ethical issues in the application of AI are to be considered [179]. As big data analytics and AI draw more attention in different segments of the industry, this study would lead to a greater interest among researchers who intend to determine what has driven the trend in healthcare and what would be the effects of the adoption of big data analytics and AI in healthcare. To investigate the potential of these advanced technologies in the healthcare domain, there is a clear need to direct more resources toward investigating the practices of mature teams [180]. Quality, affordability, and accessibility in healthcare services are the three biggest challenges faced by Indian population. A recent report ranks India at 145th place out of 195 countries based on healthcare access and quality index [181]. Most patients do not approach a physician in the initial stages, so their disease is usually diagnosed when it has reached an advanced stage. This increases the cost of treatment and reduces the likelihood of recovery [182]. The performance of such prediction models is evaluated in terms of accuracy, precision, and measure [183]. The medical practitioner shall instruct a patient with a high-risk score to consult the specialist to start the treatment promptly.

Thus, AI ensures a cost-effective way of diagnosing diseases early and can help significantly reduce medical complications in diseases like diabetes [184]. While the use of AI in medicine should enhance healthcare delivery, we must ensure meticulous design and evaluation of AI applications. The primary care informatics community needs to be proactive and guide the ethical and rigorous development of AI applications so that they will be safe and effective. AI is the ultimate goal is to develop technology that best serves humanity. The term "intelligence" does not best depict the technical need. It is not intelligence but wisdom associated with the well-being, happiness, health, and longevity of the individual and community. Thus, the future need for technology is artificial wisdom (AW). In that case, it can ensure that these technologies are designed to emulate wise humans' qualities and thus serve humanity's most significant benefit. Human wisdom is a scientific construct supported by empirical research during the last 45 years. It has a scientifically based definition, validated measurement scales, underlying neurobiology and genetics, and a relationship to aging that are all quite different from those of human intelligence. Intelligence is necessary and needed for the survival of Homo sapiens, but knowledge is critical for thriving in the modern society. The future AI technologies will require new conceptual models on human wisdom and not human intelligence. It can make humans wiser through long-term transdisciplinary collaboration, which is essential for the development of AW, that will have a far more significant impact on human well-being and technology development [185].

Similarly, the integration of IoT cloud and big data has been frequently used to monitor, to do surveillance, and to forecast the COVID-19 curve. It indicates that researchers, policymakers, and academic fraternities should continuously increase research collaborations and emphasize emerging technologies (such as 5G, DL, ML, 4D printing, and IoT) in the healthcare domain. Industry 4.0 is an essential foundation for futuristic healthcare under the global profile of technological advancements. The sustainability of supply chain management has been a critical issue in healthcare during this pandemic. The main research topics that need to be addressed are disruption propagation, global propagation, global supply chain, and disruptive risks. The future work will be extended to focus on sub-themes of Industry 4.0 and COVID-19 research [186]. The 5G network is expected to spread further the AI utilization in the healthcare service market shortly. Medical imaging devices, such as MRI, generate large files. 5G networks improve the quality and accessibility of care services through quick and accurate transmission of large-capacity medical image data. Ericsson [187], a world leader in communications, has predicted that the healthcare 5G market will make a revenue opportunity of approximately $76 billion by 2026. Beyond time and space, AI-based technology can cross the expert knowledge limits, and is breaking the boundaries of healthcare, well-being, and life itself [188]. Therefore, AI-enabled technology penetrates all aspects of healthcare and our daily lives.

12 CONCLUSION

We are in a stage of transition, and AI will never replace a commiserating clinician. The AI-enabled clinician will likely spend more time empathizing with his patient rather than getting drowned in voluminous data [189]. Healthcare professionals will have access to the blockchain to display the patient's medical records. Blockchain enables the storage of cryptographic records, which AI needs [190]. AI has exciting applications in many other biomedical areas, New AI provides novel solutions for biomedicine, and biomedicine demands new levels of AI. This match of supply and demand and coupled developments will enable both fields to advance significantly in the foreseeable future, benefiting the quality of life of people in need [191]. While much of what has been discussed may appear hyperbolic, in places optimistic and others pessimistic, it is essential to acknowledge these as the two polarized viewpoints shaping the 21st-century AI debate. The optimism is sufficiently plausible that it warrants further research, and the pessimism is such that it deserves a cautious approach. As an innovation, AI exhibits three key characteristics: self-referential, reprogrammable, and capable of pronounced generativity. While the timescales for these impacts are uncertain, we should not assume they are far away [192]. AI-enabled applications will help primary care physicians better identify patients requiring extra attention and provide personalized protocols for everyone [193]. It is noted that physicians spent 27% of their time on direct clinical face time with their patients and spent 49.2% of their office days on electronic hospital records and desk work. Some studies have documented that AI systems outperform dermatologists correctly classifying suspicious skin lesions [194]. AI-based decision-making approaches are used when experts disagree, e.g., identifying pulmonary tuberculosis on chest radiographs [195]. AI has potential, but unlikely that will replace doctors outrightly. AI will be an integral part of medicine in the future. Hence, it is crucial to train the new generation of physicians, the concepts and application of AI and work efficiently for better productivity, and empathy in them. However, the rate of technology adoption in the public health sector differs from that in other sectors. The banking, tourism, and transport sectors usually adopt newer technologies faster than the public health sector. It is different for the public health sector. We must remain patient to enjoy this technology's most exclusive benefit.

Lastly, we must recognize technological advancement. We have to use technology to prevent human suffering with proper caution. AI-enabled doctors can contribute to managing the "maldistribution" of doctors in India and addressing health problems of the community. It is high time to experiment with AI-enabled doctors in other resource-poor countries [196]. Responsible AI has now become the subject of widespread study and discussion. The 174 dyadic data findings also confirm the mediation mechanism of the patient's cognitive engagement with reliable AI solutions and perceived value, which leads to market performance [197]. Apps in medicine are based on algorithms and are getting used, especially in critical care [198], [199]. Some of these apps are time sensitive and thus have given rise to the concept of the "golden minute" and have helped reduce mortality. Unfortunately, these algorithms still need to be readily available at the bedside, especially on mobile phones. In contrast to its competitors, e.g., Algoman allows the user to create algorithms. There is no denying an e-revolution in medical education and practice [200]. The era of AI in medicine is approaching fast [35]. There is a need to navigate the increasing volumes of medical literature before making life-critical decisions in the intensive care unit (ICU) time-limited settings [199]. Computerized health diagnostics and decision-making algorithms can provide timely clinical decision support at the bedside, improve adherence to evidence-based guidelines, and be a source for education and research [199]. Healthcare professionals (HCPs) cannot interpret the data available to them. Every HCP should use AI technology in the future to analyze such data [41]. Despite this potential, only some AI healthcare solutions can impact the frontline [24] [201]. The author agreed with the proposed model of Wilson et al. [202] which may help any AI projects succeed in a clinical environment consisting of ten steps with four phases, namely, conceptualization, data acquisition and preparation (data management), AI application, and translation/deployment [202] Despite uncertainty concerning authorizations and regulations, there is a huge demand for digital transformation in healthcare and significant potential for AI solutions. Finally, they must build trust in AI by developing generalizable, interpretable, and user-focused solutions. In conclusion, primary care physicians must get well-versed with AI advances and the new world of medicine. The goal should be a delicate, mutually beneficial balance between the effective use of AI and the human physicians. It is essential because AI completely replacing humans in medicine is a concern that might otherwise hamper the benefits it can derive from it.

REFERENCES

[1] Seethalakshmi, S. and Nandan, R. "Health is the motive and digital is the instrument," *J Indian Inst Sci*, 100(4):597–602; https://doi.org/10.1007/s41745-020-00190-5, 2020.

[2] Sullivan, Frost "Artificial intelligence in healthcare takes precision medicine to the next level," *Cision: PR Newswire*, 2018. www.prnewswire.com/news-releases/artificial-intelligence-inhealthcare-takes-precision-medicine-to-the-nextlevel-300712098.html.

[3] Jean-David Zeitoun, Philippe Ravaud. "Artificial intelligence in health care: value for whom?" *The Lancet Digital Health*, 2(7):e338–e339, 2020, ISSN 2589–7500. https://doi.org/10.1016/S2589-7500(20)30141-2.

[4] Fuchs. VR. "Major concepts of health care economics," *Ann Intern Med*, 162:380–383, 2015.

[5] Ganapathy, K., Abdul, SS. and Nursetyo AA. "Artificial intelligence in neurosciences: A clinician's perspective," *Neurol India*, 66:934–939, 2018.

[6] Sun, R., Limkin, EJ., Vakalopoulou, M., et al. "A radiomics approach to assess tumour-infiltrating CD8 cells and response to anti-PD-1 or anti-PD-L1 immunotherapy: an imaging biomarker, retrospective multicohort study," *Lancet Oncol*, 19:1180–1191, 2018.

[7] Obermeyer, Z. and Emanuel, EJ. "Predicting the future—big data, ML, and clinical medicine," *N Engl J Med*, 375:1216–1219, 2016.

[8] Hinton, G. "Deep learning—a technology with the potential to transform health care," *JAMA*, 320:1101–1102, 2018.

[9] Bolukbasi, T., Chang, K.-W., Zou, J., Saligrama, V. and Kalai, A. "Man is to computer programmer as woman is to homemaker? Debiasing word embeddings," *Adv Neural Inf Process Syst*, 29:4349–4357, 2016.

[10] Norouzzadeh, M. S., et al. "Automatically identifying, counting, and describing wild animals in camera-trap images with deep learning," *Proc Natl Acad Sci USA*, 115:E5716–E5725, 2018.

[11] Goyal, J., Sharma, N., Kumar, A., Anand, A. and Prabha, C. "Classifying Diabetes Using Artificially Intelligent Techniques: A Comparative Analysis." In *2023 IEEE 2nd International Conference on Industrial Electronics: Developments & Applications (ICIDeA)* (pp. 353–358). IEEE, 2023, September.

[12] Courtland, R. "Bias detectives: The researchers striving to make algorithms fair," *Nature*, 558:357–360, 2018.

[13] Lutimath, N., Sharma, N. and Byregowda, K. "Prediction of heart disease using biomedical data through machine learning techniques." *EAI Endorsed Trans Pervasive Health Technol*, 7(29):170881, 2021 Aug 30.

[14] Ahmad Karnama, Ehsan Bitaraf Haghighi, Ricardo Vinuesa. "Organic data centers: A sustainable solution for computing facilities," *Results Eng*, 4:100063, 2019.

[15] Helbing, D. The automation of society is next how to survive the digita revolution; version 1.0, Createspace, 2015.

[16] Seo, Y., Kim, S., Kisi, O. and Singh, V. P. "Daily water level forecasting using wavelet decomposition and artificial intelligence techniques," *J Hydrol*, 520:224–243, 2015.

[17] Adeli, H. and Jiang, X. *Intelligent Infrastructure: Neural Networks, Wavelets, and Chaos Theory for Intelligent Transportation Systems and Smart Structuress*, Boca Raton: CRC Press, 2008.

[18] Nunes, I. and Jannach, D. "A systematic review and taxonomy of explanations in decision support and recommender systems," *Use Model Use Adapt Interact*, 27:393–444, 2017.

[19] Francescato, D. "Globalization, artificial intelligence, social networks and political polarization: New challenges for community psychologists," *Commun Psychol Glob Perspect*, 4:20–41, 2018.

[20] Dalenberg, D J. "Preventing discrimination in the automated targeting of job advertisements," *Comput Law Secur Rev*, 34:615–627, 2018.

[21] Vinuesa, R., Fdez. De Arévalo, L., Luna, M. and Cachafeiro, H. "Simulations and experiments of heat loss from a parabolic trough absorber tube over a range of pressures and gas compositions in the vacuum chamber," *J Renew Sustain Energy*, vol. 8(2), 2016 Mar 1.

[22] Mohamadi, A., Heidarizadi, Z. and Nourollahi, H. "Assessing the desertification trend using neural network classification and object-oriented techniques," *J Fac Istanb Univ*, 66:683–690, 2016.

[23] Kwok, R. "AI empowers conservation biology," *Nature*, 567:133–134, 2019.

[24] Panch, T., Mattie, H. and Celi, LA. "The 'inconvenient truth' about AI in healthcare," *NPJ Digit Med*, 2019(2):1–3, 2019.

[25] Vinuesa, R., Azizpour, H., Leite, I., et al. "The role of artificial intelligence in achieving the Sustainable Development Goals," *Nat Commun*, 11:233. https://doi.org/10.1038/s41467-019-14108-y, 2020.

[26] Bresnick, J. "Artificial intelligence in healthcare spending to hit \$36B," 2018. [Online]. Available: https://healthitanalytics.com/news/artificial-intelligence-in-healthcare-spendingto-hit-36b.

[27] Popov, VV., Kudryavtseva, EV., Kumar Katiyar, N., Shishkin, A., Stepanov, SI., Goel, S. "Industry 4.0 and digitalisation in healthcare," *Materials*, 15(6):2140. https://doi.org/10.3390/ma15062140, 2022.

[28] Myers, A. "Stanford's John McCarthy, seminal figure of artificial intelligence, dies at 84," April 2018. [Online]. Available: https://news.stanford.edu/news/2011/october/johnmccarthyobit102511.html.

[29] Pan, Y. "Heading toward artificial intelligence 2.0," *Engineering*, 2(4):409–413, 2016.

[30] Senders, JT., Arnaout, O., Karhade, AV., Dasenbrock, HH., Gormley, WB., Broekman, ML., et al. "Natural and artificial intelligence in Neurosurgery: A systematic review," *Neurosurgery*, 0:112, 2017.

[31] Godil, SS., Shamim, MS., Enam, SA. and Qidwai, U. "Fuzzy logic:A 'simple' solution for complexities in neurosciences?" *Surg Neurol Int*, 2:24, 2011.

[32] Arbour, D. "Artificial intelligence for authentic engagement," *Syneos Health Communic*, 147, 2018.

[33] Vosburgh, KG., Golby, A., Pieper, SD. "Surgery, virtual reality,and the future," *Studies Health Technol Inform*, 184:713, 2013.

[34] Hassabis, D., Kumaran, D., Summerfield, C. and Botvinick, M. "Neuroscienceinspired artificial intelligence," *Neuron*, 95:245258, 2017.

[35] Jiang, F., Jiang, Y., Zhi, H., et al., "Artificial intelligence in healthcare: Past, present and future," *Stroke Vasc Neurol*, 2017(2):230–243, 2017.

[36] Editorial, "Artificial intelligence in health care: Within touching distance," *The Lancet*, 390:27–39, 2017.

[37] Mesko, B. "The role of artificial intelligence in precision medicine," *Expert Review of Precision Medicine and Drug Development*, 2:239241, 2017.

[38] Powels, J., Hodson, H. "Google DeepMind and healthcare in an age of algorithms," *Health Technol (Berl)*, 7:351367, 2017.

[39] Panetta, K. "Top trends in the Gartner hype cycle for emerging technologies. 2017," 2018. [Online]. Available: https://www.gartner.com/smarterwithgartner/ top-trendsinthe-gartner-hype-cycle-foremerging-technologies-2017/.

[40] Paschen, U., Pitt, C. and Kietzmann, J. "Artificial intelligence: Building blocks and an innovation typology," *Bus Horiz.* https://doi.org/10.1016/j. bushor.2019.10.004, 2019.

[41] Topol, EJ. "High-performance medicine: the convergence of human and artificial intelligence," *Nat Med*, 2019(25):44–56, 2019.

[42] Haenssle, HA., Fink, C., Schneiderbauer, R., et al. "Man against machine: Diagnostic performance of a deep learning convolutional neural network for dermoscopic melanoma recognition in comparison to 58 dermatologists," *Ann Oncol*, 29(8):1836–1842, 2018.

[43] Rajpurkar, P., Irvin, J., Zhu, K., et al. "CheXNet: Radiologist-level pneumonia detection on chest X-rays with deep learning," *arXiv*, 2:1–58, 2017.

[44] Miotto, R., Li, L., Kidd, BA. and Dudley, JT. "Deep patient: An unsupervised representation to predict the future of patients from the electronic health records," *Sci Rep*, 6(1):26094, 2016. https://doi.org/10.1038/srep26094.

[45] Bostrom, N. *Superintelligence: Paths, Dangers, Strategies*, Oxford: OUP, 2014.

[46] Aicardi, C. Fothergill, BT., Rainey, S., Stahl, BC. & Harris, E. "Accompanying technology development in the Human Brain Project: From foresight to ethics management," *Futures,* 102:114–124, 2018. https://doi.org/10.1016/j.futures.2018.01.005.

[47] Russel, SJ., Norvig, P. *Artificial Intelligence: A Modern Approach*, Malaysia: Pearson Education Limited, 2016.

[48] Armstrong, S. "The apps attempting to transfer NHS 111 online," *BMJ*, 360:k156, 2018.

[49] Fraser, H., Coiera, E. and Wong, D. "Safety of patient-facing digital symptom checkers," *Lancet*, 392:2263–2264, 2018.

[50] Michalski, RS., Carbonell, JG. and Mitchell, TM. *Machine Learning: An Artificial Intelligence Approach*, New York: Springer Science & Business Media, 2013.

[51] Bradley, AP. "The use of the area under the ROC curve in the evaluation of machine learning algorithms," *Pattern Recognit*, 30:1145–1159, 1997.

[52] Agah, A. *Medical Applications of Artificial Intelligence.* Agah A, ed., Boca Raton: CRC Press, 2017, p. 461.

[53] Ramesh, AN., Kambhampati, C., Monson, JRT. and Drew, PJ. "Artificial intelligence in medicine," *Ann R Coll Surg Engl*, 86:334–338, 2004.

[54] J. Wells. "Canadian health system, like UK, 'Stretched to max capacity'. American Council on Science and Health," 2018. [Online]. Available: https://www.acsh.org/ news/2017/08/28/canadian-health-system-uk-stretched-max-capacity-11753.

[55] Huang, J., Jennings, NR. and Fox, J. "An agent-based approach to health care management," *Appl Artif Intell*, 9:401–420, 1995.

[56] MA., Musen. *Biomedical Informatics*, New York: Springer, 2006, pp. 698–736. [Online]. Available: http://link.springer.com/10.1007/0-387-36278-9.

[57] Amato, F., Ló pez, A., Peñ a-Méndez, EM., Vaň hara, P., Hampl, A. and Havel, J., "Artificial neural networks in medical diagnosis," *J Appl Biomed*, 11:47–58, 2013.

[58] Contreras, and Vehi. "Artificial intelligence for diabetes management and decision support: Literature review," *J Med Internet Res*, 20:e10775, 2018.

[59] Szeliski, R. *Computer Vision: Algorithms and Applications*, 1st edn, London: Springer-Verlag, 2011, p. 812.

[60] Thevenot, J., Ló pez, MB. and Hadid, A. "A survey on computer vision for assistive medical diagnosis from faces," *IEEE J Biomed Heal Informatics*, 1:1479–1511, 2018.

[61] Mintz, Y., and Brodie, R. "Introduction to artificial intelligence in medicine," *Minim Invasive Ther Allied Technol*, 28:7381, 2019.

[62] Hamlet, P., and Tremblay, J. "Artificial intelligence in medicine," *Metabolism*, 69S:S3640, 2017.

[63] Amisha, Malik, P., Pathania, M., Rathaur, VK. "Overview of artificial intelligence in medicine," *J Family Med Prim Care*, 8:2328–2331, 2019.

[64] Menzies, T. "21st-century AI: Proud, not smug," *IEEE Intell Syst*, 18(3):18–24, 2003.

[65] Millard, M. "Use your words! Sorting through the confusing terminology of artificial intelligence," 2018. [Online]. Available: www.healthcareitnews.com/news/use-your-wordssorting-through-confusing-terminology-artificial-intelligence.

[66] Lee, S. and Lee, D. "Healthcare wearable devices: An analysis of key factors for continuous use intention," *Serv Bus*, 14:503–531, 2020.

[67] Lee, S. and Lim, S. *Living Innovation: From Value Creation to the Greater Good*, Bingley, UK: Emerald Publishing Limited, 2018.

[68] Lee, D. "Effects of key value co-creation elements in the healthcare system: Focusing on technology applications," *Serv Bus*, 13:389–417, 2019.

[69] Sharma, N. and Batra, U. "A study on integrating crypto-stego techniques to minimize the distortion." In *Data Science and Analytics: 4th International Conference on Recent Developments in Science, Engineering and Technology, REDSET 2017, Gurgaon, India, October 13–14, 2017*, Revised Selected Papers 4 (pp. 608–615). Springer Singapore, 2018.

[70] Porter, M.E., and Teisberg, E. O. How physicians can change the future of health care. *Jama*, 297(10):1103–1111, 2007 Mar 14.

[71] Rigby, M. "Ethical dimensions of using artificial intelligence in healthcare," *AMA J. Ethics*, 21:E121–E124, 2019.

[72] Miyashita, M. and Brady, M. "The health care benefits of combining wearables and AI," *Harv Bus Rev*, 2019.

[73] Sharma, N. and Batra, U. "An enhanced Huffman-PSO based image optimization algorithm for image steganography." *Genet Program Evolvable Mach*, 22:189–205, 2021.

[74] Abe, M. and Abe, H. "Lifestyle medicine—An evidence-based approach to nutrition, sleep, physical activity, and stress management on health and chronic illness," *Pers Med Universe*, 8:3–9, 2019.

[75] Kagawa, R., et al. "Development of type 2 diabetes mellitus phenotyping framework using expert knowledge and machine learning approach," *J Diabetes Sci Technol*, 11:791–799, 2017.

[76] Tsirigos, NA. and Razavian, N., "Pathologists meet their match in tumour-spotting algorithm," *Nature*, 561:436–437, 2018.

[77] Schnyer, DM., Clasen, PC., Gonzalez, C. and Beevers, CG. "Evaluating the diagnostic utility of applying a ML algorithm to diffusion tensor MRI measures in individuals with major depressive disorder," *Psychiatry Res Neuroimaging*, 264:1–9, 2017.

[78] Abedi, V., Goyal, N., Tsivgoulis, G., Hosseinichimeh, N., Hontecillas, R., Bassaganya-Riera, J., Elijovich, L., Metter, JE., Alexandrov, AW., Liebeskind, DS., Alexandrov, AV, Z. R. "Novel screening tool for stroke using artificial neural network," *J Stroke*, 48:1678–1681, 2017.

[79] Lehman Constance, D., Yala Adam, Schuster Tal, Dontchos Brian, Bahl Manisha, Swanson Kyle, R. B. "Mammographic breast density assessment using deep learning: Clinical implementation," *J Radiol*, 290(1):52–58, 2019.

[80] Taylor, N. "Duke report identifies barriers to adoption of AI healthcare systems," *MedTech Dive*, 2019.

[81] Arsene, C. "Artificial Intelligence in healthcare: The Future is Amazing," *Healthcare Weekly.*, 2019.

[82] Rivers, EP., McIntyre, L., Morro, DC., R. K. "Early and innovative interventions for severe sepsis and septic shock: Taking advantage of a window of opportunity," *Can Med Assoc J*, 173:1054–1065, 2005.

[83] Costello, JC., et al. "A community effort to assess and improve drug sensitivity prediction algorithms, *Nat Biotechnol*, 32:1202–1212, 2014.

[84] Hargrave-Thomas, E. Yu, B., R. J. "Serendipity in anticancer drug discovery," *World J Clin Oncol*, 3:1–6, 2012.

[85] Abedi, V., Yeasin, M., Zand R. "Empirical study using network of semantically related associations in bridging the knowledge gap," *J Transl Med*, 11(27), 12:324, 2014.

[86] Zand, R., et al. Development of Synthetic Patient Populations and *In Silico* Clinical Trials. In Bassaganya-Riera, J. (ed) *Accelerated Path to Cures*. Springer, Cham, 2018. https://doi.org/10.1007/978-3-319-73238-1_5.

[87] V. Abedi, P., Lu, R., Hontecillas, M., Verma, G.A., Vess, C.W., Philipson, A., Carbo, A., Leber, N.T., Juni, S., Hoops, J., Bassaganya-Riera, Chapter 28 - Phase III Placebo-Controlled, Randomized Clinical Trial With Synthetic Crohn's Disease Patients to Evaluate Treatment Response, Editor(s): Quoc Nam Tran, Hamid R. Arabnia, In *Emerging Trends in Computer Science and Applied Computing, Emerging Trends in Applications and Infrastructures for Computational Biology, Bioinformatics, and Systems Biology, Morgan Kaufmann*, 2016, Pages 411-427, ISBN 9780128042038, https://doi.org/10.1016/B978-0-12-804203-8.00028-6. (https://www.sciencedirect.com/science/article/pii/B9780128042038000286)

[88] Zamiri, A., Yazdi, HS., G. S. "Temporal and spatial monitoring and prediction of epidemic outbreaks," *IEEE J Biomed Heal Inform*, 19:735–744, 2015.

[89] Kesorn, K., Ongruk, P., Chompoosri, J., Phumee, A., Thavara, U., Tawatsin, A., S. P. "Morbidity rate prediction of Dengue Hemorrhagic Fever (DHF) using the support vector machine and the Aedes aegypti infection rate in similar climates and geographical areas," *PLoS One*, 10:e0125049, 2015.

[90] Xie, W., Kantarcioglu, M., Bush, WS., Crawford, D., Denny, JC., Heatherly, R., M. B SecureMA "Protecting participant privacy in genetic association meta-analysis," *Bioinformatics*, 30:3334–41, 2014.

[91] Palanica, A., Flaschner, P., Thommandram, A., Li, M., Fossat, Y. "Physicians' perceptions of chatbots in health care: Cross-sectional web-based survey," *J Med Internet Res*, 21:e12887, 2019.

[92] Forbes, "The hospital will see you now," 2019. [Online]. Available: https://www. forbes.com/sites/insights-intelai/2019/02/11/the-hospital-will-see-you-now/ #4c9b42ae408a.

[93] Torkamani, A., Andersen, KG., Steinhubl, SR and Topol EJ. "High-definition medicine," *Cell*, 170:828–843, 2017.

[94] Park, CW., Seo, SW., Kang, N., Ko, B., Choi, BW. "Artificial intelligence in health care: Current applications and issues," *J Korean Med Sci*, 35(42):e379, 2020 Nov 2.

[95] Hu, W., Cai, B., Zhang, A., Calhoun, VD., Wang, YP. "Deep collaborative learning with application to the study of multimodal brain development," *IEEE Trans Biomed Eng*, 66(12):3346–3359, 2019.

[96] Graham, S., Depp, C., Lee, EE., et al. "Artificial intelligence for mental health and mental illnesses: An overview," *Curr Psychiatry Rep*, 21(11):116, 2019.

[97] Haleem, A., Javaid, M., Vaishya. "Effects of COVID 19 pandemic in daily life," *Curr Med Res Pract*, 10(2):78, 2020.

[98] Ai, T., Yang, Z., Hou, H., Zhan, C., Chen, C., Lv, W., Tao, Q., Sun, Z., Xia L. "Correlation of chest CT and RT-PCR testing for coronavirus disease 2019 (COVID-19) in China: a report of 1014 cases," *Radiology*. 296(2):E32-40, 2020.

[99] Haleem, A., Vaishya, R., Javaid, M., Khan, IH. "Artificial Intelligence (AI) applications in orthopaedics: An innovative technology to embrace," *J Clin Orthop Trauma*, 2019.

[100] Sohrabi, C., Alsafi, Z., O'Neill, N., Khan, M., Kerwan, A., Al-Jabir, A., Iosifidis, C., Agha, R. World Health Organization declares global emergency: A review of the 2019 novel coronavirus (COVID-19). *Int. J. Surg*, 76(1):71-76, 2020 Apr.

[101] Ting, DS., Carin, L., Dzau, V., Wong, TY. "Digital technology and COVID-19," *Nat Med*, 26(4):459-461, 2020 Apr.

[102] Gupta, R., Ghosh, A., Singh, AK., Misra, A. "Clinical considerations for patients with diabetes in times of COVID-19 epidemic. Diabetes & metabolic syndrome," *Clin Res Rev*, 14(3):211e2, 2020.

[103] Al-qaness, MAA., Saba, AI., Elsheikh, AH., Abd, M., Ewees, AA. "Efficient artificial intelligence forecasting models for COVID-19 outbreak in Russia and Brazil," *Process Saf Environ Protect*, 149(2021):399e409., 2020.

[104] Tang, Y., Schmitz, JE., Persing, DH., Stratton, CW. "Laboratory diagnosis of COVID-19: current issues and challenges," *J Clin Microbiol*, 58(6):1e9, 2020.

[105] Mushtaq, J., Pennella, R., Lavalle, S., et al. "Initial chest radiographs and artificial intelligence (AI) predict clinical outcomes in COVID-19 patients: Analysis of 697 Italian patients," *Eur Radiol*, 31(3):1770e1779, 2021.

[106] McRae, MP., Simmons, GW., Christodoulides, NJ., et al. "Clinical decision support tool and rapid point-of-care platform for determining disease severity in patients with COVID-19," *medRxiv*, 2020.

[107] Caruso, FP., Scala, G., Cerulo, L., Ceccarelli, M. "A review of COVID-19 biomarkers and drug targets: resources and tools," *Briefings Bioinf*, 22(2):701e713, 2021.

[108] Ong, E., Wong, MU., Huffman, A., He, Y. "COVID-19 Coronavirus vaccine design using reverse vaccinology and machine learning," *Front Immunol*, 11(1581):1e13, 2020.

[109] Ahuja, V., and Nair, LV. "Artificial Intelligence and technology in COVID Era: A narrative review," *J Anaesthesiol Clin Pharmacol*, 37:28–34, 2021.

[110] Swayamsiddha, S., Prashant, K., Shaw, D., Mohanty, C. "The prospective of Artificial Intelligence in COVID-19 Pandemic," *Health Technol (Berl)*, 11(6):1311–1320, 2021. https://doi.org/10.1007/s12553-021-00601-2.

[111] Saha, R., Aich, S., Tripathy, S., Kim. H-C., "Artificial intelligence is reshaping healthcare amid COVID-19: A review in the context of diagnosis & prognosis," *Diagnostics*, 11(9):1604, 2021. https://doi.org/10.3390/diagnostics11091604.

[112] Turing., A. M. "Computing machinery and intelligence," *Mind*, 49:433–60, 1950.

[113] Murdoch, TB. & Detsky, AS. "The inevitable application of big data to health care," *JAMA*, 309:1351–1352, 2013.

[114] Baxt, WG., Shofer, FS., Sites, FD., Hollander, JE. "A neural network aid for the early diagnosis of cardiac ischemia in patients presenting to the emergency department with chest pain," *Ann Emerg Med*, 40:575–83, 2002.

[115] Johnson, KW., Torres Soto, J., Glicksberg, BS., Shameer, K., Miotto, R., Ali. M., et al. "Artificial intelligence in cardiology," *J Am Coll Cardiol*, 71:2668–2679, 2018.

[116] Carneiro, G., Nascimento, JC. "Combining multiple dynamic models and deep learning architectures for tracking the left ventricle endocardium in ultrasound data," *IEEE Trans Pattern Anal Mach Intell*, 35:2592–2607, 2013.

[117] Wolterink, JM., Leiner, T., de Vos BD., van Hamersvelt, RW., Viergever, MA., Išgum, I. "Automatic coronary artery calcium scoring in cardiac CT angiography using paired convolutional neural networks," *Med Image Anal*, 34:123–136, 2016.

[118] Shahid, N., Rappon, T., Berta, W. "Applications of artificial neural networks in health care organizational decision-making: A scoping review," *PloS One*, 14(2):e0212356., 2019 Feb 19.

[119] Commission European, "Ethics guidelines for trustworthy AI | Digital Single Market," 8 April 2019. [Online]. Available: https://ec.europa.eu/digital-single-market/en/news/ethics-guidelinestrustworthy-ai.

[120] Sharma, N., Soni, M., Kumar, S., Kumar, R., Deb, N. & Shrivastava, A. "Supervised machine learning method for ontology-based financial decisions in the stock market," *ACM Trans Asian Low-Resource Lang Inf Process*, 22(5):1–24, 2023.

[121] Atun, R. "Transitioning health systems for multimorbidity," *Lancet*, 386:721–7222, 2015.

[122] Kocher, R., Sahni, NR. "Rethinking health care labor," *N Engl J Med*, 365:1370–1372, 2011.

[123] Badawi, O., Brennan, T., Celi, LA., Feng, M., Ghassemi, M., Ippolito, A., et al. "Making big data useful for health care: A summaryof the inaugural mit critical data conference," *JMIR Med Inform*, 2:e22, 2014.

[124] Jones, SS., Heaton, PS., Rudin, RS., Schneider, EC. "Unraveling the IT productivity paradox—lessons for health care," *N Engl J Med*, 366:2243–2245, 2012.

[125] Beam, A. and Kohane, I. "Big data and machine learning in health care," *JAMA*, 319:1317–1318, 2018.

[126] LeCun, Y., Bengio, Y., Hinton, G. "Deep learning," *Nature*, 521:436, 2015.

[127] Marcus, G. "Deep learning: A critical appraisal," *arXiv:1801.00631.*, 2018.

[128] Atun, R., Aydın, S., Chakraborty, S., Sümer, S., Aran, M., Gürol, I., et al. "Universal health coverage in Turkey: Enhancement of equity," *Lancet*, 382:65–99, 2013.

[129] Henglin, M., Stein, G., Hushcha, PV., Snoek, J., Wiltschko, AB., Cheng, S. "Machine learning approaches in cardiovascular imaging," *Circ Cardiovasc Imaging*, 10:e005614, 2017.

[130] Celi, LA., Moseley, E., Moses, C., Ryan, P., Somai, M., Stone, D., et al. "From pharmacovigilance to clinical care optimization," *Big Data*, 2:134–141, 2014.

[131] Panch, T., Szolovits, P., Atun, R. "Artificial intelligence, machine learning and health systems," *J Glob Health*, 8(2):020303, 2018 December. https://doi.org/10.7189/jogh.08.020303.

[132] Liu, X., Faes, L., Kale, AU., Wagner, SK., Fu, DJ., Bruynseels, A., et al. "A comparison of deep learning performance against health-care professionals in detecting diseases from medical imaging: a systematic review and meta-analysis," *Lancet Digit Health*, 1:e27–97, 2019.

[133] Mittelstadt, B. "Ethics of the health-related internet of things: A narrative review," *Ethics Informat Technol*, 19:157–175, 2017. https://doi.org/10.1007/s10676-017-9426-4.

[134] Brouillette, M. "AI added to the curriculum for doctors-to-be," *Nat Med*, 25:1808–1809, 2019. https://doi.org/10.1038/s41591-019-0648-3.

[135] Acampora, G., Cook, DJ., Rashidi, P., Vasilakos, AV. "A survey on ambient intelligence in health care, *Proc IEEE Inst Elect Electron Eng*, 101:2470–2494, 2013. https://doi.org/10.1109/JPROC.2013.2262913.

[136] Briganti, G., and Moine, O. L. "Artificial intelligence in medicine: Today and tomorrow," *Frontiers in Medicine*, 7, 2020. https://doi.org/10.3389/fmed.2020.00027.

[137] WHO, "Ethics and governance of artificial intelligence for health," World Health Organization;. Licence: CC BY-NC-SA 3.0 IGO, WHO guidance. Geneva, 2021.

[138] Powles, J., Hodson, H. "Google DeepMind and healthcare in an age of algorithms," *Health Technol (Berl)*, 7(4):351–367, 2017.

[139] Price, N. "Artificial intelligence in health care: Applications and legal issues," *Sci Tech Lawyer*, 14(1):10–13, 2017.

[140] Hoyle, P. "Health information is central to changes in healthcare: A clinician's view," *Health Inf Manag*, 48(1):48–51, 2018.

[141] Shepheard, J. "Ethical leadership and why health information management professionals need to be involved. Commentary on Health Information is central to changes in healthcare: a clinician's view," *Health Inf Manag*, 48(1):52-55, 2019.

[142] Gerke, S., Minssen, T., Cohen, G. "Ethical and legal challenges of artificial intelligence-driven healthcare," *Artif Intell Healthcare*, 295–336, 2020. https://doi.org/10.1016/B978-0-12-818438-7.00012-5.

[143] Char, DS., Abràmoff, MD., Feudtner, C. "Identifying ethical considerations for machine learning healthcare applications," *Am J Bioethics,* 20:7–17, 2020. https://doi.org/10.1080/15265161.2020.1819469.

[144] Mannes, A. "Governance, risk, and Artificial Intelligence," *AI Magazine,* 41:61–69, 2020. https://doi.org/10.1609/aimag.v41i1.5200.

[145] Henz, P. "Ethical and legal responsibility for artificial intelligence," *Discov Artif Intell,* 1:2, 2021. https://doi.org/10.1007/s44163-021-00002-4.

[146] Nelson, GS. "Bias in artificial intelligence," *North Carolina Med J,* 80:220–222, 2019. https://doi.org/10.18043/ncm.80.4.220.

[147] Naik, N., Zeeshan Hameed, B. M., Shetty, D. K., Swain, D., Shah, M., Paul, R., Aggarwal, K., Ibrahim, S., Patil, V., Smriti, K., Shetty, S., Rai, B. P., Chlosta, P., and Somani, B. K. "Legal and ethical consideration in artificial intelligence in healthcare: Who takes Responsibility?" *Frontiers in Surgery,* 14(9):266, 2022.

[148] Dignum, V. *Responsible Artificial Intelligence: How to Develop and Use AI in a Responsible Way,* Cham: Springer International Publishing, 2019.

[149] Sharma, N., Chakraborty, C. and Kumar, R. "Optimized multimedia data through computationally intelligent algorithms," *Multimedia Syst,* 29(5):2961–2977.

[150] Bhattacharya, S., Hossain, MM., Juyal, R., Sharma, N., Pradhan, KB., Singh, A. "Role of public health ethics for responsible use of artificial intelligence technologies," *Indian J Community Med,* 46:178–181, 2021.

[151] Kumar, A., Gadag, S., Nayak, UY. "The beginning of a new era: Artificial intelligence in healthcare," *Adv Pharm Bull,* 11(3):414–425, 2021 May. https://doi.org/10.34172/apb.2021.049.

[152] Jureček, M., and Lórencz, R. "Malware detection using a heterogeneous distance function," *Comput Inform,* 37(3):759–780, 2018.

[153] Spence, M. "Cost reduction, competition, and industry performance," *Econometrica,* 52(1):101–121, 1984. https://doi.org/10.2307/1911463.

[154] Amisha, et al. "Artificial intelligence," *Journal of Family Medicine and Primary Care,* 8(7):2331, July 2019.

[155] Lupton, M. "Some ethical and legal consequences of the application of Artificial Intelligence in the field of medicine," *Trends Med,* 18:1–7, 2018.

[156] Kaptchuk, T. and Miller, F. "Placebo effects in medicine," *N. Engl. J. Med,* 373:8–9, 2015.

[157] Wartman, S. and Combs, C. "Medical education must move from the information age to the age of artificial intelligence," *Acad Med,* 93(8):1107–1119, 2018.

[158] Davenport, T. and Dreyer, K. "AI will change radiology, but it won't replace radiologists," *Harvard Business Review,* 27, 2018.

[159] Kletzer, LG. "The question with AI isn't whether we'll lose our jobs —it's how much we'll get paid," November 2019. [Online]. Available: https://hbr.org/2018/01/the-questionwith-ai-isnt-whether-well-lose-our-jobs-its-how-much-well-getpaid.

[160] Del Canale, S., Louis, DZ., Maio, V., et al. "The relationship between physician empathy and disease complications," *Acad Med,* 87(9):1243–1249, 2012.

[161] Hazarika, I. "Artificial intelligence: Opportunities and implications for the health workforce," *Int Health,* 12(4):241–245, 2020. https://doi.org/10.1093/inthealth/ihaa007.

[162] Galmarini, CM., Lucius, M. "Artificial intelligence: A disruptive tool for a smarter medicine," *Eur Rev Med Pharmacol Sci,* 24(13):7462–7474, 2020. https://doi.org/10.26355/eurrev_202007_21915.

[163] Floridi, M. and Taddeo, L. "What is data ethics?," *Philos Trans A Math Phys Eng Sci,* 28;374(2083):20160360, 2016 Dec.

[164] Mehta, NDM. "Machine learning, natural language programming, and electronic health records: The next step in the artificial intelligence journey?" *J Allergy Clin Immunol,* 141, 2019–2021, 2018.

[165] Botsis, T., Hartvigsen, G., Chen, F., W. C. "Secondary use of EHR: Data quality issues and informatics opportunities," *AMIA Jt. Summits Transl Sci*, 1, 1–5, 2010.

[166] Miller, E., DD, B. "Artificial intelligence in medical practice: The question to the answer? " *Am J Med*, 131, 129–133, 2018.

[167] Kingsto, J. *Artificial Intelligence and Legal Liability. Research and Development in Intelligent Systems XXXIII*, Cham, Cambridge, UK: Springer, 2016, pp. 269–279.

[168] Lancet, T. "Artificial intelligence in health care: Within touching distance," *Lancet*, 390:2739, 2017.

[169] Caliskan, A., Bryson, JJ. and Narayanan, A. "Semantics derived automatically from language corpora contain human-like biases," *Science*, 356:183–186, 2017.

[170] Rivard, LS., Lapointe, "Getting physicians to accept new information technology: Insights from case studies," *CMAJ*, 174:1573–1578, 2006.

[171] Heston, TF. "Making health care smart" In Heston TF (ed) *eHealth - Making Health Care Smarter.* 1st edn., London: IntechOpen, 2018.

[172] Schmidt, MDN Alscher and. "The practice of medicine in the age of information technology" In *eHealth: Making Health Care Smarter.* 1st edn., London: IntechOpen, 2018. http://dx.doi.org/10.5772/intechopen.75482.

[173] Gurupur, V., Wan, TTH. "Inherent bias in artificial intelligence-based decision support systems for healthcare," *Medicina,* 56(3):141, 2020. https://doi.org/10.3390/medicina56030141.

[174] Challen, R., et al. "Artificial intelligence, bias and clinical safety," *BMJ Qual. Saf,* 28:231–237, 2019.

[175] Gurupur, V., et al. "Analysing the power of deep learning techniques over the traditional methods using medicare utilization and provider data," *J. Exp. Theor. Artif. Intell*, 31:99–115, 2019.

[176] Henriksen, K. and Kaplan, H. "Hindsight bias, outcome knowledge and adaptive learning," *Qual Saf Healthc*, 12:ii46–ii50, 2003.

[177] Wan, T.T.H. *Population Health Management for Poly Chronic Conditions: Evidence-Based Research Approaches*, New York: Springer, 2018.

[178] Johnson, S., Speedie, S., Simon, G., Kumar, V., Westra, B. "Quantifying the effect of data quality on the validity of an eMeasure," *Appl Clin Inform*, 8:1012–1021, 2017.

[179] Davenport, T., and Kalakota, R. "The potential for artificial intelligence in healthcare," *Future Healthcare Journal*, 6(2), 94–98, 2019. https://doi.org/10.7861/futurehosp.6-2-94.

[180] Nishita Mehta, Anil Pandit, Sharvari Shukla, "Transforming healthcare with big data analytics and artificial intelligence: A systematic mapping study," *J Biomed Inform*, 100:10331, 2019. https://doi.org/10.1016/j.jbi.2019.103311.

[181] Collaborators, GBD 2016 Healthcare Access and Quality. "Measuring performance on the Healthcare Access and Quality Index for 195 countries and territories and selected subnational locations: A systematic analysis from the Global Burden of Disease Study 2016," *Lancet*, 391:2236–71, 2018.

[182] WHO, "WHO global action plan for the prevention and control of non-communicable diseases 2013–2020," April 2019. [Online]. Available: http://www.who.int/nmh/events/ncd_action_plan/en/.

[183] Maini, E., Venkateswarlu, B., Gupta, A. "Applying machine learning algorithms to develop a universal cardiovascular disease prediction system," In Hemant J, Fernando X, Lafate P, Baig Z (eds) *International Conference on Intelligent Data Communication Technologies and Internet of Things ICICI 2018, Lecture Notes on Data Engineering and Communications Technologies*, 2019.

[184] Kaur, H., Kumari, V. "Predictive modelling and analytics for diabetes using a machine learning approach," *Applied Comput Inform*, 2018. https://doi.org/10.1016j.aci.2018. 12.004.

[185] Jeste, DV., Graham, SA., Nguyen, TT., Depp, CA., Lee, EE., Kim, HC. "Beyond artificial intelligence: Exploring artificial wisdom," *Int Psychogeriatr,* 32(8):993–1001, 2020. https://doi.org/10.1017/S1041610220000927.

[186] Sandeep Kumar Sood, Keshav Singh Rawat, Dheeraj Kumar, "A visual review of artificial intelligence and Industry 4.0 in healthcare," *Comput Elect Eng,* 101:107948, 2022.

[187] Kumar, R., Sharma, N. and Kumar, S. "Image intelligence in cyber security using sensing system towards the future generation intelligence," In *2022 2nd International Conference on Advance Computing and Innovative Technologies in Engineering (ICACITE)* (pp. 298–300). IEEE.

[188] Lee, S. and Lee, D. "Lessons learned from battling COVID-19: The Korean experience," *Serv Bus,* 17:7548, 2020.

[189] Ganapathy, K., Abdul, SS., Nursetyo, AA. "Artificial intelligence in neurosciences: A clinician's perspective," *Neurol India,* 66:934–939, 2018.

[190] Tagde, P., Tagde, S., Bhattacharya, T., et al. "Blockchain and artificial intelligence technology in e-Health," *Environ Sci Pollut Res,* 28:52810–52831, 2021. https://doi.org/10.1007/s11356-021-16223-0.

[191] Guoguang Rong, Arnaldo Mendez, Elie Bou Assi, Bo Zhao, Mohamad Sawan, "Artificial intelligence in healthcare: Review and prediction case studies," *Engineering,* 6(3):291–301, 2020. https://doi.org/10.1016/j.eng.2019.08.015.

[192] Arora, A. "Conceptualising artificial intelligence as a digital healthcare innovation: An introductory review," *Med Devices (Auckl),* 20(13):223–230, 2020 August. https://doi.org/10.2147/MDER.S262590.

[193] Sinsky, C., Colligan, L., Li, L., Prgomet, M., Reynolds, S., Goeders, L., et al. "Allocation of physician time in ambulatory practice: A time and motion study in 4 specialities," *Ann Intern Med,* 165:75360, 2016.

[194] Esteva, A., Kuprel, B., Novoa, RA., Ko, J., Swetter, SM., Blau, HM., et al. "Dermatologistlevel classification of skin cancer with deep neural networks," *Nature,* 542:115118, 2017.

[195] Lakhani, P. and Sundaram, B. "Deep learning at chest radiography: Automated classification of pulmonary tuberculosis by using convolutional neural networks," *Radiology,* 284:57482, 2017.

[196] Bhattacharya, S., Pradhan, KB., Bashar, MA., Tripathi, S., Semwal, J., Marzo, RR., et al. "Artificial intelligence enabled healthcare: A hype, hope or harm," *J Family Med Prim Care,* 8:3461–3464, 2019.

[197] Kumar, P., Dwivedi, Y.K. and Anand, A. "Responsible Artificial intelligence (AI) for value formation and market performance in healthcare: The mediating role of patient's cognitive engagement," *Inf Syst Front,* 2021. https://doi.org/10.1007/s10796-021-10136-6.

[198] Rajkomar, A., Dean, J., Kohane, I. "Machine learning in medicine," *New Engl J Med,* 380: 1347–1358, 2019.

[199] Schwarz, D., Štourač, P., Komenda, M., et al. "Interactive algorithms for teaching and learning acute medicine in the network of medical faculties MEFANET," *J Med Internet Res,* 15:e135, 2013.

[200] Dhir, SK., Verma, D., Batta, M., Mishra, D. "E-learning in medical education in India," *Indian Pediatr,* 54:871–877, 2017.

[201] Lyell, D., Coiera, E., Chen, J., et al. "How machine learning is embedded to support clinician decision making: an analysis of FDA-approved medical devices," *BMJ Health Care Inform,* 28:100301, 2021.

[202] Wilson, A., Saeed, H., Pringle, C., et al. "Artificial intelligence projects in healthcare: 10 practical tips for success in a clinical environment," *BMJ Health Care Inform,* 28:e100323, 2021. https://doi.org/10.1136/ bmjhci-2021-100323.

10 Security Issues and Defense Mechanism Using IoMT

Lekha Rani

1 INTRODUCTION

The Internet of Medical Things (IoMT), or the healthcare Internet of Things (IoT), has emerged as a web of interrelated medical devices and applications operating on a range of heterogeneous networks. Healthcare practitioners have availed themselves of the IoMT solutions to optimize disease management, drug administration, treatment techniques, and patient care, while curtailing costs and minimizing errors. The IoMT has grown exponentially, currently interconnecting around 10 billion IoT devices with an anticipated augmentation to 25 billion by the year 2025 [1]. The data procured is optimized for safe cloud storage, with interconnected computing devices coalescing to form a network that facilitates communication and data sharing. Significantly, during the COVID-19 pandemic, the IoMT has played a pivotal role in remote patient monitoring, telemedicine, and telehealth, effectively transforming healthcare delivery.

Nevertheless, the IoMT faces considerable security obstacles which arise from insufficient user security comprehension, substandard storage and transmission procedures, device impairment, denial-of-service assaults, and the theft and manipulation of medical records. A survey has shown that approximately 35% of IoMT users experienced a cybersecurity incident in 2016 [2]. Regrettably, a mere 17% of connected medical device makers and 15% of healthcare professionals demonstrate awareness of potential security issues, rendering regulations a necessity to ensure IoMT security [3]. Given the sensitivity of medical data and the critical nature of medical procedures, security breaches can have grave consequences such as reduced patient well-being, invasion of privacy, damaged brand reputation, business interruption, and financial instability. As such, healthcare entities must establish clear-cut security requirements and measures to safeguard the IoMT networks. In addition, those who choose to adopt IoMT solutions should have the liberty to appraise and confirm security protocols and select security features based on their particular needs and tolerance for risk.

DOI: 10.1201/9781003377818-10

2 HOW IOMT WORKS

The IoMT is a revolutionary network that brings together an array of cutting-edge medical technologies, such as devices, sensors, wearables, and implants, and connects them to the Internet, enabling the real-time collection, analysis, and sharing of patient health data. With its intricate web of interconnected devices, the IoMT can provide medical professionals with unprecedented access to vast amounts of medical data, allowing them to monitor and analyze a patient's health remotely. These IoMT devices function by collecting a vast amount of medical data from patients and then transmitting it to a local hub or gateway device, which filters and processes the data before transmitting it to a cloud-based platform. The platform then leverages sophisticated machine learning (ML) algorithms to analyze the data and detect meaningful patterns, trends, and anomalies [4]. After analysis, the platform transmits the analyzed data to healthcare providers, caregivers, and patients via web or mobile applications.

Security plays a critical role in the design and implementation of IoMT, given that it involves sensitive and confidential medical data. To ensure patient privacy is protected, robust security protocols must be put in place to prevent unauthorized access or misuse of patient data. By implementing a secure and reliable IoMT network, medical professionals can leverage the power of IoMT to improve patient outcomes through real-time monitoring and diagnosis, reduce hospitalization and readmission rates, and ultimately enhance the overall quality of patient care (refer Figure 10.1).

3 ROLE OF BIG DATA IN IOMT

The advent of the IoMT has ushered in a new era of transformation within the healthcare sector, enabling medical devices and sensors to interconnect with the internet, thereby providing healthcare professionals with unprecedented access to remote health monitoring and diagnostic capabilities. As the volume of data generated from these interconnected devices continues to increase, it has become increasingly clear that the effective management and interpretation of this data necessitates the deployment of advanced big data analytics techniques.

By leveraging big data analytics, healthcare providers can gain valuable insights and uncover patterns that would otherwise be impossible to detect. This, in turn, enables medical practitioners to identify key trends, predict potential health issues, and develop tailored treatment strategies to optimize patient outcomes. With the advent of IoMT and big data analytics, the healthcare industry has been able to leverage cutting-edge technologies to significantly enhance patient care and transform the overall healthcare experience.

Big Data in Healthcare – Big data, in the context of IoMT, refers to the massive amount of data generated by interconnected medical devices and sensors that can be analyzed to uncover patterns, trends, and valuable insights. Healthcare providers can harness the power of big data analytics to effectively collect, process, and analyze vast quantities of data from diverse sources such as medical records, wearable devices, and healthcare systems. This enables them

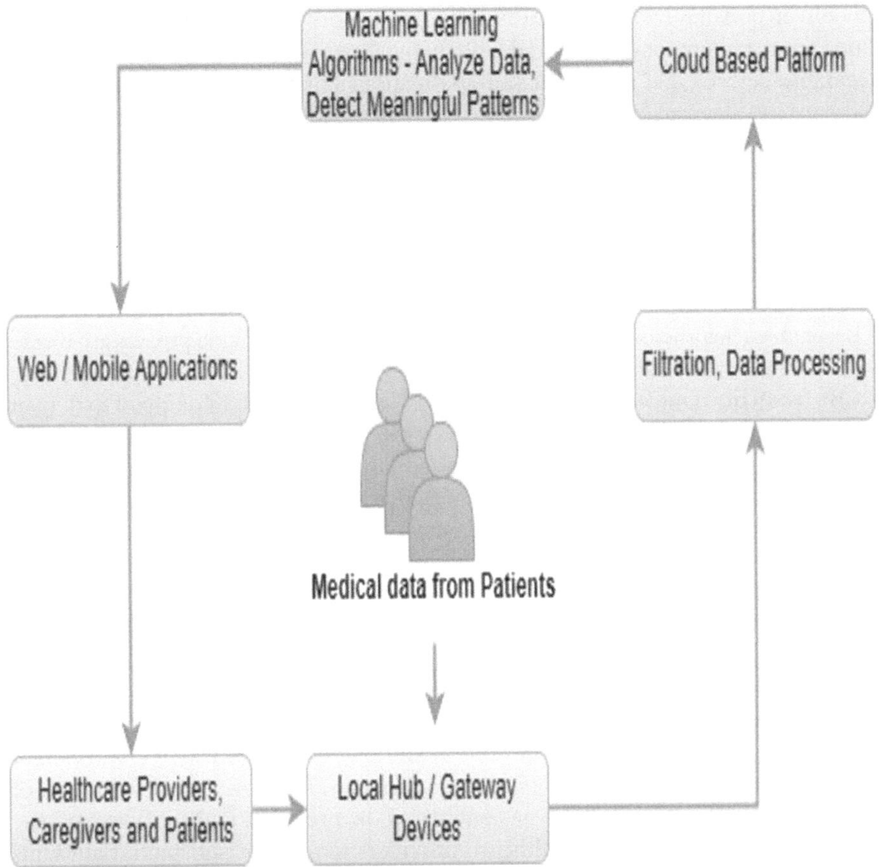

FIGURE 10.1 Explaining the Functioning of IoMT in Remote Patient Monitoring

to make informed decisions about patient care, create personalized treatment plans, and identify potential health risks. Moreover, big data analytics empowers healthcare providers to access real-time insights into patient health conditions, thereby enabling them to intervene in a timely manner and prevent the progression of diseases [5]. For instance, continuous glucose monitoring devices can gather data on patients' blood sugar levels, allowing healthcare professionals to identify patterns and trends that can inform adjustments to medication dosages or recommendations for lifestyle modifications. By utilizing big data analytics, healthcare providers can deliver better quality care and significantly enhance patient outcomes. The ability to collect, process, and analyze large volumes of data from IoMT devices provides invaluable opportunities to identify new treatment approaches, optimize patient care, and ultimately revolutionize the healthcare industry.

<u>Empowering Patients Through Personalized Care</u> – Big data analytics has revolutionized the healthcare industry, empowering healthcare providers to deliver personalized care that is tailored to individual patient needs, thereby improving patient outcomes and enhancing quality of life [6]. For example, wearable devices and mobile health applications collect data on patients' physical activity, sleep patterns, and dietary habits, enabling healthcare providers to develop personalized treatment plans that aid in managing chronic conditions such as diabetes, heart disease, and obesity.

In addition, big data analytics holds the capability to assist healthcare providers in recognizing patients who have a likelihood of developing chronic ailments. By analyzing data from multiple sources, healthcare providers can identify patterns and trends that may indicate a higher likelihood of developing certain conditions. This enables healthcare providers to intervene early and provide preventative care to reduce the risk of chronic conditions.

By using big data analytics, healthcare providers are better equipped to deliver personalized care, improve health outcomes, and enhance the overall quality of life for patients. This represents a paradigm shift in the healthcare industry, where advanced technology and data analytics are being used to address a range of health challenges, improve the efficiency of healthcare delivery, and drive better health outcomes for patients.

<u>Advancements in Disease Diagnosis</u>– The use of big data analytics has led to advancements in the diagnosis of past illnesses by providing insights into their root causes and risk factors. By examining vast amounts of data on patient health records and medical history, healthcare professionals can identify common risk factors for diseases such as cancer, heart disease [7], and Alzheimer's. This allows them to develop strategies for prevention and recommend lifestyle changes that can lower the chances of developing these illnesses. Moreover, the integration of big data analytics in healthcare has enhanced the precision and swiftness of disease diagnosis by enabling healthcare providers to analyze substantial amounts of data rapidly and efficiently. This has been particularly beneficial in areas like radiology, where ML algorithms can examine medical images and detect potential abnormalities. By utilizing big data analytics to scrutinize patient data and medical images, healthcare providers can make more accurate and timely diagnoses, leading to prompt treatment for patients.

In addition to the aforementioned examples of cancer, heart disease, and Alzheimer's, big data analytics has also aided in the diagnosis and treatment of several other diseases. For instance, in the field of infectious diseases, big data analytics has played a significant role in tracking and controlling outbreaks, as well as predicting the emergence of new pathogens [8]. The use of big data analytics in public health has helped identify patterns and clusters of infectious disease transmission, and inform targeted interventions.

Another area in which big data analytics has made a significant impact is mental health [9]. By analyzing large datasets of patient information, scientists have pinpointed novel risk elements associated with mental health disorders such as bipolar disorder, depression, and anxiety. This has enabled healthcare providers to develop personalized treatment plans that are tailored to the specific needs of individual patients.

Finally, big data analytics has been instrumental in the development of precision medicine [10], which involves tailoring treatment to individual patients based on their unique genetic and environmental profiles. By analyzing vast amounts of genomic data and health records, researchers can identify genetic mutations and other biomarkers that may indicate susceptibility to certain diseases or response to specific treatments. This has led to more effective and targeted therapies and has the potential to revolutionize the field of medicine.

<u>Cybersecurity in Smart Healthcare Systems</u>– Ensuring the safety and confidentiality of patients' information has emerged as a significant concern in the field of healthcare. The transmission and storage of medical data via wireless channels have amplified the possibility of security breaches, which could pose a serious threat to the sensitive information of patients. The careless handling of technology can lead to various security risks, putting patients' privacy and even their lives at stake. As a result, smart healthcare systems prioritize the goal of maintaining cybersecurity in emergency response and remote patient monitoring, as it is of utmost importance.

3.1 Challenges and Opportunities of Privacy and Security in Data Collection for Remote Healthcare

Remote healthcare, also known as telemedicine or telehealth, is an innovative approach that harnesses cutting-edge technology to provide healthcare services and support to patients who are unable to physically attend a medical facility. This transformative method of healthcare has garnered significant attention and popularity in recent years, primarily because of its potential to offer multiple advantages to both healthcare providers and patients.

One of the most significant benefits of remote healthcare is its ability to provide essential care to patients who require home care. Individuals suffering from chronic illnesses, disabilities, or those residing in remote areas often find it difficult to travel to a healthcare facility to receive medical attention. Remote healthcare enables these individuals to connect with healthcare providers virtually, thereby receiving medical services in the comfort of their own homes. Recent technological advancements have made remote healthcare more accessible and reliable than ever before. The use of medical devices and sensors that are linked to a patient's body has made it possible to collect and transmit large amounts of health-related data wirelessly to a central gateway unit [11]. This information may encompass critical indicators such as blood glucose levels, blood pressure, and heart rate. By using this data, healthcare providers can remotely monitor and evaluate a patient's health status, providing a higher level of care and support.

The central gateway unit is equipped with communication server software that enables the system to handle vast amounts of data from multiple patients. The software collects and processes the data, storing it in multiple databases for easy retrieval and analysis. Healthcare providers can use this platform to oversee the health condition of their patients and provide timely medical intervention, resulting in a more efficient and effective healthcare system. In addition to health-care providers, patients can also benefit significantly from remote healthcare services. Patients can use mobile applications or online platforms to connect with healthcare providers, schedule appointments, and receive feedback. This platform allows patients to communicate with healthcare providers swiftly, leading to faster diagnosis and treatment, which ultimately results in improved health outcomes.

Remote healthcare facilitates early detection and intervention of health issues. Healthcare providers can analyze the collected data to identify patterns and trends that can help detect potential health issues before they become more severe. Early detection and intervention lead to decreased healthcare expenses and better health results for patients. Another notable advantage of remote healthcare is its cost-effectiveness. Patients can save both time and money by not having to travel to a healthcare facility to receive medical attention. Similarly, healthcare providers can reduce their overhead costs by utilizing remote healthcare services, as they do not require a physical office.

3.2   PROTECTING SENSITIVE PATIENT DATA IN SMART HEALTHCARE: KEY CONSIDERATIONS AND STRATEGIES

In contemporary times, there has been an increase in the gathering of biomedical information from individuals through wireless communication and wearable technology. As a result of the delicate nature of the information and the vulnerability of communication channels in healthcare applications based on edge computing, safeguarding privacy has become more important than ever.

First, it is important to recognize the significance of safeguarding sensitive patient data, particularly with the increasing use of ML techniques for predicting heart and kidney diseases. While these methods have proven to be highly accurate in predicting medical conditions, it is crucial to prioritize the protection and security of patient data. A review of relevant literature on the use of ML in healthcare indicates that classification methods like decision trees, artificial neural networks (ANNs), and Naive Bayes are frequently employed for predicting heart and kidney diseases. Various tools and frameworks, including Spark, HDFS, and RapidMiner, are also used for data pre-processing and analysis [12].

However, the use of these techniques also carries a risk of data breaches and privacy violations, given the sensitive nature of patient data, which includes medical history, age, gender, and lifestyle habits. Misuse of such information could result in negative consequences for patients, including discrimination and stigmatization. Therefore, it is critical to implement robust data protection measures. Consequently, numerous investigations have been carried out in the area of protecting privacy and security in smart healthcare systems.

Liu et al. proposed a technique in their study for safeguarding the privacy of medical wearable devices that operate on cloud and edge computing [13]. This technique involves both controlling access to data and authenticating identity. The findings of their study indicate that this approach effectively protects the privacy of wearable devices. Similarly, Das et al. proposed a simple authentication protocol that can be used on mobile terminals, such as iOS and Android handsets, and wearable technology [14]. This protocol underwent proactive verification, including a security analysis using the AVISPA tool, which automatized the authentication of internet security protocols and applications. The researchers also looked into the computing cost and communication overhead of the protocol using the NS2 network simulator.

Diez et al. presented an authentication protocol that enables both wearable device users and other systems to mutually authenticate [15]. In addition, their research established secure connections between remote wearable devices via the internet, thus facilitating flexible data sharing. The study further examined various interactive scenarios that offer different levels of security protection, which can be adjusted according to the delicacy of the wearable devices involved.

Bhardwaj et al. discusses security issues with the IoT and suggests using Software Defined Networking (SDN) as a solution, but warns that it can create new security weaknesses. The article emphasizes the need to enhance Intrusion Detection Systems (IDS) due to their limitations in handling non-linear data sets. The focus is on the security challenges of SDN, such as DDoS attacks, susceptibility of SDN controllers to attacks, and timely detection of attacks. The article proposes that Network IDSs (NIDS) can help prevent potential attacks but require improvement [16]. Effective network anomaly detection is necessary for robust security architecture.

Zhou et al. introduced a protocol designed to safeguard the privacy of smart healthcare services, which is based on data aggregation [17]. To safeguard data aggregation, the method makes use of image feature extraction and dynamic medical text mining. Compared to other existing protocols, it demonstrated higher efficacy in terms of processing cost and communication overhead, according to the experimental results. In addition, Sprager et al. proposed an authentication protocol that relies on electrocardiogram (ECG) signals for both authentication and identity recognition [18]. This approach utilizes ECG sensors to capture heart rate and user-specific variations in ECG, and the protocol's efficacy was assessed using high-level statistics.

The use of IoMT sensors and cameras has created multimedia security concerns, as the substantial volumes of videos and visual data they capture for medical purposes put significant strain on network congestion and network overload. In response to this issue, a smart technique is proposed in this study that reduces the massive visual data into a few keyframes [19]. This method is similar to the lightweight summarization method presented in a previous study, where critical frames were chosen from a significant amount of visual data. The selected information is subsequently condensed utilizing the discrete cosine transformation method, and the picture is secured utilizing the discrete fractional random transformation method. Furthermore, the writers suggest a secure IoT platform for intelligent healthcare surveillance that employs Fully Homomorphic Encryption (FHE) to execute analytical services in an encrypted domain [20]. Based on the research findings, the suggested structure preserves a significant level of analytical precision and data confidentiality. The study concludes by stating that additional methods will be explored as part of the ongoing project.

3.3 MITIGATING CYBERSECURITY RISKS IN SMART HEALTHCARE SYSTEMS THROUGH INTRUSION DETECTION AND ML

With the integration of wireless technologies, IoMT devices, and cloud computing are now capable of performing remote patient analysis and diagnosis in the medical sector. Nevertheless, the system generates a vast amount of data due to the constant communication among different medical biosensors and actuators, which can make it challenging to manage and analyze the data. For instance, a patient with a pacemaker can generate data on heart rhythm, heart rate, blood pressure, and other vital signs, all of which must be accurately collected and analyzed by the e-healthcare system to ensure optimal treatment outcomes. This immense amount of data generated by the system can pose a significant challenge, making it complex to process and manage effectively. Thus, an IDS capable of detecting abnormal operations carried out in the edge network of the intelligent healthcare system is critical for maintaining the security of the system and the safety of patients. Additionally, it is vital that healthcare professionals receive the appropriate training to use this technology properly and safely to avoid any misuse or malfunctions that could endanger patients. As the medical sector continues to embrace wireless technologies, it is imperative to prioritize patient safety by developing and implementing robust security measures and providing healthcare professionals with the necessary training and tools to navigate this complex system.

A prior method was developed to securely and efficiently transmit accurate patient details to healthcare professionals without interference or manipulation [21]. To achieve this, a scalable architecture was designed with significant security mechanisms to identify any malevolent actions on the wireless communication occurring at the edge node. The primary objective was to provide a secure mechanism that could be implemented on diverse edge nodes, including those in patients' homes, hospitals, or ambulances.

ML was used at the edge to analyze data collected from various IoMT sensors through IoMT gateways [21], which underwent extensive analysis and processing before being sent to medical professionals for diagnosis. The IoMT gateway accepted data from sub-IoMT gateways or IoMT devices directly, which was further analyzed and stored in the edge cloud. In the past, the IoMT gateway was a vulnerable point for attackers who could manipulate patient information or launch denial-of-service attacks, which put patients' lives at risk. To prevent these malevolent activities, a multilayer intrusion detection model was enforced on the edge nodes of the healthcare system.

An efficient and secure architecture was designed to transmit accurate patient details to healthcare professionals, using a multilayer intrusion detection model to prevent any malicious activities. The system relied on ML at the edge to analyze data from various IoMT sensors and detect abnormal wireless traffic. The primary goal was to implement a secure IDS on the edge node of the healthcare system to prevent attackers from accessing patient information, ensuring patient safety, and protecting the healthcare system from potential cyberattacks.

4   ML-BASED ATTACKS

The IoMT communication environment is confronted with a significant security challenge posed by malicious attacks, namely malware botnets and poisoning attacks. These poisoning attacks involve the introduction of fraudulent data into a system with the intention of hindering its operation and causing a considerable decrease in performance. These kinds of attacks can be executed through various methods, including the use of malware, Trojan attacks, and other similar techniques. It is imperative to ensure that the IoMT environment is protected against these types of attacks as they have the potential to seriously jeopardize the privacy, resilience, and availability of IoMT capabilities. Indications of such attacks may include unusual behavior of devices or networks, irregular data patterns, or unexplained downtime. Consequently, a collection of security protocols has been created to counter these attacks and safeguard the security of the IoMT. In general, safeguarding the security of IoMT is extremely crucial to ensure the secure and efficient utilization of interconnected medical apparatus and technologies.

4.1   POISONING ATTACKS

Poisoning attacks are a type of cyber-attack that involves the injection of false data or commands into a computer or network system with the goal of disrupting its functioning and decreasing its performance. This type of attack can be particularly detrimental in critical areas such as the healthcare industry, where patient data and care systems rely on accurate and timely information to function effectively (refer Figure 10.2).

There are several strategies or methods that attackers can use to perform poisoning attacks. These include:

1. **DNS Poisoning**–Domain Name System (DNS) poisoning involves the modification of DNS server settings to redirect users to a fraudulent website. Attackers can change the IP address of a legitimate website to that of a malicious one, leading users to believe they are accessing the correct site. Once the user is on the fake website, the attacker can harvest sensitive information such as login credentials, financial information, or personal data.

2. **ARP Poisoning**– Address Resolution Protocol (ARP) poisoning is a technique used to intercept network traffic between two devices by modifying the MAC address table in a router or switch. By doing so, the attacker can redirect network traffic to their device, enabling them to steal sensitive information or launch further attacks on the network.

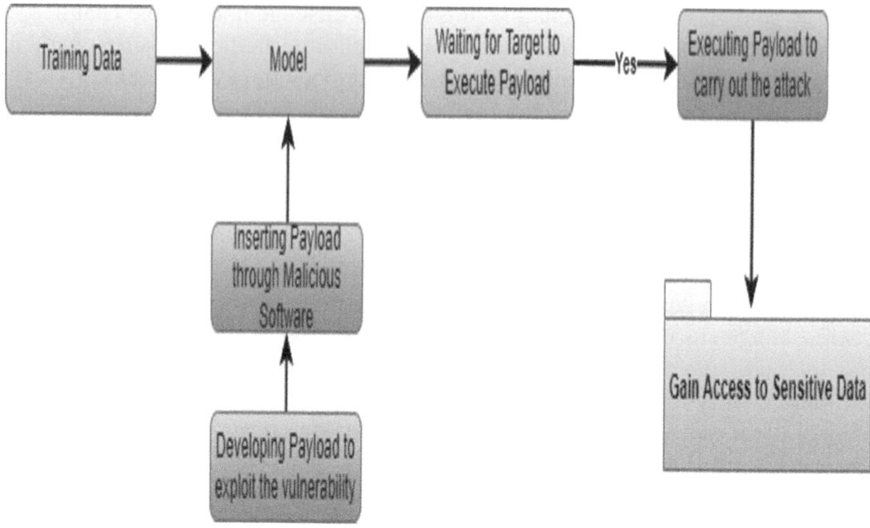

FIGURE 10.2   Flowchart Illustrating Poisoning Attacks: Understanding the Process and Impacts

3. **<u>Watering Hole Attacks</u>**– Watering hole attacks involve compromising a legitimate website that is known to be frequented by a target group of users. The attacker injects malicious code into the website that downloads malware onto the user's device when they visit the site. This type of attack can be particularly effective in the healthcare industry, where attackers can target websites that are frequently visited by medical professionals.

4. **<u>Malware Injection</u>**– Malware injection involves injecting malicious code into a legitimate piece of software, often through vulnerability in the software itself. Once the software is infected, the malware can spread throughout the system and cause significant damage.

5. **<u>SQL Injection</u>**– SQL injection denotes a sort of assault that capitalizes on the susceptibilities present in the SQL database of a website. The attacker injects SQL code into the website's search field or login page, allowing them to retrieve sensitive information from the database or execute malicious code.

To protect against poisoning attacks, several strategies can be employed. These include:

1. **<u>Implementing Access Controls</u>**–Access controls can be used to restrict access to sensitive systems and data, limiting the potential impact of a poisoning attack.

2. **<u>Network Segmentation</u>**– By segmenting networks, an attack on one part of the system can be isolated, preventing the attacker from accessing other parts of the system.

3. __Regular Patching__–Guaranteeing the software and systems are updated with the most recent security patches can assist in thwarting the exploitation of vulnerabilities.
4. __User Education__– Educating users on the risks of poisoning attacks and how to identify and report suspicious activity can help to prevent attacks from being successful.

4.2   Malware Attacks

Malware is a type of software designed to infiltrate and damage computer systems without the user's knowledge or consent. In the context of IoMT, malware can be classified into several categories (refer Figure 10.3).

1. __Viruses__– A virus is a malicious program that can replicate itself and infect other files on a system. In the case of IoMT, viruses can infect medical devices and applications, causing them to malfunction or leak sensitive patient information. This can lead to serious consequences, such as incorrect diagnosis or treatment, which can endanger patient lives.
2. __Trojans__–A Trojan refers to a kind of malicious software that camouflages itself as a genuine program with the intention of infiltrating a computer system. Upon gaining entry, it can carry out a diverse array of malevolent activities like purloining data, altering system configurations, or installing supplementary malware. In the context of IoMT, Trojans can infiltrate medical devices and steal sensitive patient information or cause physical harm by modifying the device's settings.
3. __Ransomware__–Ransomware is a classification of malevolent software that encrypts a sufferer's data and demands recompense in return for the decryption code. These attacks can be incredibly ruinous in the healthcare industry, as they can prevent access to critical patient data, which can affect treatment and decision-making processes.
4. __Spyware__– Spyware is a type of malware that tracks a victim's online activity and collects sensitive data, such as login credentials, credit card information, or personal health information (PHI). In the context of IoMT, spyware can infiltrate medical devices and steal sensitive patient data, which can be used for identity theft, fraud, or other malicious purposes.

Symptoms of Malware Attacks:

1. __Slow system performance__– Malware can cause a computer system to slow down, as it consumes system resources to perform its malicious actions. In the context of IoMT, slow system performance can affect the accuracy and reliability of medical devices, which can have serious consequences for patient care.
2. __Unusual network activity__– Malware can generate unusual network activity, such as sending or receiving data to suspicious IP addresses. In the context of IoMT, unusual network activity can indicate that a

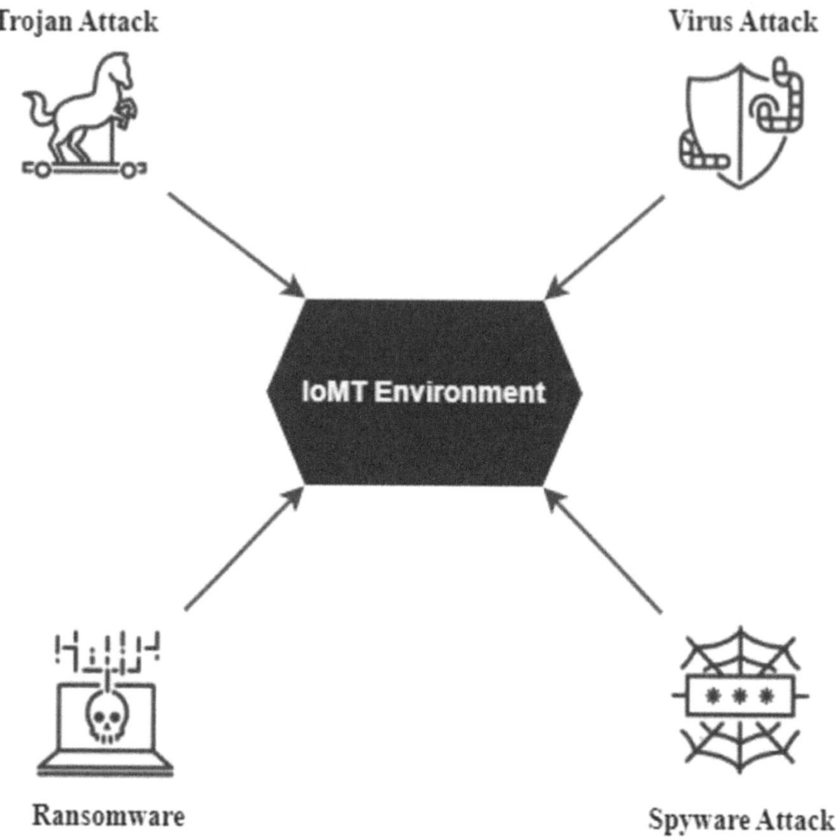

FIGURE 10.3 Types of Malwares

medical device has been compromised and is communicating with a malicious actor.

3. **<u>Pop-up ads</u>**– Malware can generate pop-up ads that are difficult to close, even after clicking the "X" button. In the context of IoMT, pop-up ads can indicate that a medical device has been compromised and is displaying malicious content to the user.

4. **<u>System crashes</u>**– Malware can cause a computer system to crash or freeze, making it difficult to perform basic tasks. In the context of IoMT, system crashes can affect the operation of medical devices and can prevent healthcare professionals from accessing critical patient data.

5. **<u>Unauthorized access</u>**– Malware can grant unauthorized access to a computer system, allowing an attacker to remotely control the device or steal sensitive data. In the context of IoMT, unauthorized access can lead to the theft of sensitive patient data or the manipulation of medical devices, which can endanger patient lives.

Strategies Used to Perform Malware Attacks:

1. **Phishing**–Phishing denotes a social engineering technique that leverages electronic mail or other modes of communication to deceive a victim into opening an attachment or clicking on a link containing malware. In the context of IoMT, phishing assaults can be directed toward healthcare practitioners or patients via fraudulent emails or messages that seem to originate from a genuine source.
2. **Supply Chain Attacks**– Supply chain attacks occur when malware is introduced into a system through a third-party vendor or service provider that has access to the system. In the context of IoMT, supply chain attacks can target medical device manufacturers, software vendors, or healthcare providers that use third-party services for data storage or other purposes.
3. **Exploiting vulnerabilities**– Attackers can exploit vulnerabilities in software or hardware to obtain entry to a system or device without proper authorization. In the context of IoMT, attackers can exploit vulnerabilities in medical devices or applications that are not patched or updated regularly, allowing them to gain access to sensitive patient data or manipulate the device's settings.
4. **Malvertizing**– Malvertizing is a type of attack that uses malicious ads to infect a victim's computer with malware. In the context of IoMT, malvertizing can target medical websites or applications, displaying ads that contain malware or redirecting users to malicious websites.
5. **Brute force attacks**– Brute force attacks are a type of attack that uses automated tools to guess login credentials or passwords. In the context of IoMT, brute force attacks can target medical devices or applications that have weak or default login credentials, allowing an attacker to gain unauthorized access to the device or its data.

Prevention and Mitigation Strategies:

1. **Regular software updates**–Frequent software updates can aid in the prevention of malware attacks by patching vulnerabilities and fixing bugs in the system. In the context of IoMT, medical device manufacturers and software vendors should ensure that their products are regularly updated to prevent vulnerabilities from being exploited.
2. **Strong authentication**–Robust authentication mechanisms, including dual-factor authentication or biometric authentication, may assist in preventing unauthorized entry to medical devices and applications. Healthcare providers should ensure that their systems and devices are protected by strong authentication mechanisms that cannot be easily bypassed.
3. **Employee education**– Employee education and training programs can help prevent social engineering attacks, such as phishing or malvertizing.

Healthcare providers should ensure that their employees are trained to recognize and report suspicious emails or messages.

4. **<u>Network segmentation</u>**– Network segmentation can help prevent malware from spreading across the network by isolating compromised devices from the rest of the network. Healthcare providers should ensure that their networks are segmented and that medical devices are isolated from other systems and data.

5. **<u>Incident response planning</u>**– Incident response planning can help healthcare providers respond quickly and effectively to malware attacks. Healthcare providers need to establish an incident response plan that specifies the necessary actions to be taken in the occurrence of a malware attack and guarantees the safeguarding of essential patient data.

4.3   Trojan Attacks

Trojan attacks are a type of cyber-attack where a malicious code or software is hidden within a legitimate program, leading to the unauthorized access and manipulation of data or systems. This type of attack is particularly difficult to detect, as the Trojan appears to be a legitimate program and can evade detection by antivirus software and other security measures. The name "Trojan" comes from the Trojan horse in Greek mythology, which was a deceptive gift used to gain access to a city. The reason why Trojan attacks are so difficult to detect is because the malicious code is hidden within a seemingly legitimate program. This means that the Trojan can evade detection by antivirus software and other security measures, as it appears to be a legitimate program. In addition, Trojans can be designed to disable or circumvent security measures, making them even harder to detect.

One common example of Trojan attacks in the IoMT field is the case of medical devices that are compromised by Trojans. Medical devices are increasingly connected to the Internet, and this connectivity can make them vulnerable to cyberattacks. In some cases, attackers have been able to compromise medical devices by inserting Trojans into the devices' software. This can allow attackers to gain access to patient data, manipulate medical devices, or even cause harm to patients.

ANNs are also vulnerable to Trojan attacks. ANNs are a type of ML algorithm that can be used in a wide range of applications, includingnatural language processing, image recognition, and speech recognition. Trojans can be inserted into ANNs during the training process and can then be activated later by an attacker. This can allow the attacker to manipulate the output of the ANN, leading to incorrect predictions or decisions (refer Figure 10.4).

There are several techniques that can be used to protect against Trojan attacks. One approach is to use hardware-based security measures, such as secure enclaves or trusted execution environments. These hardware-based security measures can protect against attacks that attempt to bypass software-based security measures. Another approach is to use software-based security measures, such as runtime monitoring or code obfuscation. Runtime monitoring can detect anomalous

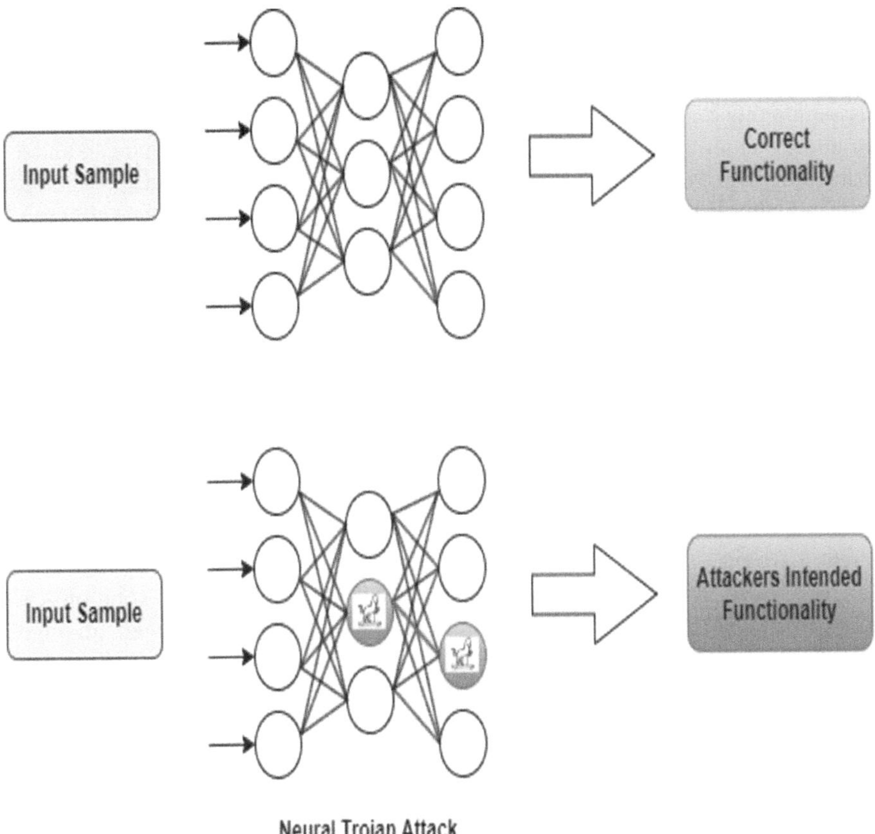

FIGURE 10.4 When the input image detects the Trojan trigger, the Trojaned ANN produces an inaccurate output.

behavior in software, which can be a sign of a Trojan attack. Code obfuscation can make it more difficult for attackers to reverse-engineer software and identify vulnerabilities.

5   SAFEGUARDING IOMT SYSTEMS FROM ML-BASED ATTACKS

The healthcare sector is becoming more and more reliant on IoT technologies to improve the efficacy and productivity of healthcare services. IoMT has revolutionized the healthcare industry by enabling connected devices to gather and share data in real-time, improving patient care, reducing cost, and quality. IoMT devices are helping healthcare providers to remotely monitor patients' health conditions, track medication adherence, and facilitate timely interventions, thus improving the overall health outcomes of patients. However, this progress comes with potential risks of cybersecurity attacks, which can lead to data breaches, compromised patient information, and even loss of life.

ML has risen as a potent technique in the cybersecurity arsenal, and attackers are increasingly using it to infiltrate IoMT networks. ML-based attacks can penetrate the security protocols of IoMT devices, collect sensitive data, and perform unauthorized actions. These attacks can target various components of IoMT systems, including sensors, network protocols, and cloud services, and can undermine the integrity, confidentiality, and accessibility of healthcare data. Therefore, securing IoMT from ML-based attacks is crucial for ensuring the safety and security of patients and their data.

To secure IoMT from ML-based attacks, healthcare providers need to implement a robust security strategy that includes several layers of protection. One of the most crucial steps in securing IoMT is to ensure that all connected devices are secured and up-to-date with the latest security patches. Additionally, healthcare providers need to implement advanced (IDS/IPS) in order to identify and prevent any unauthorized activity on the network. They should also implement secure data transmission protocols to prevent unauthorized access to data in transit. Another important measure is to deploy advanced ML-based security solutions to detect and prevent ML-based attacks. ML algorithms can analyze network traffic patterns, identify anomalies, and identifying possible security risks in a timely manner as they occur. For instance, some ML-based security solutions can analyze system logs and identify suspicious activity that might indicate an ongoing attack. These solutions can also learn from previous attacks and adjust their algorithms to prevent similar attacks in the future.

Furthermore, healthcare providers need to implement access control mechanisms to guarantee that confidential information is accessed only by authorized personnel. This includes limiting the number of users with privileged access, requiring multifactor authentication, and implementing role-based access control (RBAC) mechanisms. Additionally, healthcare providers should conduct regular security audits and risk assessments to identify vulnerabilities and develop strategies to mitigate them.

Examples of Connected Medical Devices in the Healthcare Industry:

1. **Implantable Cardioverter Defibrillators (ICDs) – Risk Factor: High-Type: Invasive**

   ICDs are implantable devices that regulate heart rhythms and are surgically implanted in the chest. They are considered invasive because they require a surgical procedure for implantation and are directly connected to the patient's heart.

2. **Infusion Pumps – Risk Factor: Medium-Type: Stationary/Portable**

   Infusion pumps are devices that deliver fluids, including medications and nutrients, to patients in a controlled manner. They can be either stationary or portable, depending on the use case. Stationary infusion pumps are typically used in hospital settings, while portable infusion pumps are designed for patients to use at home.

TABLE 10.1

Instances of IoMT System Utilized Medical Equipment

Connected Medical Devices	Type	Working	Risk Factor
Implantable Cardioverter Defibrillators (ICDs)	Invasive	Regulate heart rhythms	High
Infusion pumps	Stationary/Portable	Deliver fluids, including medications and nutrients, to patients in a controlled manner	Medium
Blood glucose monitors	Non-Invasive	Measure their blood glucose levels	Low to Medium
Medical imaging devices	Non-Invasive	Use radiation or magnetic fields to create images of the body	Low

3. **Blood Glucose Monitors – Risk Factor: Low to Medium-Type: Non-Invasive**

   Blood glucose monitors are devices used by patients to measure their blood glucose levels. They are typically non-invasive, meaning that they do not require a surgical procedure or penetration of the skin. Instead, they use a small lancet to prick the skin and obtain a blood sample.

4. **Medical Imaging Devices – Risk Factor: Low-Type: Non-Invasive**

   Medical imaging devices include a variety of non-invasive devices, such as MRI machines, CT scanners, and X-ray machines. These devices use radiation or magnetic fields to create images of the body, without the need for invasive procedures. They are typically used in hospital or clinical settings as in Table 10.1.

5.1 ADVANCED THREAT DETECTION FOR IoMT DEVICES USING ML

ML is a branch of artificial intelligence (AI) that empowers computer systems to learn and enhance themselves based on experience without any direct programming. The key advantage of ML is its capability to recognize patterns and identify anomalies in extensive data sets, thereby enhancing the precision and efficacy of security measures. Unlike conventional security methods, which rely on predefined rules and patterns, ML algorithms can adjust to new circumstances and dynamic risks, making them more efficient in detecting and managing security hazards.

In the realm of IoMT security, ML offers several benefits. To begin with, ML algorithms have the capacity to scrutinize vast quantities of data instantly, rendering it simpler to recognize and counter possible security risks. Furthermore, ML can uncover patterns in data that might not be apparent to human analysts. This capability can be helpful in detecting slight variations in device activity that might indicate a security breach [22]. Lastly, ML can aid in developing prognostic models that foresee forthcoming security threats and pre-emptively manage them before they materialize.

There are different types of ML algorithms and we can see how they are used to solve problems in IoMT security:

- **Anomaly detection** – Anomaly detection is a method utilized to recognize deviations from typical actions in IoMT devices. ML algorithms can be trained on extensive datasets of device behavior to recognize unusual activities that may signify a security breach. One instance of this is utilizing an ML algorithm to identify a sudden increase in network traffic from an IoMT device, which may suggest that the device has been compromised. Other examples of anomalous behavior in IoMT devices could include a device sending or receiving data at odd times, transmitting data to an unexpected location, or performing actions that are not typical for the device's intended use. By detecting and addressing these anomalies early, security breaches can be prevented, and patient safety can be ensured.
- **Deep learning** –Deep learning is a subfield of ML that excels in processing unstructured data, such as videos and images. When applied to the realm of IoMT security, deep learning algorithms can be utilized to scrutinize medical images to detect potential security breaches like tampering or forgery. As an illustration, a deep learning algorithm can be implemented to detect slight alterations in a medical image that may suggest that the image has been manipulated. Further examples of security threats in medical images that deep learning algorithms could detect may include missing or added components, hidden messages, or inconsistencies in the image's metadata. By leveraging the power of deep learning techniques in IoMT security, potential threats can be detected and addressed promptly, ensuring the integrity of medical images and, consequently, patient safety.
- **Decision Trees** – Decision trees are a type of ML algorithm that can be used to classify data into different categories based on a set of predefined criteria. In the context of IoMT security, decision trees can be used to classify IoMT device behavior into different categories such as normal or suspicious. For example, a decision tree could be used to classify a network packet from an IoMT device as normal or suspicious based on its characteristics.
- **Support Vector Machines** – Support Vector Machines (SVM) are a type of ML algorithm that excels in recognizing patterns in data that may not be immediately evident. When applied to the realm of security,

SVM algorithms can be utilized to examine large datasets of device behavior to detect potential security threats. For instance, an SVM algorithm can be implemented to scrutinize network traffic from an IoMT device to detect patterns that may suggest a security breach. Other examples of security threats in IoMT device behavior data that SVM algorithms can detect include unusual data transfer or usage patterns, unexpected device behavior, and suspicious application usage. By utilizing SVM algorithms in IoMT security, potential security threats can be identified early on, and appropriate action can be taken to prevent harm to patients and ensure the security of medical devices.

- **Adversarial ML** – Adversarial ML is a technique that focuses on identifying and mitigating attacks that aim to manipulate or fool ML models. In the context of IoMT security, adversarial ML can be used to protect medical devices from attacks such as data poisoning or model evasion. For example, an adversarial ML algorithm could be used to detect and block attempts to modify the data collected by a medical device to manipulate its behavior.
- **Reinforcement learning** – Reinforcement learning is an ML algorithm that instructs machines on how to make decisions based on rewards or penalties associated with particular actions. In the field of IoMT security, reinforcement learning algorithms can be utilized to train medical devices to promptly detect and respond to security threats in real-time. For example, a reinforcement learning algorithm can train a medical device to detect and react to a security breach by implementing specific measures such as deactivating the device or alerting security personnel.
- **Natural Language Processing** – Natural Language Processing (NLP) is a field of ML that is focused on the processing and analysis of human language. Within the context of IoMT security, NLP techniques can be employed to scrutinize and categorize text-based data, such as medical records or security reports, to detect potential security threats. For instance, an NLP algorithm can be utilized to analyze security reports regarding IoMT devices and recognize patterns that may suggest a security breach.
- **Ensemble Methods** – Ensemble methods are a group of ML algorithms that combine the results of multiple algorithms to produce more accurate and robust predictions. In the context of IoMT security, ensemble methods can be used to improve the accuracy of security threat detection by combining the results of multiple ML algorithms. For example, an ensemble method could be used to combine the results of an SVM algorithm and a decision tree algorithm to identify potential security threats in IoMT device behavior.

5.2 IoMT Security Models

5.2.1 The Ontology-Based IoMT Security Model

The ontology-based IoMT security model is a cutting-edge approach to securing the vast network of medical devices and systems that are connected to the

Internet. This model is built on the foundation of ontology, a branch of philosophy that deals with the study of existence and the nature of things. In the context of IoMT security, ontology refers to a formal representation of the concepts and relationships that exist within the healthcare domain [23].

The use case for this model in the healthcare sector is numerous and varied. One such use case is in the area of patient monitoring. With the advent of wearable devices and sensors, patients can now be monitored in real time from the comfort of their own homes. This has the capacity to enhance patient results and decrease expenses related to healthcare. However, it also presents a significant security challenge. The ontology-based IoMT security model can help to address this challenge by providing a framework for securing these devices and the data they generate. Another use case for this model is in the area of medical imaging. Medical imaging is an essential tool for diagnosing and treating a wide range of medical conditions. However, the images generated by these systems can be sensitive and must be protected. The ontology-based IoMT security model can help to ensure that these images are only accessible to authorized personnel and that they are not tampered with or altered in any way.

5.2.1.1 Description of the Ontology-Based IoMT Security Model

<u>Stakeholders</u> –The stakeholders in this model include healthcare providers, device manufacturers, patients, and regulatory agencies. Healthcare providers are responsible for implementing the security measures outlined in the model to protect their patients' data. Device manufacturers must ensure that their products comply with the security requirements outlined in the model. Patients have a vested interest in the security of their medical data and must be informed about the measures being taken to protect it. Regulatory agencies are responsible for enforcing compliance with the security requirements outlined in the model.

<u>Security Protocol</u> – The ontology-based IoMT security model provides a comprehensive solution to the security challenges associated with the IoMT. It includes a set of security requirements, protocols, and best practices that can be customized to meet the specific needs of a healthcare organization. This model can help to prevent unauthorized access to sensitive medical data, ensure the integrity of medical images, and provide a secure environment for remote patient monitoring.

<u>Components</u> – The components of this model include the ontology itself, which provides a formal representation of the concepts and relationships within the healthcare domain. The model also includes a set of security requirements that are based on the ontology, as well as a set of protocols and best practices for implementing these requirements. Finally, the model includes a set of tools and technologies that can be used to implement and enforce the security requirements.

<u>Issue Handling</u>– Some of the issues that the ontology-based IoMT security model can handle include data breaches, unauthorized entry to medical information, and tampering with medical images. By providing a comprehensive framework for securing the IoMT, this model can help to address these issues and ensure the safety and privacy of patients' medical data.

5.2.1.2 Ontology Approach

The ontology-based IoMT security model is constructed on the foundation of the ontology approach, which is a technique for producing precise and structured depictions of concepts and connections within a particular domain [24]. In the healthcare field, an ontology is capable of representing an array of concepts, including diseases, symptoms, treatments, and medications, as well as the relationships that exist among them. The approach can also account for instances, which refer to particular examples of concepts, such as a diabetic patient. Axioms are other crucial components of ontology, serving as statements that describe the relationships between concepts, including their properties and classification. The ontology approach is notably useful in portraying intricate relationships between concepts and entities, making it possible to examine and reason over large datasets. By implementing this approach within the IoMT environment, it becomes feasible to create a structured representation of healthcare concepts and relationships, thereby laying the groundwork for a secure and effective medical data management system.

5.2.2 Biometric-Based IoMT Security Model

Biometric-based IoMT security systems have emerged as a cutting-edge technology that utilizes biometric authentication to ensure the safety and security of medical data transmitted through the IoMT. These systems can significantly reduce the risk of data breaches and unauthorized access, which are prevalent issues in the healthcare industry [25]. They offer a more secure and efficient way of identifying and verifying the identity of patients and healthcare professionals, improving patient outcomes and enhancing the overall quality of care.

The use cases of biometric-based IoMT security systems in the healthcare sector are numerous. One such use case is the identification of patients. Biometric identification systems can reduce the risk of medical errors that arise from misidentification, improving patient outcomes. Additionally, biometric authentication can improve the security of electronic medical records (EMRs), allowing only authorized personnel to access sensitive patient information. Another use case of biometric-based IoMT security systems is for tracking medication administration. Biometric authentication can be used to ensure that only authorized healthcare professionals administer medication to patients, reducing the risk of medication errors and adverse drug events. Moreover, biometric-based IoMT security systems can be used for tracking the attendance of healthcare professionals, ensuring that only authorized personnel have access to sensitive medical data. Biometric authentication can also help prevent fraud and misuse of healthcare resources.

There are two categories of biometric-based IoMT security systems, namely unimodal biometric systems and multimodal biometric systems. Unimodal biometric systems use a single biometric identifier, such as fingerprints, facial recognition, or iris scans, to authenticate an individual's identity. On the other hand, multimodal biometric systems employ a combination of two or more biometric identifiers to enhance accuracy and reliability in the authentication process.

Multimodal systems can include a combination of fingerprints, facial recognition, voice recognition, and other biometric modalities.

Unimodal biometric system– Unimodal biometric systems work by scanning a single biometric trait and comparing it against a pre-existing database to determine the identity of an individual. For instance, fingerprint scanners capture a person's unique fingerprint pattern, which is then compared with pre-existing records to verify their identity. Similarly, facial recognition systems capture an individual's facial features and compare them with existing records to authenticate their identity.

Multimodal biometric system – Multimodal biometric systems, on the other hand, employ a combination of biometric identifiers to authenticate an individual's identity [26]. For example, a multimodal system might require a fingerprint scan and facial recognition before granting access to medical data. The system compares the collected data against a pre-existing database to verify the individual's identity.

5.2.2.1 Description of the Biometric-Based IoMT Security Model

Stakeholders – The various stakeholders in biometric-based IoMT security systems include healthcare providers, medical device manufacturers, and patients. Healthcare providers rely on these systems to ensure that patient data is secure and to improve patient outcomes. Medical device manufacturers develop biometric sensors and algorithms to implement biometric authentication in medical devices. Patients benefit from the increased security and accuracy provided by these systems, ensuring the privacy and confidentiality of their medical information.

Security Protocol – The solution provided by biometric-based IoMT security systems is improved security and efficiency in the healthcare industry. These systems reduce the risk of data breaches, improve patient identification, and prevent unauthorized access to medical data. Additionally, biometric authentication ensures that only authorized healthcare professionals access sensitive patient information, reducing the risk of medical errors and improving patient outcomes.

Issue Handling – Biometric-based IoMT security systems can address various issues in the healthcare industry. One such issue is the high prevalence of data breaches, which can lead to medical identity theft and other fraudulent activities. Biometric authentication can significantly reduce the risk of data breaches, ensuring the privacy and confidentiality of patient data.

5.2.2.2 Biometric Approach

The biometric approach is based on the concept that every individual has unique biological traits that can be used for identification and authentication. These biological traits can include fingerprints, facial features, voice, patterns, iris scans, and other physical and behavioral characteristics. These traits are used as instances or samples to create a biometric template that is unique to each individual. Biometric systems utilize axioms, such as enrollment, verification, and identification, to ensure the accuracy and reliability of the authentication process.

Enrollment is the process of capturing an individual's biometric data and creating a template for future authentication. During enrollment, the system collects several instances of the individual's biometric trait to create a comprehensive and accurate template. Verification is the process of comparing a person's biometric template with a pre-existing template to confirm their identity. Identification is the process of searching a biometric database for a match to an individual's biometric data, even if they are not enrolled in the system.

5.2.3   Risk-Based IoMT Security Model

The risk-based IoMT security model is an advanced and sophisticated security framework designed specifically for the healthcare sector. It is a comprehensive solution that can help to safeguard sensitive patient data and protect against cyberattacks in the increasingly connected world of the IoMT [27]. The risk-based IoMT security model is a robust and scalable approach that can be tailored to meet the specific security needs of different healthcare organizations.

One of the key advantages of the risk-based IoMT security model is its ability to address various use cases in the healthcare sector. For example, it can be used to secure medical devices, electronic health records, and other digital health technologies. It can also be used to protect against cyberattacks on hospitals and other healthcare providers, as well as to ensure compliance with data privacy regulations.

5.2.3.1 Description of the Risk-Based IoMT Security Model

Stakeholders – The risk-based IoMT security model has a variety of stakeholders, including healthcare providers, medical device manufacturers, patients, and regulatory bodies. Healthcare providers can benefit from the security model by enhancing their security posture and protecting patient data. Medical device manufacturers can use it to build more secure products that can withstand cyberattacks. Patients can benefit from the security model by knowing that their medical data is safe and secure. Regulatory bodies can use it to ensure that healthcare organizations are complying with security and privacy regulations.

Security Protocol – One of the key solutions provided by the risk-based IoMT security model is the ability to identify and prioritize security risks. This is done through a comprehensive risk assessment process that takes into account the unique characteristics of each healthcare organization. The model then provides guidance on how to mitigate those risks, including recommendations for specific security controls and best practices.

Components – The risk-based IoMT security model is composed of several components, including risk assessment, risk management, and risk monitoring. The risk assessment component involves identifying and assessing potential security risks, while the risk management component involves implementing appropriate security controls to mitigate those risks. The risk monitoring component involves ongoing monitoring and management of security risks to ensure that the security posture remains effective over time.

<u>Issue Handling</u> – The risk-based IoMT security model is designed to handle a variety of issues related to cybersecurity in the healthcare sector. This includes protecting against data breaches, malware attacks, and other forms of cyber threats. The model can also help to ensure compliance with data privacy regulations, such as the Health Insurance Portability and Accountability Act (HIPAA) and the General Data Protection Regulation (GDPR).

5.2.3.2 Risk-Based Approach

There are several instances where the risk-based approach has been used effectively. For instance, healthcare organizations can use the risk-based approach to identify and prioritize the risks associated with medical devices, such as the potential for cyberattacks or unauthorized access to patient data. They can then develop strategies to mitigate these risks, such as implementing security controls and conducting regular vulnerability assessments.

There are also several axioms associated with the risk-based approach. One of these is that all risks cannot be eliminated, and therefore resources should be focused on mitigating the most significant risks. Another axiom is that risk assessments should be based on sound scientific and technical principles, as well as expert judgment. Finally, regularly evaluating and revising risk management techniques are important to ensure their continued efficacy.

5.2.4   Blockchain-Based IoMT Security Model

The blockchain-based IoMT security model is an innovative approach to enhancing the security of the IoMT through the integration of blockchain technology. Incorporating blockchain technology in the healthcare sector has the capacity to transform the industry by offering a secure and transparent means of sharing data, improving patient outcomes, and reducing healthcare costs. This model is designed to address the increasing need for secure and private healthcare data sharing among healthcare providers, patients, and other stakeholders [28].

One of the use cases of the blockchain-based IoMT security model in the healthcare sector is the secure sharing of patient data between healthcare providers. With this model, healthcare providers can easily share and access patient data securely and efficiently. This helps to improve patient outcomes and reduces the likelihood of medical errors. Another use case is the tracking and monitoring of medical devices. The model allows medical devices to be tracked and monitored in realtime, reducing the likelihood of device failure and improving patient safety.

5.2.4.1 Description of the Blockchain-Based IoMT Security Model

<u>Stakeholders</u> – The stakeholder in the blockchain-based IoMT security model is the patient. Patients have the right to access their healthcare data securely and easily. The model provides patients with complete control over their healthcare data, allowing them to securely share their data with healthcare providers and other stakeholders. This helps to improve patient engagement and increases patient satisfaction.

<u>Security Protocol</u> – The solution provided by the blockchain-based IoMT security model is the secure and transparent sharing of healthcare data. The model utilizes blockchain technology to provide a decentralized and secure platform for data sharing. The data shared on the platform is encrypted and stored in a tamper-proof manner, ensuring that only authorized stakeholders can access the data.

<u>Components</u> – The components of the blockchain-based IoMT security model include the blockchain network, smart contracts, and decentralized applications (dApps). The blockchain network is responsible for storing and securing healthcare data. Smart contracts are used to automate processes and enforce rules on the network. dApps are used to provide users with a user-friendly interface for accessing and interacting with the blockchain network.

<u>Issue Handling</u> – The blockchain-based IoMT security model can handle a wide range of issues in the healthcare sector, including data privacy and security, interoperability, and patient engagement. The model addresses these issues by providing a secure and transparent platform for data sharing, promoting interoperability between different healthcare providers, and increasing patient engagement.

5.2.4.2 Blockchain-Based Approach

In terms of the blockchain-based approach, the concept revolves around the idea of a decentralized and secure platform for data sharing. The blockchain network is a distributed ledger that is shared by all participants in the network. Each block in the blockchain contains a unique cryptographic hash, ensuring the integrity and security of the data [29]. Instances of the blockchain technology in healthcare include secure data sharing, tracking, and monitoring of medical devices, and improving the supply chain for pharmaceuticals.

The axioms of the blockchain-based approach include transparency, immutability, and decentralization. Transparency ensures that all transactions on the blockchain network are visible to all participants, promoting trust and accountability. Immutability ensures that after a block is added to the blockchain, any changes or removal of it is not possible, providing a tamper-proof platform for data sharing. Decentralization ensures that the network is distributed across multiple nodes reducing the likelihood of a single point of failure and providing increased security (refer Table 10.2).

6 TYPOLOGY OF INFORMATION PROTECTION PROTOCOLS

Within the realm of computer security, an extensive array of security protocols has been developed to safeguard computer systems against potential threats and attacks. These protocols incorporate various techniques such as encryption, digital signatures, firewalls, and IDSs, among others. The classification of security protocols, also known as the taxonomy of security protocols, aims to organize these protocols based on their intended use, features, and efficacy. The primary objective of the taxonomy of security protocols is to establish a comprehensive

TABLE 10.2

A Brief Overview of Different Security Models and their Characteristics

Type of Model	Stakeholders	Issues Handled	Security Protocol
Ontology-based IoMT security model	Healthcare Providers, Device Manufacturers, Patients, and Regulatory Agencies	Unauthorized entry to medical information, and tampering with medical images	Security can be customized to meet the specific needs of a healthcare organization
Biometric-based IoMT security model	Medical Device Manufacturers, Healthcare Providers, and patients	Data breaches, improve patient identification, and prevent Unauthorized entry to medical information	Only authorized healthcare professionals access sensitive patient information
Risk-based IoMT security model	Medical Device Manufacturers, Healthcare Providers, patients, and Regulatory Bodies	Data Breaches, Malware attacks, and other forms of Cyber threats	Risk assessment process
Blockchain-based IoMT security model	Patients	Data security and Privacy, Interoperability, and Patient Engagement	Provide a decentralized and secure platform for data sharing

comprehension of the diverse types of security protocols available and their potential applications for shielding computer systems (refer Figure 10.5).

6.1 User Authentication

User authentication is a fundamental security protocol that serves to validate a user's identity. This process involves confirming that the user is indeed the individual they assert themselves to be, and it typically involves a combination of a username and password. The importance of user authentication cannot be overstated, as it ensures that only authorized users can gain access to a given system. Beyond the traditional username and password approach, there are numerous other forms of user authentication that can be employed, such as biometric identification, two-factor authentication, and smart cards.

6.2 Confidentiality

Confidentiality is a security measure that aims to safeguard sensitive information from unauthorized access. To achieve this, encryption is often utilized, which obfuscates the data in a way that only individuals with authorized access can interpret it. The role of confidentiality in shielding confidential information, such as financial data, personal details, and intellectual property, is of paramount importance to ensure their protection.

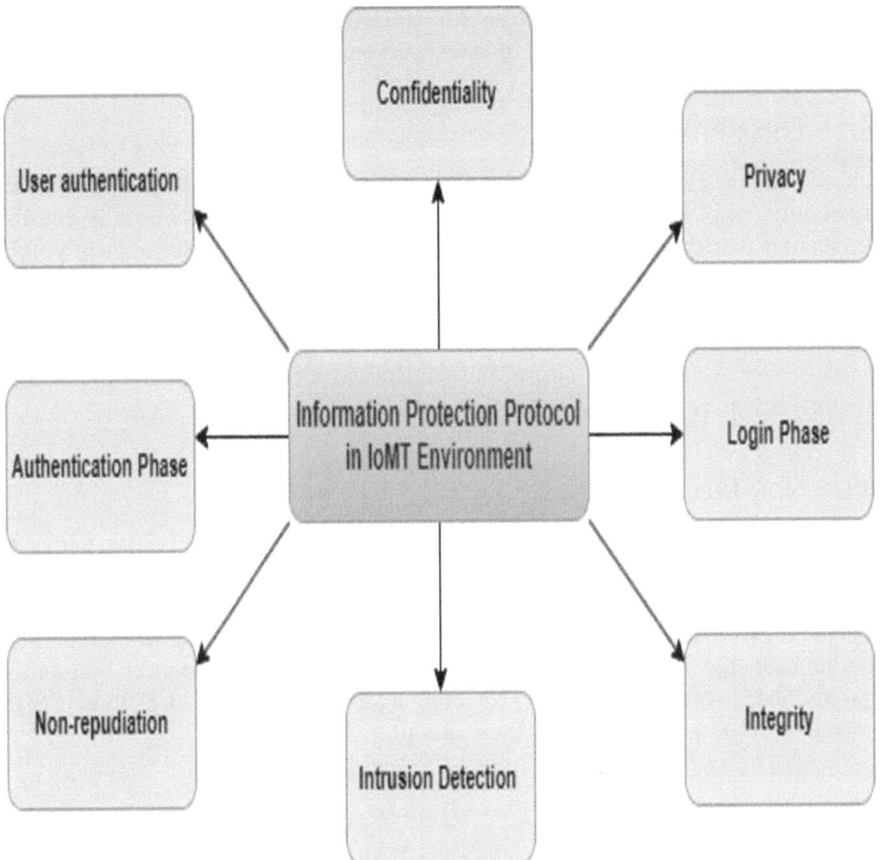

FIGURE 10.5   Topology of Information Protection Protocols

6.3 INTEGRITY

Integrity, as a security protocol, aims to guarantee that data is not modified or interfered with in any way. This is typically accomplished through the use of digital signatures, which confirm the validity and authenticity of the information. Maintaining the integrity of data is of utmost importance to ensure that it is trustworthy and precise, and this is essential for upholding the faith and confidence of users in the information. Preserving the integrity of information is critical for the credibility and reliability of the data.

6.4 PRIVACY

Privacy, as a security protocol, serves to safeguard users' personal information. This objective is usually accomplished through encryption, which guarantees that sensitive data remains inaccessible to unauthorized users. The importance of privacy cannot be overstated, as it is crucial in protecting confidential information, such as medical records, financial details, and personal communications, from unauthorized access or misuse. Maintaining privacy is paramount to guarantee the privacy and protection of users' personal data.

6.5 LOGIN PHASE

The login phase represents a crucial element of user authentication, which is the procedure, employed to verify the identity of a user. This phase usually entails requesting that the user enter their username and password. Subsequently, the system verifies the accuracy of the entered information, and if it is validated, grants the user access to the system. The login phase plays an essential role in guaranteeing that the system only permits access to authorized users. The login phase serves as an integral part of the security protocol to ensure the protection and privacy of a system.

6.6 NON-REPUDIATION

Non-repudiation is a security mechanism intended to prevent users from denying their involvement in a particular action. This is typically accomplished through the use of digital signatures, which serve to confirm that a user has indeed performed a given action. Non-repudiation is crucial in establishing accountability among users for their actions. Its role in cybersecurity is paramount in maintaining the integrity of a system and protecting against potential risks or threats that may arise from users' denials of their actions.

6.7 AUTHENTICATION PHASE

The authentication phase is the process of confirming the identity of an individual, which is a critical component of user authentication. During the authentication phase, the system verifies the identity of the user using a variety of different methods, including biometric identification, two-factor authentication, and smart cards. The authentication phase is critical in ensuring that only authorized users have access to the system.

6.7.1 Two-Factor Authentication

Two-factor authentication is a security protocol that requires two distinct methods of identification to confirm the identity of a user. Typically, in this method a multifactor authentication system employs a combination of factors including something the user is aware of, such as a password, and something the user possesses, such as a smart card or mobile device, to achieve secure access.

6.7.2 Biometric Identification

Biometric identification is a security protocol that uses unique physical characteristics of a user to verify their identity. This can include fingerprints, facial recognition, iris scanning, and voice recognition.

6.7.3 Single Sign-On

The security protocol known as "single sign-on" enables users to access various systems using only one set of login credentials. This approach simplifies the login process and enhances the user experience by providing easy access to the necessary systems.

6.7.4 Federated Identity

Federated identity is a security protocol that allows users to use their login credentials from one system to access other systems. This can improve the user experience and reduce the burden of managing multiple sets of login credentials.

6.8 IDS

IDS is a security protocol that is designed to detect unauthorized access to a computer system. It is typically achieved through the use of software that monitors the system for signs of suspicious activity. IDSs are critical in identifying and responding to security threats, and they are an essential component of any comprehensive security strategy.

6.8.1 Host-Based IDSs

Host-based IDSs are software that monitors individual computers or servers for suspicious activity, such as unauthorized access or changes to critical system files, to quickly detect potential security threats and alert system administrators.

6.8.2 Network-Based IDSs

Network-based IDSs are hardware-based systems that monitor network traffic for signs of suspicious activity. They can identify and block unauthorized access attempts, as well as identify patterns of behavior that may indicate a security threat.

6.8.3 Signature-Based IDSs

IDSs that rely on attack signatures are referred to as signature-based systems. These systems maintain a database of known attack signatures to compare against incoming traffic and identify potential security threats. When a signature matches an attack, the system can respond by blocking the traffic or alerting the security team.

6.8.4 Behavior-Based IDSs

Behavior-based IDSs are systems that use ML algorithms to identify patterns of behavior that may indicate a security threat. These systems can identify potential threats that may not match known attack signatures, making them a valuable addition to any comprehensive security strategy.

6.8.5 Intrusion Prevention Systems

Intrusion prevention systems are systems that can identify and block potential security threats before they can cause harm to the system. They can automatically respond to security threats, such as blocking traffic or shutting down connections, to prevent attackers from gaining access to the system.

7   CONCLUSION

In conclusion, the deployment of IoMT has drastically transformed the healthcare landscape by furnishing patients with tailored and streamlined healthcare services. Nonetheless, the implementation of IoMT also poses significant security risks that must be addressed to safeguard the privacy and safety of patients. The abundant sensitive patient information generated and transmitted through IoMT devices can be alluring to cyber criminals. To mitigate these risks, defense mechanisms, including encryption techniques, access control measures, and network security protocols, are fundamental to securing IoMT data. However, the effectiveness of these security measures is contingent on the security awareness of healthcare personnel and vendors. Thus, comprehensive education and training programs must be developed to promote security awareness among all individuals involved in IoMT, ensuring that they are equipped with the necessary knowledge to recognize and mitigate security threats.

8   FUTURE SCOPE

To advance research in this area, it is crucial to explore the integration of emerging technologies like blockchain and AI, to fortify the security and privacy of IoMT. Furthermore, further inquiries can assess the efficacy of the current defense mechanisms and pinpoint any deficiencies that require attention. Given the rapid expansion of IoMT, it is imperative to stay attuned to the constantly evolving security threats and deploy robust security measures to ensure the safeguarding of patient data at all times.

REFERENCES

[1] Yuehong, Y.I.N., Zeng, Y., Chen, X. and Fan, Y., 2016. The internet of things in healthcare: an overview. *Journal of Industrial Information Integration*, *1*, pp. 3–13.

[2] Cyber Risk Services | Deloitte US | Enterprise risk services. https://www2.deloitte.com/us/en/pages/risk/solutions/cyber-risk-services.html

[3] Synopsys and Ponemon Study Highlights Critical Security Deficiencies in Medical Devices. https://www.prnewswire.com/news-releases/synopsys-and-ponemon-study-highlights-critical-security-deficiencies-in-medical-devices-300463669.html

[4] Venkatesh, D.A.N., 2019. Reimagining the future of healthcare industry through internet of medical things (IoMT), artificial intelligence (AI), machine learning (ML), big data, mobile apps and advanced sensors. *Artificial Intelligence (AI), Machine Learning (ML), Big Data, Mobile Apps and Advanced Sensors (October 28, 2019)*.

[5] Dash, S., Shakyawar, S.K., Sharma, M. and Kaushik, S., 2019. Big data in healthcare: management, analysis and future prospects. *Journal of Big Data*, *6*(1), pp. 1–25.

[6] Adewole, K.S., Akintola, A.G., Jimoh, R.G., Mabayoje, M.A., Jimoh, M.K., Usman-Hamza, F.E., Balogun, A.O., Sangaiah, A.K. and Ameen, A.O., 2021. Cloud-based IoMT framework for cardiovascular disease prediction and diagnosis in personalized E-health care. In (Eds.) Arun Kumar Sangaiah and Subhas Mukhopadhyay. *Intelligent IoT Systems in Personalized Health Care* (pp. 105–145). Academic Press.

[7] Bajeh, A.O., Abikoye, O.C., Mojeed, H.A., Salihu, S.A., Oladipo, I.D., Abdulraheem, M., Awotunde, J.B., Sangaiah, A.K. and Adewole, K.S., 2021. Application of computational intelligence models in IoMT big data for heart disease diagnosis in personalized health care. In (Eds.) Arun Kumar Sangaiah and Subhas Mukhopadhyay. *Intelligent IoT Systems in Personalized Health Care* (pp. 177–206). Academic Press.

[8] Jain, S., Nehra, M., Kumar, R., Dilbaghi, N., Hu, T., Kumar, S., Kaushik, A. and Li, C.Z., 2021. Internet of medical things (IoMT)-integrated biosensors for point-of-care testing of infectious diseases. *Biosensors and Bioelectronics, 179,* p. 113074.

[9] Gupta, D., Bhatia, M.P.S. and Kumar, A., 2021. Resolving data overload and latency issues in multivariate time-series IoMT data for mental health monitoring. *IEEE Sensors Journal, 21*(22), pp. 25421–25428.

[10] Lee, H.Y., Lee, K.H., Lee, K.H., Erdenbayar, U., Hwang, S., Lee, E.Y., Lee, J.H., Kim, H.J., Park, S.B., Park, J.W. and Chung, T.Y., 2023. Internet of medical things-based real-time digital health service for precision medicine: empirical studies using MEDBIZ platform. *Digital health, 9,* p. 20552076221149659.

[11] Hensen, B., Mackworth-Young, C.R.S., Simwinga, M., Abdelmagid, N., Banda, J., Mavodza, C., Doyle, A.M., Bonell, C. and Weiss, H.A., 2021. Remote data collection for public health research in a COVID-19 era: ethical implications, challenges and opportunities. *Health Policy and Planning, 36*(3), pp. 360–368.

[12] Lutimath, N., Sharma, N. and Byregowda, K., 2021. Prediction of heart disease using biomedical data through machine learning techniques. *EAI Endorsed Transactions on Pervasive Health and Technology, 7*(29), p. 170881.

[13] Das, A.K., Wazid, M., Kumar, N., Khan, M.K., Choo, K.K.R. and Park, Y., 2017. Design of secure and lightweight authentication protocol for wearable devices environment. *IEEE Journal of Biomedical and Health Informatics, 22*(4), pp. 1310–1322.

[14] Diez, F.P., Touceda, D.S., Camara, J.M.S. and Zeadally, S., 2015. Toward self-authenticable wearable devices. *IEEE Wireless Communications, 22*(1), pp. 36–43.

[15] Zhou, J., Cao, Z., Dong, X. and Lin, X., 2015. PPDM: privacy-preserving protocol for dynamic medical text mining and image feature extraction from secure data aggregation in cloud-assisted e-healthcare systems. *IEEE Journal of Selected Topics in Signal Processing, 9*(7), pp. 1332–1344.

[16] Šprager, S., Trobec, R. and Jurič, M.B., 2017, May. Feasibility of biometric authentication using wearable ECG body sensor based on higher-order statistics. (Ed.) Petar Biljanovic In *2017 40th International Convention on Information and Communication Technology, Electronics and Microelectronics (MIPRO)* (pp. 264–269). IEEE, Opatija, Croatia.

[17] Bhardwaj, A., Tyagi, R., Sharma, N., Khare, A., Punia, M.S. and Garg, V.K., 2022. Network intrusion detection in software defined networking with self-organized constraint-based intelligent learning framework. *Measurement: Sensors, 24,* p. 100580.

[18] Peng, G., Zhou, G., Nguyen, D.T., Qi, X., Yang, Q. and Wang, S., 2016. Continuous authentication with touch behavioral biometrics and voice on wearable glasses. *IEEE Transactions on Human-machine Systems, 47*(3), pp. 404–416.

[19] Hou, D., Miao, Z., Xing, H. and Wu, H., 2019. V-RSIR: an open access web-based image annotation tool for remote sensing image retrieval. *IEEE Access, 7,* pp. 83852–83862.

[20] Tabassum, A., Erbad, A. and Guizani, M., 2019, June. A survey on recent approaches in intrusion detection system in IoTs. In *2019 15th International Wireless Communications & Mobile Computing Conference (IWCMC)* (pp. 1190–1197). IEEE.

[21] Unal, D., Bennbaia, S. and Catak, F.O., 2022. Machine learning for the security of healthcare systems based on Internet of Things and edge computing. In (Ed.) Ahmed A. Moustafa. *Cybersecurity and Cognitive Science* (pp. 299–320). Academic Press.

[22] Papaioannou, M., Karageorgou, M., Mantas, G., Sucasas, V., Essop, I., Rodriguez, J. and Lymberopoulos, D., 2022. A survey on security threats and countermeasures in internet of medical things (IoMT). *Transactions on Emerging Telecommunications Technologies, 33*(6), p. e4049.

[23] Alsubaei, F., Abuhussein, A. and Shiva, S., 2019. Ontology-based security recommendation for the internet of medical things. *IEEE Access, 7*, pp. 48948–48960.

[24] Sharma, N., Soni, M., Kumar, S., Kumar, R., Deb, N. and Shrivastava, A., 2023. Supervised machine learning method for ontology-based financial decisions in stock market: ontology-based financial decisions in stock market. *ACM Transactions on Asian and Low-Resource Language Information Processing, 22*(5), 1–24.

[25] Pirbhulal, S., Wu, W. and Li, G., 2018, November. A biometric security model for wearable healthcare. In *2018 IEEE International Conference on Data Mining Workshops (ICDMW)* (pp. 136–143). IEEE.

[26] Xin, Y., Kong, L., Liu, Z., Wang, C., Zhu, H., Gao, M., Zhao, C. and Xu, X., 2018. Multimodal feature-level fusion for biometrics identification system on IoMT platform. *IEEE Access, 6*, pp. 21418–21426.

[27] Mustafa, M., Alshare, M., Bhargava, D., Neware, R., Singh, B. and Ngulube, P., 2022. Perceived security risk based on moderating factors for blockchain technology applications in cloud storage to achieve secure healthcare systems. *Computational and Mathematical Methods in Medicine, 2022.*

[28] Pelekoudas-Oikonomou, F., Zachos, G., Papaioannou, M., de Ree, M., Ribeiro, J.C., Mantas, G. and Rodriguez, J., 2022. Blockchain-based security mechanisms for IoMT Edge networks in IoMT-based healthcare monitoring systems. *Sensors, 22*(7), p. 2449.

[29] Jeyavel, J., Parameswaran, T., Mannan, J.M. and Hariharan, U., 2021. Security vulnerabilities and intelligent solutions for IoMT systems. *Internet of Medical Things: Remote Healthcare Systems and Applications*, pp. 175–194.

11 Threat Modeling in Health Care Systems

Gurpreet Singh, Kriti Sharma,
Mamta, and Rajwinder Kaur

1 INTRODUCTION

Threat modeling is the way to analyze the security gaps existing in different health care systems. These security gaps need to be addressed due to the crucial nature of health-related data or complete information [1]. The other aspect related to health care data is the bulky nature of the data itself. This kind of information may lead to the huge amount of data storage to reflect the number of hidden facts or parametric values. The major data types in case of health care systems can be considered as clinical data, medical devices-oriented data or information, supply chain information, and different claims made by patients. According to the above-mentioned data types related to health care systems, it can be observed that the nature of data involved is bulky [2], [3]. To analyze the different sources which are vulnerable due to the huge amount of information involved is a challenging task and it requires a different kind of model to deal with the situation. The different methods involved in managing these threats can be categorized as STRIDE, PASTA, TRIKE, and VAST. The approach STRIDE was introduced by Microsoft to deal with the identification of security threats present in the data used for different computations. PASTA is another model used for threat modeling. It represents the process for attack simulation and threat modeling. This kind of threat model is basically used for business applications where large amount of data entries or information is involved [4], [5]. It basically worked with seven-step architecture by considering the risk centric algorithmic approach. On the other hand TRIKE methodology is used for threat modeling for the purpose of security audits after some given regular intervals. The main purpose of TRIKE is to access the risk involved with different valuable assets. It is used to calculate the risk involved at the level of identified assets, the roles assigned to different users, acceptable actions performed over the bulky data, and the risk exposure defined for each asset. Visual Agile Simple Threat (VAST) is another aspect of threat modeling which is involved in the contribution where the scalable environment has to be considered [6]. It mainly refers to VAST model. The main aim of this model is to scale up the process at any level of software development lifecycle model; either it can be the requirement specification and freezing phase or it

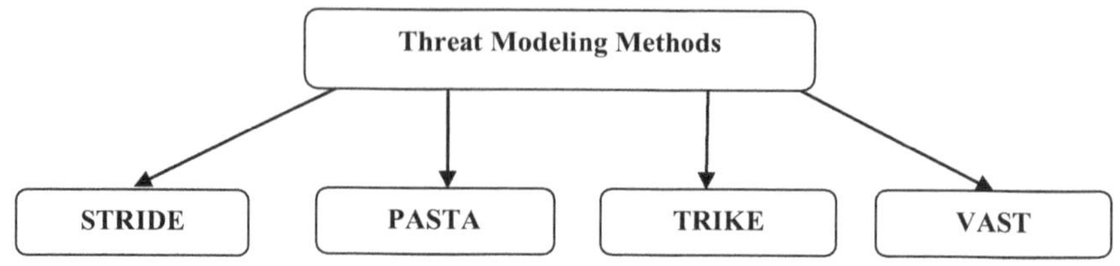

FIGURE 11.1   Threat Modeling Methods According to the Type of Risk Involved

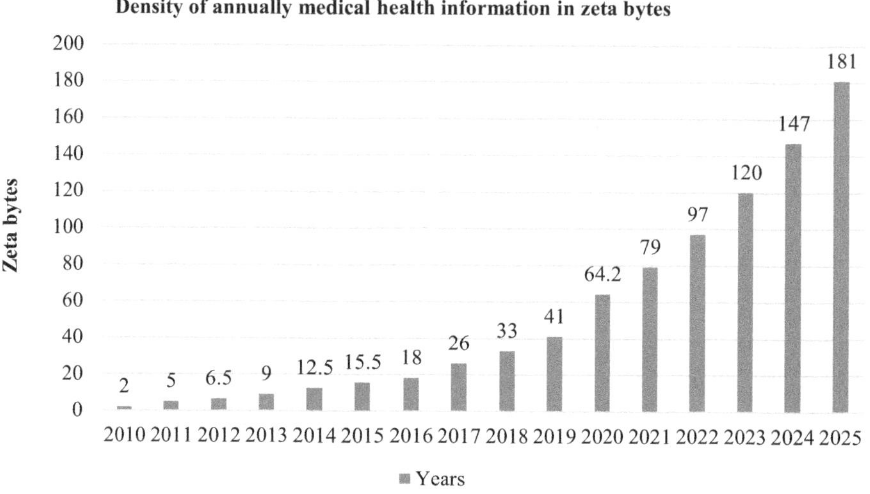

FIGURE 11.2   Annual Growth of Health Information Datasets Over the Years in Zeta Bytes

can be the feasibility study phase of the software or it can be the deciding phase which is reflecting the design of the system where the different modules can be identified and the relationship among modules in terms of their contributions can be decided. Figure 11.1 is reflecting the different methods of threat modeling.

In case of health care systems the data involved under the different categories can be identified as patient health records, device parameters, patient claim records, etc. [7]. The overall growth of the data related to this field is considered to be exponential. Day by day these records are increasing in number and also affecting the overall density of the database. The requirements of data retrieval for these applications need optimized search to fetch techniques and provide quick access to information. Figure 11.2 is representing the growth of health care data with respective years and reflected the exponential growth of this data for the purpose of further analysis. The overall growth of the data is represented in zeta bytes. This exponential growth shows the requirement of handing this huge information from intruders due to the sensitive nature of medical history or normal data.

The next part of this chapter presented the literature related to threat modeling by focusing on the need of different models and the existing techniques in the field of threat modeling and medical applications. After checking the current state of the art, the data analysis aspect of threat modeling has been presented. The next part of the research presented the methodology section. This section highlighted the different threat analysis issues in case of medical data and the solution of these issues in the form of STRIDE modeling. The last part of this chapter will represent the discussion about the proposed solution and its affects.

2 LITERATURE REVIEW

Cagnazoo et al. [1] highlighted the security challenges in the field of mobile health care due to the introduction of technologies like Internet of Things (IoT). The authors also proposed the solutions to address different challenges. The main methodology to deal with the security-related threats to the health care system was STRIDE, according to the authors. The authors also highlighted the different levels of risks involved with the bulky data storage of health care system. All these challenges were affecting the data analysis part of mobile health care systems. The authors defined various threat categories according to the perspective of mobile health care data. The authors also observed the priority nature of the threats. They found some threats which can cause some mental as well as physical harm to the patient. They suggested solutions to these stress categories on a priority basis. They also considered the scenario that there may be a case when the device of high priority may be offline and how that kind of situation can be virtually managed to maintain the security of the system.

Seeam et al. [2] worked on the concept of providing a threat modeling in the area of IoT. They performed the academic audits of research papers and industry papers for the same. The authors discussed various systems such as smart homes, smart city, wearable and health care systems, smart retail, and connected cars. The different profile categories considered by the authors were input validation, the authenticity of the authors, data sensitivity, and manipulation parameters. They proposed to work over the standardization of devices in case of IoT environment.

Almohri et al.,[3] worked on the concept of Medical Cyber-Physical Systems (MCPS). The authors checked the various threat conditions over MCPS and highlighted some security concerns regarding the same. They observed the threats and put them into three main categories: confidentiality, integrity, and availability. The authors proposed the scenario where collective efforts of industry and academia are required to address this issue.

Almulhem [4] worked on a technology which is handling threat modeling. The technique proposed by them was "attack tree". They worked on the system, where the attacks can be considered under the different categories like at the level of client, at the level of server, or at the level of the entire network. Different countermeasures like authentication of users, authorization of users, auditing, detection of malware, timeout policies, server security and encryption, etc. The authors proposed that the early analysis of attacks can prevent the occurrences of these kinds of events.

Lagerstrom and Xiong [5] presented a review on threat modeling concept. During the study part, they focused on the new research done in the field of threat recognition, existing work related to this field of research, and the articles representing an in-depth knowledge of threat modeling concept. The authors observed from the vast literature they considered that many of the proposed models were not implemented in real-time environment and no such validated proofs of the suggested methods were recorded. This means many theoretical models have been proposed with some promising results, but at the ground level, the work still needs to be done. Many future research directions were also highlighted in the presented article.

Omotosho et al. [6] proposed a threat model of IoT devices. For the purpose of handling threat modeling, the authors used STRIDE threat model and for the purpose of providing ranking to different risks involved, they used DREAD. For generating a constraint environment, the authors also proposed some list of selective risks on different IoT devices used during their experimental setup. The authors also made claims that their said model improves the performance of various health devices involved by providing a kind of user interface to the different users to view different types of risks involved in the system. The different categories of users considered by the authors are classified as manufacturers, stakeholders, medical professionals, researchers, and administrators.

Gholami et al. [7] proposed a threat modeling concept for Bio-bank clouds. The authors worked over the different risk strategies related to Bio-bank services. They focused over various requirements of the devices which were must to build a threat model. The authors claimed that the direct benefit of their study is to the researchers working in the field of threat modeling. CPTM threat model was used during the implementation process. The target achieved by this research was the identification and handling of risk involved by checking the proposed ranking model. The authors considered various levels of privacy requirements such as lawfulness, informed concepts, purpose binding, data minimization, data accuracy, transparency, data security, etc.

Gupta et al. [8] proposed a machine learning- and deep learning-based approach for handling threat modeling. The main purpose of the said technique was to detect and address both kinds of threats as known and unknown. Unknown threats can be addressed by using the power of machine learning to deal with extracted knowledge from various patterns observed. The concept of secured data analytics (SDA) was also suggested by the authors to deal with the different patterns present. The authors proposed various SDA proposals as the solution to threat management issues. The extensive comparison of these proposals was also discussed in detail by them. The authors considered different levels of attacks also during their research. The addressed attacks were classified under the different categories like data fabrication attacks, data modification attacks, attacks related to the availability of data, attacks related to communication link during data traveling, etc.

Rizvi et al. [9] proposed a device-level threat model for IoT devices. The authors performed the analysis of different IoT devices for the purpose of finding the points which reflected the vulnerability of these devices against various attacks. They also proposed a threat vector by considering the scenario at three different levels: health care sector, commerce, and home security. In health care sector they focused over the devices like pacemaker, RFID tags, NFC terminal, IP camera, etc. The different types of attacks observed by the research fall under the categories like poor encryption storage, proper authentication of PPD in the case of pacemakers, access of firmware in the case of RFID tags, extraction of memory and control access for NFC terminals, default passwords and back door effects for IP camera, etc.

3   HEALTH CARE DATA ANALYSIS

The major part of health care data analytics can be divided into four major functions. These functions can be categorized as descriptive analysis, predictive analysis, prescriptive analysis, and discovery analysis as represented in Figure 11.3. The major role of descriptive analysis is to get an idea about the historical information related to the health diseases of the patient [8], [9]. This kind of information can be generated from the recorded information about the different medical reports of the patients. This huge information may lead to the security threats. This information can be fetched by the intruders and can be misused for any purpose. So handling this kind of data is one of the major security concerns. The other kind of health care analysis can be performed in the capacity of predictive analysis where from the stored information of medical backgrounds of different persons the idea about the health conditions can be predicted with the involvement of some experts in the medical field. During predictive analysis the completeness of data is the most important concern. The complete information about the predictive function parameters will help during the cause of decease estimation process. The other aspect of health care analysis is prescriptive analysis. During prescriptive analysis again there is a need to

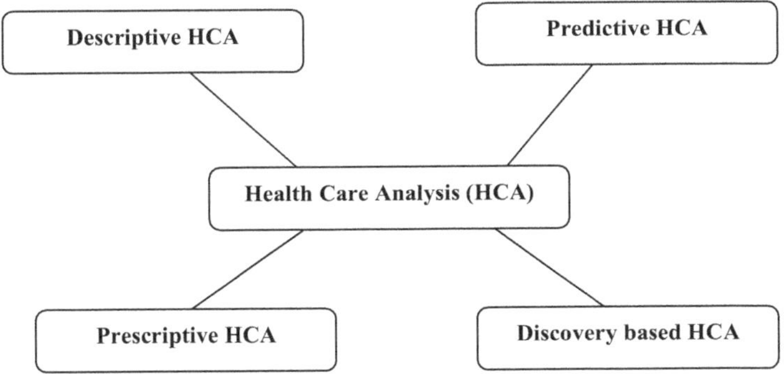

FIGURE 11.3   Types of Health Care Data Analytics

maintain a knowledge-based system reflecting bulky records. These records of the knowledge-based system further help in providing the solutions/suggestions in the form of medicines or some kind of physical exercises based on the values of available parameters [10], [11]. The final aspect of the health care data analysis is to discover the new knowledge based on the existing parameters. This knowledge will help to provide the solution to the problems which are embedded in nature. These kinds of problems are very complex in nature and large in size too. It requires experienced team to solve these kinds of problems. To find out or to discover the new knowledge, very rigid constrains must be imposed to the system.

4   METHODOLOGY

For handling the issue of health care analysis and to deal with the different threats existing in this field the model proposed in this research is STRIDE [12–15]. The major roles performed by this model or the attacks handled by this model are listed as: spoofing, tempering, repudiation, information disclosure, denial of services, and elevation of privileges. All these aspects are represented with the help of Figure 11.4 and are directly concerned with the security of the entire system or the data used. To initiate the process of STRIDE, the entire system is decomposed into smaller units and then a thorough investigation of each subunit has been performed.

The criteria of decomposing these bigger data modules into smaller modules can depend on different isolation factors of different modules like historical information only, medical prescriptions, different claims made by different persons, etc. [39].

Further, spoofing deals with the identification of unauthenticated access. If there is any false identity found with the system, then it is the responsibility of STRIDE model to identify this and handle this threat to prevent any kind of data loss or information hiding [16–18]. This process under STRIDE model is

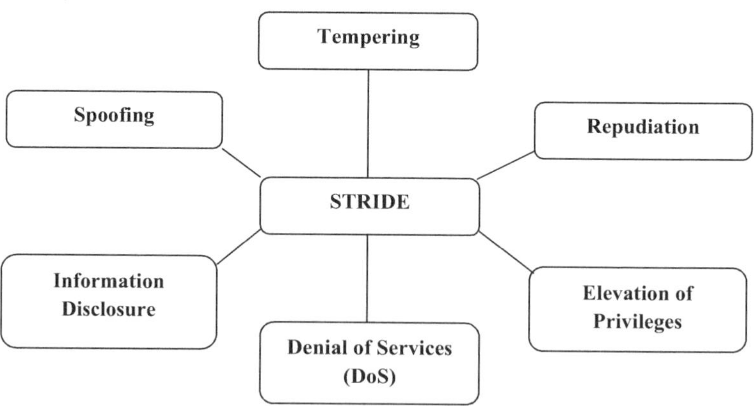

FIGURE 11.4   Risk Categories Associated with STRIDE Threat Model

involved in the functionality of providing authenticity to the users. According to the prospective of medical health security, the different attackers with the help of spoofing can access sensitive medical health information. Most of the time the attackers use the false email credentials of false males to get the authenticated user credentials and then those credentials further can be used to temper the stored information. In the STRIDE model, the following are considered to be the counter measures of the spoofing problem.

- Strong authentication
- Encrypted data storage
- Use of cryptographic algorithms or protocols

During the implementation of strong identification, the user needs to practice with somehow complex credentials or strong credentials which must not be easy to crack by the intruder. Here, the use of biometric credentials is also proposed for making strong passwords. Multi-model authentication or pattern-based authentication can also be implemented to generate strong credentials. In case of encrypted data storage, the sensitive medical information can be used in the form of some encoded data [19–23]. This data cannot be easily understood by the intruder.

To convert the normal sensitive information to some coded form, various encoding strategies can be used like cipher text approach using key strategies. Different cryptographic protocols can also be used to convert the sensitive medical information to some encoded form. Transport layer security protocol or SSL strategies can be used to convert the simple text information to the coded one.

STRIDE model worked over the part of data tempering also. During the process of data tempering, the modifications may be performed on sensitive medical data by any intruder and that modification may result in some loss of important information or may mislead the overall process of medical treatment. Tempering can be performed on data either when the data is at rest (stored only) or during the communication, when the data is traveling from a channel. The major impact created by the tempering effect is to reduce the integrity of a system. If the data is not integrated then it leads to more than one different instances of the same record over different storage spaces. To handle the issue of data tempering, the different approaches proposed by the STRIDE model can be categorized as:

- Impactful authentications
- Hash storage along with digital signatures
- Authenticated communication links

During the implementation of impactful authentication process, STRIDE tried to provide unique credentials to the different valid users of the system to prevent the sensitive medical information from unauthorized access. The user's identity also helps in keeping the track about different update operations performed on the dataset. If any sort of log is required to be checked and that which user updated different parameters of the dataset and when, all these records can be easily fetched from the system [24, 25]. The role of hash storage and digital signature also added more impactful mechanism to find out the user's identity and his/her activity record over the dataset containing sensitive medical histories of persons or other bulky records in the form of prescriptions and claim histories. Digital signatures have been used as a kind of identity proof in digital systems. Generating authentic communication links is also a kind of solution provided by the STRIDE environment where in case of data sending from any remote locations then the sensitive nature of the data can be preserved by establishing a smooth and secure link between the sender and the receiver. Again during this sort of communication, encryption at the sender end and decryption at the receiver end must have to be performed to keep the data as such. Different protocols can be used to ensure this secure communication. The end result of all these steps always increases the integrity of the medical data which is much required and also maintains the confidentiality of the information stored or communicated.

The next aspect of STRIDE model is repudiation. The process of repudiation in this model is concerned more with the protection mechanism from the internal authentic users of the system [26–28]. This deals with the power of denying the occurrence of any event in the system. These events must be performed by authentic users but must not harm the overall sensitive medical information. These events can be categorized as illegal operations performed by some authentic users of the system. These kinds of things can be handled by the different timely audits performed in the system and STRIDE always give this provision. Maintaining different data logs and maintaining the information about the different authentic users who have modified the medical records will help to undo all the affects performed by these operations on the dataset [29]. So, mainly this process of repudiation deals with denying the effects of some of the illegal operations performed by the authentic users of the system.

Information disclosure concerned with threat modeling in health care sector deals with information or data leak. This data leaks can be done in all the three different cases like the leak that can be performed on the data present in the dataset or database itself when it is not in use during any kind of processing. Second, data leak can be performed when some sort of processing over the same data is going on. This means at the time when the data is fetched from the dataset and used with the help of any data structure. Then the attack to leak information over the data structure used is considered under the concept of information disclosure. The final level of information disclosure is the attack on the information when that information or data is traveling through a communication link during any remote communication [30–34]. This part of the data leak or information leak again can either be handled by providing strong authentications to all the valid users or by using the methods of encoding or decoding always at the level of saving information in dataset/database or when passing through the communication link [35], [36]. The use of these encryption decryption protocols leads to the part of confidentiality.

Denial of services (DoS) is one of the major threats which can be imposed by any attacker over the bulky medical datasets containing sensitive information. This attack mainly causes the effect of unavailability of necessary services to the authentic users. As the information stored in case of medical records is sensitive in nature and the unavailability of this information due to the ban of services by any attacker can lead to the major loss either in terms of data and information which was required on time or in terms of major life risks too. STRIDE model handles this kind of security threat by addressing the individual problem based on the category of threat as a software threat or a hardware threat [37–38].

Elevation of privileges is the opposite of DoS attack. During this process of elevation of privileges, the attacker gains access to the different privileges granted initially to the authentic user. After gaining the access to these privileges, again the attacker can perform unauthorized operations on the sensitive datasets. The system in this may fail to recognize the attacker as unauthorized user. STRIDE provides two strategies in this case, first is by providing the role based on the authentication to different users which specifies only specific roles to the users and the tracker can easily track the activities of each user. Secondly by using the principle of providing leas privileges to the user as per the requirement of user. If a user wants to retrieve the information from the dataset/database, there is no need to give full permission to the user to perform write operations on the dataset. Only the required permission can be provided to the user. This criterion of minimum required access to the user will help in improving the overall performance of the STRIDE threat modeling system.

5 CONCLUSION AND DISCUSSIONS

The concept of threat modeling related to medical data has been discussed in this research [7], [8]. Due to the bulky nature of data related to medical health field, the risk of data alteration which results in the loss of data is considered to be high. The major categories of risks have been considered as, risk at the level of communication link during the online transportation of medical records for the purpose of some kind of consultancy or help regarding different recommendations, the risk factor involved in case of authentic information loss due to the involvement of any unauthorized person's attack, and the change or modification of information by the intruder [20]. To deal with the different threats involved in the field of health care system, the STRIDE model for threat analysis has been discussed in this research. The different levels of risks involved in this study have been considered under the categories like spoofing where the unauthorized persons may track the sensitive medical information and may use that information for any other unethical purposes. Data tempering is another issue addressed in this direction. During this period where there is risk factor, the data no longer can be considered as reliable. The tempering on data may lead to miscommunication of treatment or consultancy. The repudiation part of the security threats has also been addressed in this research, and during this risk management strategy, sometimes the denial of any event happening can be one of the solutions to maintain the integrity of data present in the system. Information disclosure aspect of the system also has been covered during the discussions as sometimes because of some privacy reasons the information stored must have to be hidden from the other users using the same system. STRIDE also helps in this and provides the solution accordingly [30–32]. Elevation of privileges and DoS are the other security threats which are handled by the STRIDE model. The different solutions proposed by the STRIDE model comes under the categories like: strong authentications for valid users, encrypted data storage or the storage of data in coded form, use of cryptography algorithms as data communication protocols for secure communication, hash storage for speedy access, etc. For further reference in future, the machine learning and deep learning models along with STRIDE mechanism can help to formulate solutions which may be based on some biometric approaches for better clarity.

REFERENCES

[1] M. Cagnazzo, M. Hertlein, T. Holz, and N. Pohlmann, "Threat modeling for mobile health systems," *2018 IEEE Wirel. Commun. Netw. Conf. Work. WCNCW 2018*, pp. 314–319, 2018, doi:10.1109/WCNCW.2018.8369033.

[2] A. Seeam, O. S. Ogbeh, S. Guness, and X. Bellekens, "Threat modeling and security issues for the internet of things," *2nd Int. Conf. Next Gener. Comput. Appl. 2019, NextComp 2019- Proc.*, pp. 1–8, 2019, doi:10.1109/NEXTCOMP.2019.8883642.

[3] H. Almohri, L. Cheng, D. Yao, and H. Alemzadeh, "On Threat Modeling and Mitigation of Medical Cyber-physical Systems," *Proc. -2017 IEEE 2nd Int. Conf. Connect. Heal. Appl. Syst. Eng. Technol. CHASE* 2017, pp. 114–119, 2017, doi:10.1109/CHASE.2017.69.

[4] A. Almulhem, "Threat modeling for electronic health record systems," *J. Med. Syst.*, vol. 36, no. 5, pp. 2921–2926, 2012, doi:10.1007/s10916-011-9770-6.

[5] W. Xiong and R. Lagerström, "Threat modeling – a systematic literature review," *Comput. Secur.*, vol. 84, pp. 53–69, 2019, doi:10.1016/j.cose.2019.03.010.

[6] A. Omotosho, B. Ayemlo Haruna, and O. Mikail Olaniyi, "Threat modeling of Internet of things health devices," *J. Appl. Secur. Res.*, vol. 0, no. 0, pp. 1–16, 2019, doi:10.1080/19361610.2019.1545278.

[7] A. Gholami, A. S. Lind, J. Reichel, J. E. Litton, A. Edlund, and E. Laure, "Privacy threat modeling for emerging biobankclouds," *Procedia Comput. Sci.*, vol. 37, pp. 489–496, 2014, doi:10.1016/j.procs.2014.08.073.

[8] R. Gupta, S. Tanwar, S. Tyagi, and N. Kumar, "Machine learning models for secure data analytics: a taxonomy and threat model," *Comput. Commun.*, vol. 153, pp. 406–440, 2020, doi:10.1016/j.comcom.2020.02.008.

[9] S. Rizvi, R. Pipetti, N. McIntyre, J. Todd, and I. Williams, "Threat model for securing internet of things (IoT) network at device-level," *Internet of Things (Netherlands)*, vol. 11, p. 100240, 2020, doi:10.1016/j.iot.2020.100240.

[10] C. Wang, Y. Shen, and L. Ji, "Geometry attention transformer with position-aware LSTMs for image captioning," *Expert Syst. Appl.*, vol. 201, pp. 1–22, 2022.

[11] P. Anderson et al., "Bottom-up and top-down attention for image captioning and visual question answering," *Proc. IEEE Comput. Soc. Conf. Comput. Vis. Pattern Recognit.*, pp. 6077–6086, 2018.

[12] J. Lu, C. Xiong, D. Parikh, and R. Socher, "Knowing when to look: adaptive attention via a visual sentinel for image captioning," *Proc. -30th IEEE Conf. Comput. Vis. Pattern Recognition, CVPR 2017*, vol. 2017-Jan, pp. 3242–3250, 2017.

[13] P. Sharma, N. Ding, S. Goodman, and R. Soricut, "Cc3M," *ACL 2018–56th Annu. Meet. Assoc. Comput. Linguist. Proc. Conf., Long Pap.*, vol. 1, pp. 2556–2565, 2018.

[14] G. Singh and M. K. Sachan, "Data capturing process for online Gurmukhi script recognition system," in *2015 IEEE International Conference on Computational Intelligence and Computing Research*, ICCIC 2015, 2016.

[15] G. Singh and K. Sachan, "A bilingual (Gurmukhi-Roman) online handwriting identification and recognition system," *IJRTE*, vol. 8, no. 1, pp. 2936-2952, 2019.

[16] G. Singh and M. K. Sachan, "An unconstrained and effective approach of script identification for online bilingual handwritten text," *Natl. Acad. Sci. Lett.*, vol. 43, no. 5, pp. 453–456, 2020.

[17] G. Singh and M. K. Sachan, "Performance comparison of classifiers for bilingual gurmukhi-roman online handwriting recognition system," *Int. J. Eng. Adv. Technol.*, vol. 8, no. 5, pp. 573–581, 2019.

[18] L. Huang, W. Wang, J. Chen, and X. Y. Wei, "Attention on attention for image captioning," *Proc. IEEE Int. Conf. Comput. Vis.*, vol. 2019-Oct, pp. 4633–4642, 2019.

[19] S. J. Rennie, E. Marcheret, Y. Mroueh, J. Ross, and V. Goel, "Self-critical sequence training for image captioning," *Proc. -30th IEEE Conf. Comput. Vis. Pattern Recognition, CVPR 2017*, vol. 2017-Jan, pp. 1179–1195, 2017.

[20] G. Singh and M. Sachan, "A framework of online handwritten Gurmukhi script recognition," *IJCST*, vol. 6, no.3, pp. 52–56, 2015.

[21] B. Charbuty and A. Abdulazeez, "Classification based on decision tree algorithm for machine learning," *J. Appl. Sci. Technol. Trends*, vol. 2, no. 1, pp. 20–28, 2021.

[22] I. M. Apriliani, N. P. Purba, L. P. Dewanti, H. Herawati, and I. Faizal, "Open access Open access," *Citizen-based Mar. Debris Collect. Train. Study case Pangandaran*, vol. 2, no. 1, pp. 56–61, 2021.

[23] M. Batra and R. Agrawal, "Comparative analysis of decision tree algorithms," *Adv. Intell. Syst. Comput.*, vol. 652, pp. 31–36, 2018.

[24] S. Kanwar, M. Sachan, and G. Singh, "N-grams solution for error detection and correction in hindi language," *Int. J. Adv. Res. Comput. Sci.*, vol. 8, no. 7, pp. 667–670, 2017.

[25] N. Dogru and A. Subasi, "Traffic accident detection using random forest classifier," *2018 15th Learn. Technol. Conf. L. T.*, vol. 2018, pp. 40–45, 2018.

[26] A. Paul, D. P. Mukherjee, P. Das, A. Gangopadhyay, A. R. Chintha, and S. Kundu, "Improved random forest for classification," *IEEE Trans. Image Process.*, vol. 27, no. 8, pp. 4012–4024, 2018.

[27] D. Petkovic, R. Altman, M. Wong, and A. Vigil, "Improving the explainability of random forest classifier – user centered approach," *Pacific Symp. Biocomput.*, vol. 0, no. 212669, pp. 204–215, 2018.

[28] R. Kaur, G. Singh, and P. K. Gaur, "Hybrid classification method for the human activity detection," in *2021 2nd Global Conference for Advancement in Technology*, GCAT, 2021.

[29] V. K. Chauhan, K. Dahiya, and A. Sharma, "Problem formulations and solvers in linear SVM: a review," *Artif. Intell. Rev.*, vol. 52, no. 2, pp. 803–855, 2019.

[30] R. J. Simes, "Treatment selection for cancer patients: application of statistical decision theory to the treatment of advanced ovarian cancer," *J. Chronic Dis.*, vol. 38, no. 2, pp. 171–186, 1985.

[31] D. A. Otchere, T. O. Arbi Ganat, R. Gholami, and S. Ridha, "Application of supervised machine learning paradigms in the prediction of petroleum reservoir properties: comparative analysis of ANN and SVM models," *J. Pet. Sci. Eng.*, vol. 200, p. 108182, 2021.

[32] N. Sharma, C. Chakraborty, and R. Kumar. "Optimized multimedia data through computationally intelligent algorithms," *Multimedia Systems*, vol. 29, no. 5, pp. 2961–2977, 2023.

[33] H. A. Abu Alfeilat et al., "Effects of distance measure choice on K-nearest neighbor Classifier Performance: A Review," *Big Data*, vol. 7, no. 4, pp. 221–248, 2019.

[34] W. Gao, S. Oh, and P. Viswanath, "Demystifying fixed κ-nearest neighbor information estimators," *IEEE Trans. Inf. Theory*, vol. 64, no. 8, pp. 5629–5661, 2018.

[35] S. Chauhan and G. Singh. Hybrid approach for path discovery in VANETs. In: Gupta, D., Khanna, A., Hassanien, A.E., Anand, S., Jaiswal, A. (eds) *International Conference on Innovative Computing and Communications. Lecture Notes in Networks and Systems*, vol 492. Springer, Singapore, 2023. https://doi.org/10.1007/978-981-19-3679-1_48

[36] V. Kukreja, A. Marwaha, B. Sareen, and A. Modgil, "AFTSMS:automatic fleet tracking & scheduling management system," *2020 8th International Conference on Reliability, Infocom Technologies and Optimization (Trends and Future Directions) (ICRITO)*, Noida, India, 2020, pp. 114–118, doi:10.1109/ICRITO48877.2020.9197819.

[37] B. Sharma and D. Koundal. "Cattle health monitoring system using wireless sensor network: a survey from innovation perspective." *IET Wirel Sens Syst*, vol. 8, no. 4, pp. 143–151, 2018.

[38] R. Kumar, N. Sharma, and S. Kumar, "Image intelligence in cyber security using sensing system towards the future generation intelligence," in *2022 2nd International Conference on Advance Computing and Innovative Technologies in Engineering (ICACITE)*, 2022, pp. 298–300, doi:10.1109/ICACITE53722.2022.9823549.

[39] N. Sharma, M. Soni, S. Kumar, R. Kumar, N. Deb, and A. Shrivastava. "Supervised machine learning method for ontology-based financial decisions in the stock market. *ACM Trans. Asian Low-Resour. Lang. Inf. Process*, vol. 22, no. 5, pp. 1–24, 2023.

12 Use of Blockchain Technology for Privacy and Threat Detection

*M Rashmi, D K Girija, H K Shilpa,
and N Yogeesh*

1 INTRODUCTION

Blockchain technology is a decentralizing and distributed database that allows transparent and secured transactions. The technology provides a unique combination of decentralization, transparency, and immutability, making it suitable for privacy protection and threat detection. Blockchain-based privacy solutions offer advantages such as decentralization, transparency, and immutability, which enhance privacy protection in various applications, including identity verification, data sharing, and secure communication. Blockchain-based threat detection solutions offer real-time monitoring, enhanced data security, and reduced false positives. The use of blockchain technology for threat detection has gained significant attention in domains such as fraud detection, malware analysis, and intrusion detection. Hybrid solutions that combine blockchain technology with other privacy and threat detection techniques have also been proposed. These solutions aim to address the limitations of blockchain technology, such as scalability and performance overhead, by combining it with other techniques such as machine learning, cryptography, and zero-knowledge proofs. This part is responsible for an outline of the use of blockchain technology for privacy and threat detection. The first section describes blockchain-based privacy solutions, including their advantages, use cases, and limitations. The second section discusses blockchain-based threat detection solutions, including their advantages, use cases, and limitations. The third section presents hybrid solutions that combine blockchain technology with other privacy and threat detection techniques. This section highlights the benefits and challenges of combining blockchain with other techniques. The fourth section discusses the future of blockchain technology for privacy and threat detection. This section presents emerging trends and potential future applications for blockchain in privacy and threat detection. As a final point, the conclusion abridges the key points of this chapter and highlights the implications for the future of privacy and threat detection.

DOI: 10.1201/9781003377818-12   255

2 BLOCKCHAIN

Blockchain is a distributed digital hyperledger that may retain data records of transactions in an immutable and unalterable format, free from the threat of hacking or other forms of malicious activity. A distributed database is one that is not well-ordered by a solo entity but rather by a decentralized network of computers called nodes. The core concept underlying blockchain is the development of a distributed public ledger that can be used to safely and efficiently record data and verify transactions. As well as a timestamp and transaction information, every single block in the blockchain also includes a cryptographic hash of the preceding block [3].

Each block is connected to the one before it, creating a chain that cannot be broken and contains an immutable record of all transactions. By offering a decentralized and transparent method for recording and verifying transactions, blockchain facilitates confidence between parties who may not know each other personally. This makes it ideal for usage in areas like voting systems, supply chain management, and monetary exchanges. Although Bitcoin and other cryptocurrencies have helped bring blockchain technology to the forefront, the technology's potential uses extend far beyond digital currency. Smart contracts, digital identity networks, and information exchange infrastructures are just a few examples. It's conceivable that blockchain technology will have far-reaching effects on many sectors of industry and culture as it develops and matures. As a form of distributed ledger technology, blockchain ensures the safe and public storage of information across a distributed network of computers.

Healthcare is only one of the many fields where it can be put to use. Blockchain technology has the ability to improve healthcare in a number of ways, including patient confidentiality and the identification of potential dangers. Blockchain technology's ability to deliver protected and see-through access to patient data can help alleviate privacy concerns in the healthcare industry as shown in Figure 12.1. Blockchain technology allows for the decentralized and secured storage of patient data, protecting it from prying eyes. Patients can have more say in who sees and uses their health records with the help of blockchain technology. Blockchain technology has applications beyond protecting user privacy; it can also be used to improve healthcare danger detection. Cybercriminals may aim their attention at healthcare databases due to the high value of the evidence they contain. The use of blockchain technology in the healthcare industry makes patient records more secure from intrusion by malicious parties [13,22]. Blockchain's distributed nature also makes it easy to see when someone tries to make unauthorized modifications to the data, which helps in identifying vulnerabilities and breaches in a system more quickly. Nevertheless, there are several advantages to implementing blockchain technology in healthcare, such as improved privacy and danger detection. Secure and transparent data management solutions will become increasingly important as the healthcare industry continues to digitize and retain more data. This issue may be resolved with the usage of blockchain technology, which is likely to gain traction in the healthcare industry in the near future.

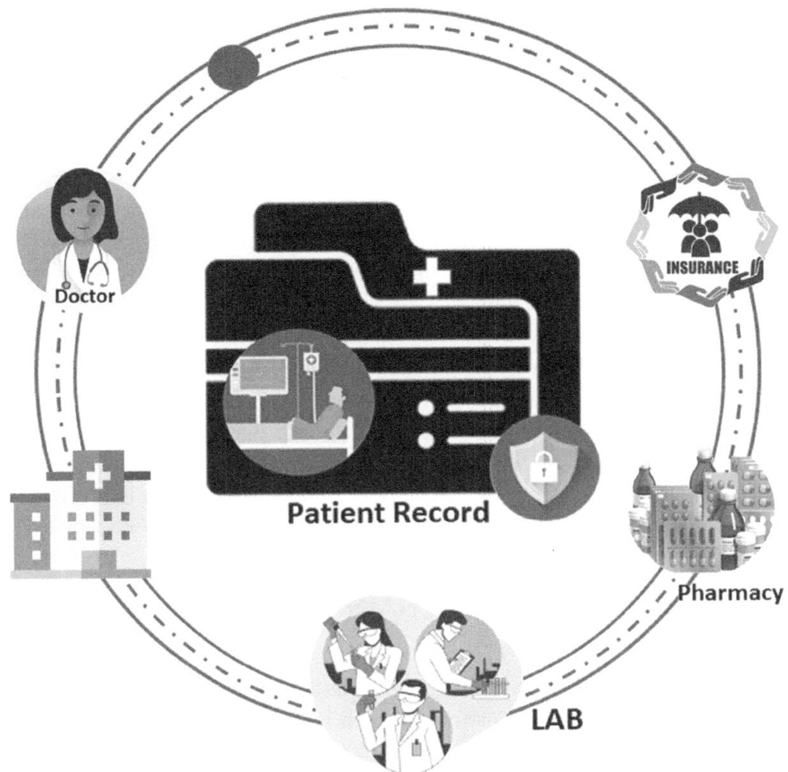

FIGURE 12.1   Healthcare Blockchain. Figure by Author.

3   EVOLUTION OF BLOCKCHAIN TECHNOLOGY

Blockchain technology has progressed significantly since its introduction in 2008 as the foundational technology behind the cryptocurrency Bitcoin. Here are some of the key milestones in the evolution of blockchain:

- **Bitcoin:** In 2008, the pseudonymous creator Satoshi Nakamoto introduced the concept of a decentralized digital currency called Bitcoin, which used blockchain technology to keep a secure ledger of all transactions.
- **Altcoins:** In the years following Bitcoin's introduction, other cryptocurrencies, known as altcoins, began to emerge. These included Litecoin, Ripple, and Ethereum, each with its own unique features and use cases [21].
- **Smart Contracts:** In 2014, Ethereum is made known to the perception of smart contracts, which are self-executing contracts with the rapports of the bargain directly written into code on the blockchain.
- **Enterprise Blockchain:** As the potential applications of blockchain technology became apparent, major corporations began exploring its

use for their own purposes, leading to the development of enterprise blockchain solutions such as Hyperledger and Corda.

- **Interoperability:** With so many different blockchain platforms and applications in use, the need for interoperability between them became clear. Projects such as Polkadot and Cosmos have emerged to address this challenge.
- **DeFi:** In recent years, decentralized finance (DeFi) has emerged as a major use case for blockchain technology. DeFi platforms allow for decentralized lending, borrowing, and trading of cryptocurrencies, with no need for intermediaries.
- **NFTs:** Non-fungible tokens (NFTs) have become popular applications of blockchain technology in the art and entertainment industries. NFTs permit for the manufacture of unique digital monies that can be bought, sold, and traded on blockchain-based marketplaces. The evolution of blockchain technology has been characterized by increasing sophistication and diversification, as developers and entrepreneurs explore new applications and use cases for this revolutionary technology.

4   APPLICATIONS OF BLOCKCHAIN TECHNOLOGY

Due to its ability to provide immutable, auditable, and decentralized ledgers, blockchain technology may well usher in a paradigm shift in many sectors and procedures. The following are examples seen in Figure 12.2 of how blockchain technology can be used:

- **Cryptocurrency:** Bitcoin, the most well-known cryptocurrency, is based on a distributed ledger called a blockchain. As a result, users can send money to one another safely and privately, without relying on any central bank or clearinghouse.
- **Supply Chain Management:** Blockchain technology can be utilized to build a trustworthy and open supply chain management system. It can be used to monitor product distribution from factory to store shelf.
- **Identity Management:** Secure digital identities for individuals can be generated using blockchain technology, which opens up new possibilities for identity management. By doing so, personal information and identity theft can be protected.
- **Voting Systems:** When it comes to voting systems, blockchain technology can be utilized to ensure both security and transparency. It can guarantee honest and unchangeable vote tallies.
- **Smart Contracts:** Self-Enforcing Contracts (also known as "Smart Contracts") are legal agreements that can be written on a blockchain and then executed mechanically. This has the potential to streamline operations and cut down on the number of middlemen involved.
- **Real Estate:** The real estate market could benefit from the usage of blockchain technology, which could help make transactions more open

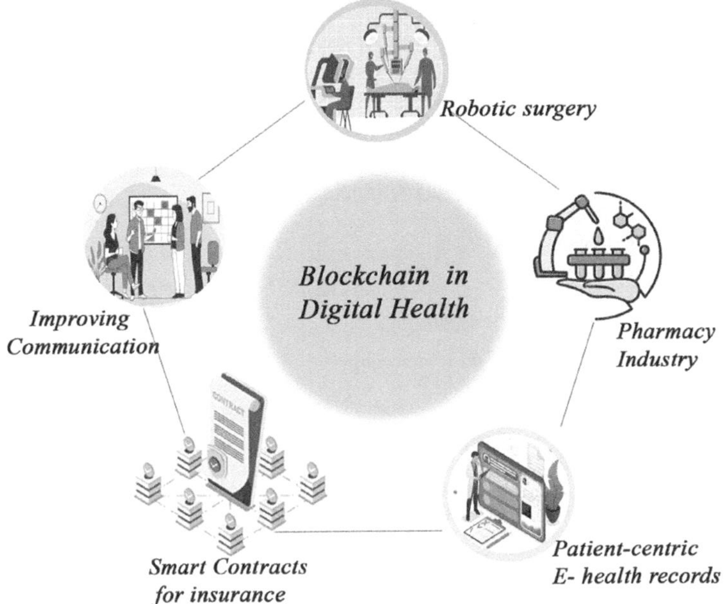

FIGURE 12.2   Applications of Blockchain. Figure by Author.

and safer. In this way, property fraud can be avoided and the correct owners can be identified.

- **Healthcare:** In the healthcare sector, blockchain technology can be utilized to produce trustworthy and traceable patient records. In healthcare, it can help make sure that information is up-to-date and easily transferred between facilities.
- **Energy Management:** Blockchain technology can be utilized to build a decentralized energy management system. You may save money on energy and resources by using it effectively.

In general, blockchain technology has a wide range of possible uses. It's conceivable that as the technology advances, it will find applications in a wider variety of contexts.

5   CHALLENGES OF BLOCKCHAIN TECHNOLOGY

While blockchain technology has many potential benefits, there are also several challenges that organizations face when implementing it. Here are some of the main challenges encountered while implementing blockchain:

- **Complexity:** Blockchain technology can be complex to understand and implement. It requires specialized skills, including knowledge of cryptography, distributed systems, and programming languages.

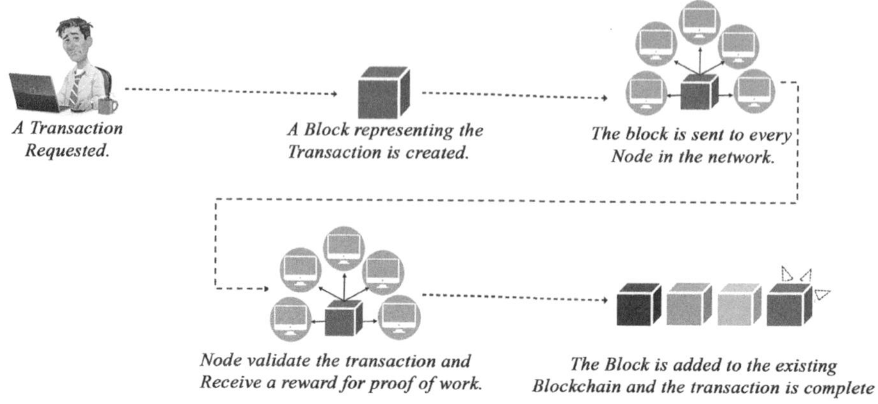

FIGURE 12.3   Challenges of Blockchain. Figure by Author.

Additionally, it can be difficult to integrate blockchain with existing systems.

- **Scalability:** Blockchain technology is still in its early stages, and there are challenges in scaling the technology to support large-scale use cases. Currently, most blockchain networks have limited transaction throughput and can become slow and congested during periods of high usage.
- **Interoperability:** There are currently many dissimilar blockchain platforms, each one with its own exclusive features and capabilities. This can make it challenging to create applications that work across multiple platforms.
- **Regulatory Issues:** Blockchain technology is still subject to a patchwork of regulatory frameworks, which can create uncertainty and legal risks for organizations using the technology [23].
- **Security Risks:** While blockchain technology is inherently secure, there are still risks associated with the use of the technology. These include potential vulnerabilities in the code, the risk of 51% attacks, and the risk of human error.
- **Cost:** Implementing blockchain technology can be expensive, both in terms of the technology itself and the specialized skills needed to develop and maintain blockchain-based systems.

Overall, while blockchain technology holds great promise, organizations face many challenges when implementing it, as shown in Figure 12.3. These challenges will need to be addressed in order for blockchain to reach its full potential as a transformative technology.

6   BLOCKCHAIN IN DIGITAL HEALTH

Staff properties are depleted and patient care is delayed as a result of the lengthy process of obtaining admittance to a patient's medical records. In order to

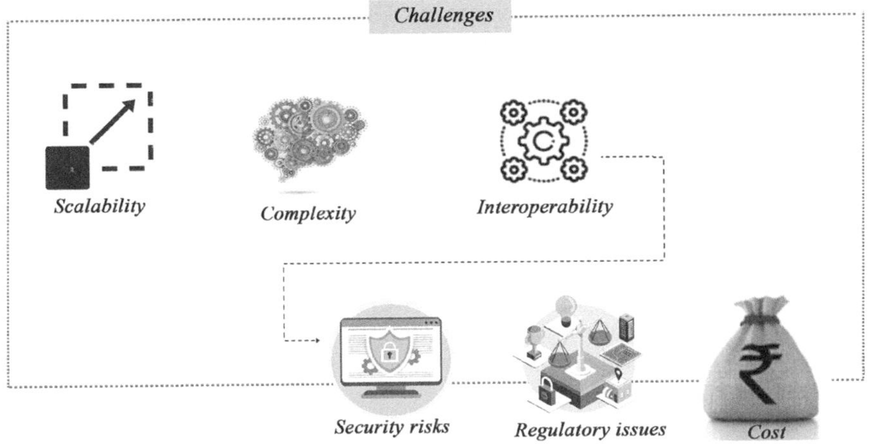

FIGURE 12.4 Blockchain in Digital Health. Figure by Author.

alleviate these problems, blockchain-based healthcare records are being developed. Due to the distributed nature of the system, all healthcare providers, facilities, and other caregivers will have access to the same unified patient record, seen in Figure 12.4. With the help of the blockchain, doctors can more accurately diagnose patients and create individualized treatment plans for them.

- **Blockchain in Pharmacy Industry:** Every day, the pharmaceutical industry faces a new wave of counterfeit drug problems. The pharmaceutical industry includes,
  - Drug Discovery.
  - Drug Manufacturing.
  - Drug Distribution.

So, it's hard to keep track of drugs the whole way through. Because of blockchain's immutability and traceability, it can be used to track pharmaceuticals from their point of production all the way to their final destination. Let's talk about how the healthcare industry could be used as an example of an Internet of Things (IoT) blockchain application. To what extent can Mediledger revolutionize the pharmaceutical sector? Mediledger is an IoT use case built on the blockchain to record the transfer of ownership of prescription drugs. When it comes to tracking potentially dangerous pharmaceuticals, full disclosure and audit trails are mandatory [12,21]. Manufacturers, Distributors, Retailers, and Consumers all have access to the immutable and time stamped data stored on the distributed ledger. Mediledger is a blockchain-based system that can,

- Simplify payment procedures.
- Limit user access.
- Prevent the primer of fake drugs into the supply chain.

Blockchain in Patient-Centric Electronic Health Records: Healthcare systems around the world are plagued by data silos, which have led to incomplete patient and doctor records. Implementing a blockchain-based medical record system that is compatible with existing electronic medical record software may solve this problem. A unique hash function, a short string of letters and numbers that cannot be duplicated and is not stored in the blockchain, is generated from each new record, such as a doctor's note, prescription, or lab result. Hash functions are unbreakable unless the creator of the function has the secret key. The patient agrees to have their data collected and used, making them the legal owner of the information.

Blockchain in Smart Contracts for Insurance and Supply Chain Settlements: Many organizations in the healthcare industry, including manufacturers of pharmaceuticals and medical devices, distributors, insurers, and direct service providers, as well as government agencies, rely on insurance firm-provided blockchain-based systems to verify the legitimacy of their business dealings, record the terms of contracts between themselves, and keep tabs on the delivery and payment status of various products and services [8]. Beyond just supply chain management, this kind of setting also paves the way for trading partners and insurance providers in the healthcare industry to operate on the basis of fully digital and in some cases automated contract terms. Disagreements over expense chargeback prerogatives for prescription medications and other goods can be greatly abridged if all parties involved in the supply chain use a single, centralized digital contract that is stored in a distributing ledger system, like the blockchain.

Blockchain in Improving Communication and Efficiency: Healthcare globally underutilizes blockchain technology. It can make healthcare data communication efficient, transparent, safe, and effective. Tokenization and smart contracts can eliminate healthcare pre-authorization. Blockchain-based health documentation solutions use secure encryption to protect individuals' data when communicating. Tokenization, smart contracts, and blockchain network encryption will drastically reduce pre-authorization, allowing patients to receive timely and informed care. The healthcare provider can now quickly access relevant information instead of relying on the patient or files mailed or emailed from local physicians, labs, etc. Tokenize can improve patient-provider communication and healthcare provider-insurance company communication [20].

Blockchain in Robotic Surgery: Surgeons can perform complicated procedures using small Internet-connected robots inside the body. Blockchain technology with AI and IoT allows small IoT devices to perform robotic surgeries, reducing incision size and speeding patient recovery. These devices must be minor and dependable for minimally invasive surgical procedure. They must also construe complex body situations to make the right surgical decisions. IoT robots are hand-me-down for surgery, proving these challenges can be overcome.

7   BLOCKCHAIN ENHANCEMENT IN DIGITAL HEALTH

Blockchain technology has the impending to transform the digital health industry by refining data security, interoperability, and transparency. Here are some future trends of blockchain in digital health:

- **Improved Data Sharing and Interoperability:** Blockchain technology can help create a more unified and secure system for sharing medical data among healthcare providers, researchers, and patients. Blockchain-based systems can allow for the secure sharing of data across multiple platforms and institutions, creating a more connected and interoperable system.
- **Personalized Medicine:** By leveraging blockchain technology, healthcare providers can collect and analyze patient data to create personalized treatment plans. This can help improve patient outcomes by tailoring treatment plans to individual patients based on their specific needs and medical histories.
- **Improved Drug Supply Chain Management:** Blockchain can be used to pathway and monitor the entire drug supply chain, from manufacturing to distribution to patients. This can help prevent counterfeit drugs from entering the market and ensure that patients receive authentic medications.
- **Increased Cybersecurity:** Blockchain technology can improve the security of digital health records by providing a tamper-proof and transparent system for storing and sharing data. By using blockchain-based systems, healthcare organizations can reduce the risk of data breaches and protect patient privacy.
- **Streamlined Medical Billing:** Blockchain can streamline the medical billing process by providing a secure and transparent system for processing payments. By using blockchain-based systems, healthcare providers can reduce administrative costs and improve the accuracy of medical billing [19].

Blockchain technology has the budding to transmute the digital health industry by refining data security, interoperability, and transparency. As the technology continues to develop, we can expect to see more widespread adoption of blockchain-based systems in healthcare.

8   WORKING OF BLOCKCHAIN TECHNOLOGY

Transactions made using blockchain technology are both safe and easily verifiable. It eliminates the need for intermediaries like banks to facilitate communication between parties. In blockchain technology, computers known as nodes verify and authenticate each and every transaction. A "blockchain" is created when each transaction is recorded as a separate "block" and then cryptographically connected to the one before it.

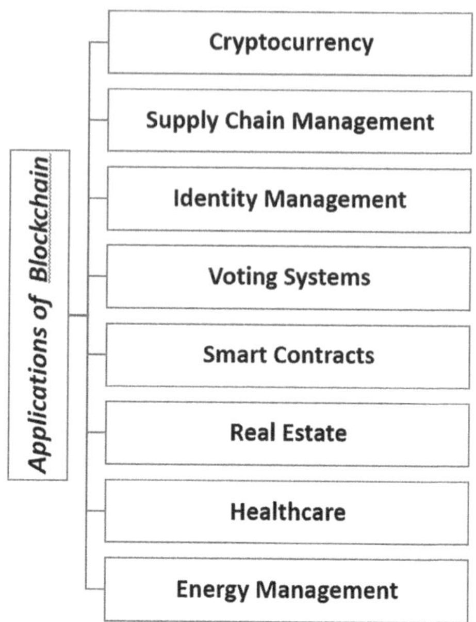

FIGURE 12.5   Working of Blockchain Technology. Figure by Author.

The process begins with a user creating a transaction that is then broadcast to the linkage of nodes. These nodes authenticate the transaction by checking its authenticity, ensuring that the sender has enough funds to complete the transaction, and confirming that the transaction is not a duplicate [2]. Once the transaction is validated, it is added to a block and broadcast to the network.

Once a block is additional to the blockchain, it cannot be reformed or deleted. This is because every single block contains an exclusive code called a hash, which is generated using complex mathematical algorithms. Any attempt to change the data in a block would vary its hash, which would, in turn, invalidate the entire blockchain, pictorially shown in Figure 12.5. This ensures that the facts stored in the blockchaining are tamper-proof and secure.

In addition, blockchain technology is often designed with consensus mechanisms, which allow the nodes on the linkage to approve on the state of the blockchaining. There are dissimilar types of harmony mechanisms, including proof-of-work (PoW), proof-of-stake (PoS), and delegated proof-of-stake (DPoS), among others. Overall, blockchain technology enables secure, transparent, and decentralized transactions, making it a valuable tool for a variety of industries and applications [18].

9   SIGNIFICANCE OF BLOCKCHAIN TECHNOLOGIES

Both public and private blockchain networks are in development, although they serve different purposes. The term "public blockchain technology" is used to describe a blockchain network in which anybody can validate and verify transactions. Cryptocurrencies like Bitcoin rely on these kinds of networks, which are powered by a decentralized system of nodes that validate and record transaction information [2]. Bitcoin and Ethereum are two illustrations of public blockchain networks.

Private blockchaining technology, on the other hand, is a network that only a select few people have access to and manage their own data. Businesses and other organizations frequently use such networks to simplify processes, boost productivity, and fortify safety. Private blockchain networks restrict access to just those with permission, and only a small set of validators verify transactions. Hyperledger and Corda are two examples of private blockchain networks. One major distinction between public and private blockchain networks is the degree to which trust is distributed or centralized. Private blockchains require trusted parties for network management, while public blockchains are built to be trusted less by not requiring a central authority or intermediary to verify transactions [1].

Also, whereas public blockchain networks are commonly linked with cryptocurrency, private blockchain networks are used in a wide variety of applications, such as supply chain management, healthcare, and financial services. To recapitulate, there are key distinctions between public and private blockchain systems in terms of accessibility, decentralization, and potential applications. Private blockchain networks serve the needs of a single company or organization and are not accessible to the public on the whole.

Organizations and smaller communities often adopt private blockchain solutions to ensure the confidentiality of their data and transactions. They provide more options for tailoring the network to meet unique business requirements and more granular control over who has access to the system. Hyperledger Fabric, Corda, and Quorum are all private blockchain technologies.

In contrast, public blockchain technologies are distributed ledgers where anybody can join and conduct transactions without the intervention of a right-hand third party. Everyone may access the network's transaction history and the information kept on a public blockchain cannot be changed once it has been recorded. Bitcoin, Ethereum, and Litecoin are all public blockchaining technology. To sum up, private blockchain technologies are used in closed networks where all users are known and trusted, while public blockchain technologies are utilized in open networks where anybody can join and participate [17].

10 NEED OF BLOCKCHAIN FOR DATA PRIVACY-SECURITY

Blockchain technology offers a decentralized and secure way of storage and conveying data, producing it as an ideal tool for improving privacy and security in various applications. Here are some ways in which blockchain can help enhance privacy and security [6]:

- **Data encryption:** With blockchain, data is encrypted, and users can only access it with a private key. This ensures that sensitive information remains secure, and it is not visible to unauthorized parties.

- **Decentralization:** In a blockchain, data is stored on numerous nodes, making it difficult for hackers to tamper with the system. This ensures that the network is not controlled by a single entity, reducing the risk of data breaches [3].
- **Immutable Records:** Blockchain records are tamper-proof, making it difficult to alter data once it has been added to the network. This ensures that records are accurate and cannot be manipulated.
- **Smart Contracts:** Blockchain empowers the conception of smart contracts, which are self-executing indentures that spontaneously execute when certain circumstances are met. This reduces the risk of fraud and ensures that parties can trust that the terms of the contract will be fulfilled.
- **Anonymous Transactions:** With blockchain, transactions can be made anonymously, providing an additional layer of privacy for users.

Overall, blockchain technology affords a sheltered and transparent way of storage and conveying data, making it an ideal tool for improving privacy and security in various applications.

11   DATA PRIVACY-SECURITY IMPORTANCE

Data privacy, often known as information privacy, refers to the practice of safeguarding private information. To ensure correct data management, data privacy regulations have been put in place to govern data collection, processing, and storage. A company's data is its most valuable asset. Today, businesses recognize the importance of amassing and disseminating information. The company had to follow the law when it came to collecting, storing, and using customer information. In order to ensure that data privacy is described in legislation, businesses working with sensitive data should think about the legal parameters. Identifying the various parties involved is crucial for establishing responsibilities and rights. The parties involved have been classified as:

- A company is considered the data controller if and only if it gathers user information in a voluntary, opt-in manner.
- Trusted Data Handlers who either initiate data collection or specify its intended use.
- Data Principal- Since to the decentralized structure of the network, there is no centralized authority to request consent or to whom consent should be addressed; hence, anonymization could be employed to secure data on the network.

An individual or entity that processes data on behalf of a controller may be a natural person, legal entity, public authority, agency, or other organization. As the number of participants is limited and the central authority can establish and govern the protocol, it is easier to implement regulations in a private blockchain. Nevertheless, with a public blockchain, where there is no central authority, this becomes extremely challenging for anyone taking part in the blockchain [16].

Pruning is employed when data blocks older than a specified time period can be safely removed, but doing so in a blockchain network would require changing a significant number on each node, which is impractical. If a block has been altered or destroyed, forking will begin a new chain of transactions independently of the original chain. If no personally identifiable information (PII) is at stake, then there is no privacy concern; if PII is involved, then one may be subject to the General Data Protection Regulation, which makes it illegal to process PII without a legal reason to do so. The majority of information is restricted, with a few exceptions. Some current tendencies in data privacy legislation include:

The increasing danger of fake news: As people hunker down at home during the pandemic, they are more likely to turn to the Internet as their primary source of information, creating a favorable environment for the proliferation of false information. Monitoring staff members puts companies at risk in court: The company's management felt uneasy about allowing employees to work from home because they couldn't see or hear their workers [12].

The ongoing legal dispute over end-to-end encryption: The Department of Justice has made it clear that they view end-to-end encryption as a serious threat to the security of public keys. To avoid potential lawsuits, businesses will stop gathering as much customer information. The most successful companies keep extensive records on their target audiences. The organization is able to set limits on data collecting because of the stricter legal framework.

12   CIA MODEL FOR PRIVACY-SECURITY

The CIA model, which stands for Confidentiality, Integrity, and Availability, is a widely used model for evaluating the security of an information system. In the context of blockchain technology, the CIA model can be applied to assess the security and privacy of blockchain-based systems.

1. **Confidentiality:** In blockchain technology, confidentiality refers to the ability to safeguard that only official parties have admittance to sensitive information facts. With the use of cryptographic techniques, such as encryption and digital signatures, blockchain technology can provide a high level of confidentiality. Additionally, access controls can be employed at the submission level to avoid unapproved access to penetrating data.
2. **Integrity:** In the context of blockchain, integrity refers to the ability to ensure that data stored on the blockchain is accurate and has not been tampered with. The immutability and traceability of blockchain technology make it an ideal platform for ensuring data integrity. The decentralized nature of blockchain also makes it difficult for any one party to alter the data without the agreement of the majority of the network.

3. **Availability:** Availability in blockchain technology refers to the ability of the network to remain operational and accessible to authorized users. The distributed nature of blockchain technology makes it impervious to single point failures and DDoS attacks, which can impact availability. The availability of a blockchain network can be further enhanced through the use of consensus machineries, such as PoW or PoS, which ensure that the network can continue to operate even in the event of a malicious attack [15].

The CIA model provides a useful framework for assessing the safekeeping and privacy of blockchain technology. By ensuring that confidentiality, integrity, and availability are properly addressed, organizations can build secure and reliable blockchain-based systems.

13 STUDY ON BLOCKCHAIN IN DATA PRIVACY-SECURITY

Governments and corporations alike have started placing a premium on cyber security. A subset of cybersecurity, known as information security, is concerned with safeguarding information at every stage of its lifecycle, from collection to storage to processing. Data security is the result of concerted efforts of humans, business processes, and technological infrastructures.

The number of privacy breaches is increasing despite improvements in security technology. The amount of compromised records in 2020 topped 37 billion, a rise of 141% over 2019. Millions of user details, including names, emails, and passwords, and in some cases even addresses, dates of birth, and financial information, have been leaked due to data breaches [14].

When hackers gain illegal access to a company's database, they can steal sensitive information facts such user names, passwords, credit card numbers, social security numbers, and bank account details. Credit card fraud and identity theft are two ill repercussions of these well-documented security holes, and repairing the damage to a victim's credit can take months or even years. The 2013–2014 Yahoo database breach is among the largest and most recent cyber intrusions; it is believed to have been a state-sponsored strike and affected more than 3 billion subscribers. User names, email addresses, phone numbers, birthdays, hashed passwords, and unencrypted answers to security questions were all stolen by the hackers.

An estimated 143 million people were impacted by a cyberattack on credit reporting firm Equifax in 2017. During two months, no one noticed anything out of the ordinary, and even after they did, it was another month before the breach was reported. Experts suspect that Chinese government-backed hackers were responsible for the hack that compromised Equifax. These incidents demonstrate the potential risk when PII are held in a centralized data base; however, the total financial cost to victims and the security and strategic damage to the state are unknown.

Governments and corporations have amassed vast amounts of PII, and it is their responsibility to keep it safe. In the meantime, these businesses may be

Annual Number of Data Breaches and Exposed Records in the United States from 2010-2019		
Year	Num of Data Breaches	Millions of Records Exposed
2010	662	16.2
2011	419	22.9
2012	447	17.3
2013	614	91.98
2014	783	85.61
2015	784	169.07
2016	1106	36.6
2017	1632	197.61
2018	1257	471.23
2019	1506	164.68

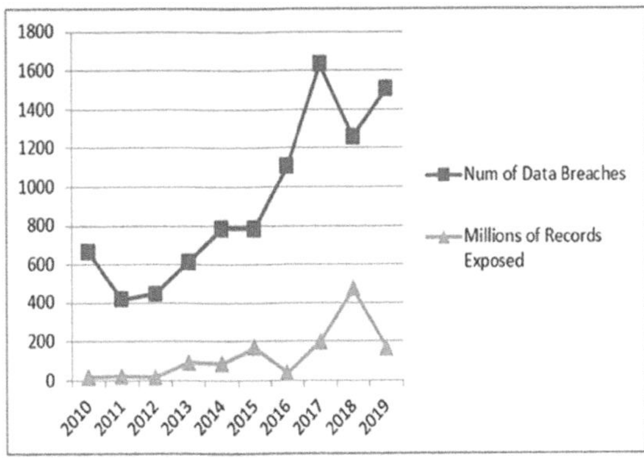

FIGURE 12.6 Annual Number of Data Breaches and Exposed Records. Figure by Author.

making money off of these datasets by either incorporating them into their own services or products or selling them to others. Users are leaving increasingly large digital footprints as the amount of data generated and gathered grows exponentially. Data aggregators can integrate information from several databases in ways neither the original data providers nor the data's end users could have foreseen.

Statista provided the data used to create Figure 12.6, which depicts the financial burden of compiling such massive databases. Cybersecurity incidents and trends are monitored by Statista, a statistics research organization. These incidents have been on the rise, especially over the past five years, as a new analysis from Statista shows, highlighting the importance of bolstering data security measures. It's worth noting that if Russia is indeed behind a large cyberattack in 2020, we might see far higher statistics, especially in the records exposed category. As of this writing, the scope of the breach is still being assessed.

Saluja et al. [25] conducted a literature study in 2022 to explore the application of blockchain technology for big data in collaborative edges. They proposed a framework for secure and efficient data sharing using blockchain technology. Bhardwaj et al. [26] also presented a research paper in 2022, where they proposed a self-organized constraint-based intelligent learning framework for network intrusion detection in software-defined networking. They demonstrated the effectiveness of their approach in detecting network intrusions in real time.

In another study, Sharma et al. [27] presented computationally intelligent algorithms for optimized multimedia data in 2022. They also discussed the use of blockchain technology for secure multimedia data sharing, highlighting its potential in ensuring data security. Furthermore, Kumar et al. [28] proposed a sensing system for image intelligence in cyber security in 2022. They emphasized the potential of blockchain technology in ensuring the security and privacy of sensitive image data.

Hence, the literature indicates a growing interest in using blockchain technology for privacy and threat detection. Researchers are exploring different approaches, such as hybrid solutions that combine blockchain with other techniques, to address the limitations of blockchain technology. The future of blockchain technology in privacy and threat detection looks promising, with emerging trends and potential future applications.

14   PROS OF USING BLOCKCHAIN IN PRIVACY-SECURITY

- **Decentralization:** Blockchain technology is decentralized, which means that it operates without a central authority. This makes it more difficult for hackers to launch cyberattacks or manipulate data since there is no single idea of failure.
- **Immutable:** Once data is recorded on the blockchain, it cannot be altered or deleted. This ensures data integrity, which is particularly important in areas such as financial transactions or legal contracts.
- **Transparency:** Transactions on the blockchain are transparent and publicly visible, which can help prevent fraud or corruption. This feature can also help with regulatory compliance.
- **Security:** Blockchain uses advanced cryptographic techniques, such as encryption and digital signatures, to guarantee the security and privacy of data. This makes it an ideal platform for storing sensitive information.

15   CONS OF USING BLOCKCHAIN IN PRIVACY-SECURITY

- **Reliance on Private Keys:** Private keys are essential for accessing and encrypting data on a blockchain. However, if these keys are lost or stolen, access to the encrypted data may be permanently lost, leading to a potential loss of valuable information. It is important to have proper key management procedures in place to minimize this risk.
- **Scalability:** Blockchain technology has significant difficulties in terms of scalability. The size of the ledger increases as more transactions are put to the blockchain, which slows down the processing of transactions.
- **Complexity:** Blockchain technology is difficult, and its implementation and upkeep call for specific knowledge and skill. Because of this, it may be difficult for small enterprises and other organizations with low resources to embrace the technology.
- **Energy Consumption:** Blockchain relies on complex computational processes to validate transactions, which can be energy-intensive. This can lead to significant environmental impacts, particularly if the majority of the energy used comes from non-renewable sources.
- **Regulatory Challenges:** The decentralized nature of blockchain technology can create challenges for regulators and law enforcement agencies. This is particularly true in areas such as financial transactions, where there are strict regulations governing the handling of sensitive information.

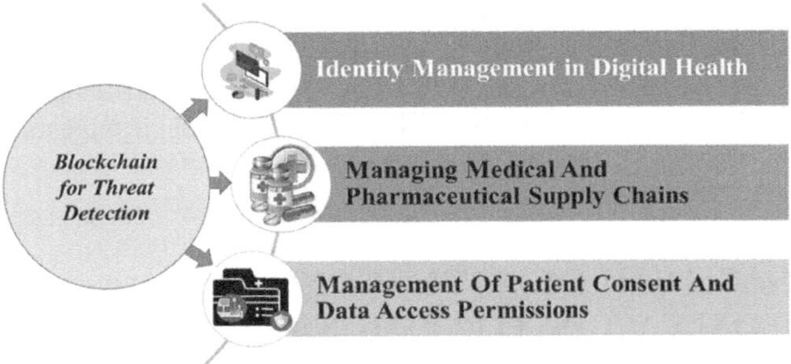

FIGURE 12.7 Blockchain for Threat Detection. Figure by Author.

16 BLOCKCHAIN FOR THREAT DETECTION

The sensitive and valuable nature of patient data makes the healthcare business a prominent target for cyberattacks. Those in the medical field must always be on the lookout for any signs of security breaches or dangers within their networks. Fortunately, blockchaining technology can help identify and avert such dangers. Blockchaining is a decentralized, secure, and immutable ledger system. Data on the network is protected from tampering because of the technology's decentralized design. Figure 12.7 shows, by keeping track of all network activities in a distributed ledger, blockchaining technology can be put to use in the healthcare industry to monitor and identify potential dangers.

17 IDENTITY MANAGEMENT IN DIGITAL HEALTH

For the purpose of identity management in the digital health industry, blockchain technology can provide substantial benefits. Good healthcare outcomes rely on accurate identification of patients, providers, and organizations; blockchain technology has the impending to increase integrity, transparency, and security in this regard. By keeping an immutable record of each time, a data record is viewed or modified, and blockchain technology can help healthcare providers ensure that their patients' records are always up-to-date and accurate. This can be especially useful when trying to connect information gathered by wearable medical devices and the IoT with an individual's electronic medical records. The KSI blockchain system has been implemented in Estonia to secure sensitive government data containing electrical health records from external cyberattacks and unauthorized internal access [9]. Any changes made to a record may be double-checked using independent Bldent electronic records, and the system offers security without compromising data privacy. This makes it easier to detect harmful activity and stop it in its tracks.

The real value of blockchain technology in a health information system comes from integrating it with other technologies, as the transactional footprint of blockchain instructions is rather modest in comparison to the actual health information held off-chain. Identity management in the digital health industry can greatly benefit from the increased integrity, transparency, and security that blockchain technology can bring. Improving healthcare outcomes requires accurate patient and provider identification, which can be achieved through the establishment of an immutable log of data access and revisions.

18 MANAGEMENT OF PATIENT CONSENT AND DATA ACCESS PERMISSIONS

Consent and authorization management for accessing patient data is an integral part of the healthcare ecosystem. There has been growing interest in using blockchain to provide patients with a trustworthy, verifiable, and secure means of controlling their own health information in recent years. By providing a distributed and irreversible ledger, blockchain technology may be used to manage dynamic consent and permissions, giving users full say over their data and who has access to it. Blockchain technology's capacity to provide dynamic consent is a major advantage when it comes to patient consent and authorization for accessing data. Dynamic consent enables individuals to give or remove access to their data on an as-needed basis, as opposed to the blanket or once-only nature of other permission models. In the healthcare industry, where electronic data can be reused indefinitely for new research topics, this is of paramount importance [7].

The MedRec system, created by the MIT media lab, is one example of a blockchain-enabled system for maintaining patient consent. MedRec makes use of blockchain smart contracts to retain track of interactions between patients and healthcare providers, as well as to link medical records to permissions and instructions for retrieving data from third-party sources [11]. A provider's note is considered legitimate only after it has been checked and the patient has given permission for others to examine it. An automated alert and encrypted link to the updated medical record are sent to the designated recipient. With the permissions recorded on the blockchain, patients can view and manage their own data. The Dwarna system at the Malta biobank is another application of blockchain technology for managing patient rights and data access. Dwarna uses a blockchain to produce an immutable record of consent, which increases the confidence in the biobank by giving donors more say over which research they participate in and whether or not their biospecimens are destroyed if they change their minds [4].

As another application of blockchain technology, safeguarding the authenticity of medical imaging records is possible. By leveraging blockchain technology, RadBit ensures that patients always have full control over and access to their medical photos. Users of the blockchain can generate tokens that temporarily grant access to healthcare providers and insurance firms. The token has no relation to the data itself; it merely contains permission commands that are checked and validated by being appended to a chain, at which point the necessary reports are sent out. Blockchain technology offers the pharmaceutical sector a safe method of managing the transfer of sensitive personal data during the recruitment phase of clinical trials. Two significant blockchain-backed initiatives in the pharmaceutical ecosystem are the Innovative Medicines Initiative (IMI) Blockchain-Enabled Healthcare Project and the Pharmaceutical Users Software Exchange (PhUSE) Blockchain Project [7]. Individuals can maintain control over their data by keeping it secluded until an agreement is made, and research teams can be certain that they are gaining access to genuine and meaningful information thanks to blockchain technology.

The new blockchain application known as Research Foundry facilitates the administration of rights and access to health research materials such as data, metadata, software code, and other items tied to health research, such as those conducted in response to the COVID-19 epidemic [5]. Its goal is to make international collaboration easier in a way that doesn't break any data privacy laws. With this approach, each node in the network can decide for itself which pieces of information to make available to the rest of the network. The healthcare industry is ripe for a blockchain-powered overhaul of how permits for patient data are managed. Blockchain technology has the potential to enhance patient autonomy, recruitment and retention in biomedical research, and data integrity by providing a transparent, auditable, and secure method for individuals to handle their own health data. Blockchain technology will play an increasingly crucial role in the healthcare business as it continues to digitize and generate enormous volumes of data, ensuring that this data is managed securely and reliably [10].

19 MANAGING MEDICAL AND PHARMACEUTICAL SUPPLY CHAINS

Supply chain management for healthcare and pharmaceutical items is benefiting from the widespread adoption of blockchain technology. Identification, tracking, verification, notification, and actionable data on purchases are just some of the perks it provides. These advantages address problems with confidence that result from disruptions in supply chains and worries about non-compliant items, counterfeiting, and fraud. The COVID-19 epidemic has brought into focus the importance of blockchain-enabled supply chains for verifying supplier legitimacy and monitoring shipments [5]. IBM Rapid Supplier Connect, for instance, is a blockchain-enabled network that brings together non-traditional suppliers of equipment, devices, and supplies with government and healthcare organizations to combat the spread of the COVID-19 virus. Chinese hospitals are using blockchain technology to keep track of COVID-19 patients' prescription orders and promptly ship them to their homes.

Protection of intellectual property, quality control, counterfeiting, and illegal sales of drugs all pose trust concerns in the pharmaceutical sector. Drug shortages can be avoided with the help of blockchain technology, which can verify the identities of sellers and buyers, as well as date and track goods. The

Hyperledger Counterfeit Pharmaceuticals Project illustrates how products can be timestamped and put on a blockchaining for pursuing and verification purposes. A similar set of challenges, including high-risk equipment with an antiquity of security vulnerabilities, affects medical device supply chains. After agreed upon standards and protocols have been established, blockchaining technology can be used to increase the safety, openness, and credibility of these endeavors. The availability of personnel, hospital beds, intensive care unit beds, and other essentials must be coordinated across numerous hospitals and health authorities during the COVID-19 epidemic. Blockchaining is a viable option since it can fix problems with trust and information sharing. Supply chain management for healthcare and pharmaceutical items can benefit greatly from blockchaining technology [24]. In doing so, it addresses issues of confidence and concerns about non-compliant products, counterfeiting, and fraud by providing transparency, immutability, and security. Blockchaining technology is likely to play a larger role in supply chain management in the healthcare business as it continues to develop.

20 CONCLUSION AND FUTURE LOOKUP

Furthermore, by solving problems with data security, interoperability, and care coordination, blockchaining technology has the potential to completely transform the healthcare system. Blockchain's decentralized and immutable nature can improve the accuracy, efficiency, and cost-effectiveness of medical care while minimizing the dangers associated with conventional client-server and cloud-based approaches. Although there are still technological hurdles to jump, like slow processing speed and lack of scalability, the field is advancing rapidly and these problems should be solved soon. In addition, the expansion of blockchaining technology into the healthcare sector may provide new avenues for investigation, especially in the realm of medical study. Age, gender, familiarity, and other contextual factors may all have a role in the acceptance and deployment of blockchaining technology in healthcare, thus future research should focus on these and other characteristics. By fixing these problems, blockchaining technology in healthcare can go even further, which in turn will benefit patients. It is anticipated that blockchaining will play an increasingly crucial role in enhancing the quality and efficiency of patient care as the healthcare industry continues to develop and realize its huge potential.

As blockchain technology continues to evolve and become more prevalent in various industries, including finance, healthcare, and supply chain management, security remains a critical concern. Here are some future trends of blockchain security:

- **Greater Use of Encryption:** Encryption is essential for protecting data stored on a blockchain. As the technology continues to advance, we can expect to see more sophisticated encryption algorithms that can provide even greater security.

- **Improved Access Control:** Blockchain-based systems can benefit from access control mechanisms that limit who can access the data and perform transactions. This can help avert unauthorized access and decrease the risk of data breaches.
- **Blockchain Interoperability:** The ability to link multiple blockchains together can help improve security by creating a more decentralized system that is more resilient to attacks. This can also enable more efficient and secure data exchange across different blockchain networks.
- **Privacy Enhancing Technologies:** With concerns around data privacy and confidentiality, blockchaining developers are increasingly exploring privacy augmenting technologies such as zero-knowledge proofs and homomorphic encrypting to secure penetrating data.
- **Consensus Algorithms:** The consensus algorithm is an essential component of blockchaining technology, and developers are continually exploring new algorithms that can improve security while maintaining scalability and speed.

Overall, blockchain security is an ever-evolving field, and as the technology continues to mature, we can expect to see ongoing improvements in security measures. However, it's important to note that blockchain security is a complex topic, and continued research and development will be necessary to keep pace with the evolving security threats.

REFERENCES

[1] Mukhopadhyay U, Skjellum A, Hambolu O, Oakley J, Yu L, & Brooks R (2016). "A brief survey of cryptocurrency systems." In *2016 14th annual conference on privacy, security and trust (PST)*, pp. 745–752. IEEE, 2016.

[2] Angeletti F, Chatzigiannakis I & Vitaletti A (2017). The Role of Blockchain and IoT in Recruiting Participants for Digital Clinical Trials 2017. In *25th International Conference on Software, Telecommunications and Computer Networks (SoftCOM), Split* (pp. 1–5).

[3] Yogeesh N & Chenniappan PK (2013). Study on intuitionistic fuzzy graphs and its applications in the field of real world. *International Journal of Advanced Research in Engineering and Applied Sciences*, 2(1), 104–114.

[4] Wust K & Gervais A (2017). Do you need a blockchain? *IACR Cryptology ePrint Archive*, 2017(2017), 375.

[5] Clauson KA, Breeden EA, Davidson C & Mackey TK (2018, March 23). Leveraging blockchain technology to enhance supply chain management in healthcare. *Blockchain in Healthcare Today*, 1. https://doi.org/10.30953/bhty.v1.20

[6] Yogeesh N & Chenniappan PK (2012). A conceptual discussion about an intuitionistic fuzzy-sets and its applications. *International Journal of Advanced Research in IT and Engineering*, 1(6), 45–55.

[7] Ting DSW, Carin L, Dzau V & Wong TY (2020). Digital technology and COVID-19. *Nature Medicine*. https://doi.org/10.1038/s41591-020-0824-5

[8] Li Y, Marier-Bienvenue T, Perron-Brault A, Wang X & Par G (2018). Blockchain technology in business organizations: a scoping review.

[9] Vazirani AA, O'Donoghue O, Brindley D & Meinert E (2019, February 12). Implementing blockchains for efficient health care: systematic review. *Journal of Medical Internet Research*, 21(2). Retrieved from https://www.ncbi.nlm.nih.gov/pubmed/30747714

[10] Hussain A, Malik A, Halim MU & Ali AM (2014). The use of robotics insurgery: a review. *International Journal of Clinical Practice*, 68(11), 1376–1382.

[11] Mamo NMG. (2019). Dwarna: a blockchain solution for dynamic consent in biobanking. *European Journal of Human Genetics*. https://doi.org/10.1038/s41431-019-0560-9

[12] Mettler M (2016). Blockchain technology in healthcare: the revolution starts here. *IEEE 18th International Conference on e-Health Networking. Applications and Services (Healthcom)*, 1–3. https://doi.org/10.1109/HealthCom.2016.7749510

[13] Pilkington M (2016). Blockchain technology: principles and applications. In *Research handbook on digital transformations* (pp. 225–253). Edward Elgar Publishing.

[14] Azaria A, Ekblaw A, Vieira T, Lippm an A & Medrec (2016). *Using blockchain for medical data access and permission management. In 2016 2nd international conference on open and big data (OBD)* (pp. 25–30). IEEE press.

[15] Bhme R, Christin N, Edelman B & Moore T (2015). Bitcoin: economics, technology, and governance. *Journal of economic Perspectives*, 29(2), 213–238.

[16] Gupta K, Choubey S, Yogeesh N, William P, Vasanthakumari TN &, Chaitanya PK (2023). Implementation of motorist weariness detection system using a conventional object recognition technique. In *2023 International Conference on Intelligent Data Communication Technologies and Internet of Things (IDCIoT)* (pp. 640–646). Bengaluru, India: IEEE. https://doi.org/10.1109/IDCIoT56793.2023.10052783

[17] Sallstrom L, Morris O & Mehta H (2019). Ethical considerations: artificial intelligence in Africa's healthcare: ethical considerations. *ORF Issue Brief* 312, 1–11.

[18] Bush J (2018). How AI is taking the scut work out of health care. *Harvard Business Review*, 5.

[19] World Health Organization. Draft global strategy on digital health 2020–2024. https://apo.org.au/node/237341

[20] Guo J &, Li B (2018). The application of medical artificial intelligence technology in rural areas of developing countries. *Health Equity*, 2(1), 174–181.

[21] Caprara R, Obstein KL, Scozzarro G, Di Natali C, Beccani M, Morgan DR, Valdastri P (2015). A platform for gastric cancer screening in low- and middle-income countries. *IEEE Transactions on Biomedical Engineering*, 62(5) (2014), 1324–1332.

[22] Hunter J, Cookson J & Wyatt J (1989). *Second European Conference on artificial intelligence in medicine, London, August 29th–31st 1989. Proceedings*. In Lecture Notes in Medical Informatics, Vol. 38. Berlin, Heidelberg: Springer Berlin Heidelberg. AIME 89.

[23] Alami H, Lehoux P, Auclair Y, de Guise M, Gagnon MP, Shaw J, Roy D, Fleet R, Ag Ahmed MA & Fortin JP (2020). Anticipating a new level of complexity. *JMIR*, 22(7), e17707. PMID: 32406850.

[24] Moyo S, Doan TN, Yun JA & Tshuma N (2018). Application of machine learning models in predicting length of stay among healthcare workers in underserved communities in South Africa. *Human Resources for Health*, 16, 1-9.

[25] Saluja, Kamal, Sunil Gupta, Amit Vajpayee, Sanjoy Kumar Debnath, Ankit Bansal, and Neha Sharma (2022). Blockchain technology: Applied to big data in collaborative edges. *Measurement: Sensors*, 24, 100521.

[26] Bhardwaj, Anurag, Ritu Tyagi, Neha Sharma, Akhilendra Khare, Manbir Singh Punia, and Vikash Kumar Garg (2022). Network intrusion detection in software defined networking with self-organized constraint-based intelligent learning framework. *Measurement: Sensors* 24, 100580.

[27] Sharma, Neha, Chinmay Chakraborty, and Rajeev Kumar (2022). Optimized multimedia data through computationally intelligent algorithms. *Multimedia Systems* 29(5), 2961-2977.

[28] Kumar, Rajeev, Neha Sharma, and Sandeep Kumar (2022). Image Intelligence in Cyber Security using Sensing System towards the Future Generation Intelligence. In *2022 2nd International Conference on Advance Computing and Innovative Technologies in Engineering (ICACITE)* (pp. 298-300). IEEE.

13 Blockchain-Based Decentralized Biometric Authentication System for Vulnerability Analysis

Gurpreet Singh, Sunil Kumar Chawla,
Pradeepta Kumar Sarangi, Neha Sharma,
and Divyanshu Ranjan

1 INTRODUCTION

Blockchain is one of the developing technologies with a relatively robust cryptographic base, allowing applications to use its characteristics to achieve resilient security solutions [1]. Blockchain technology creates an immutable and decentralized data registry that can optionally execute distributed safe code. The origin of blockchain technology is linked to the Bitcoin cryptocurrency dating back in 2009. The earliest instances of its usage are found in solving an old problem in the cryptographic community that has been open since the 1980s. To the center of the blockchain technology is the design of a consensus-based distributed algorithm on financial transactions without the human intervention, even for verification and auditing. Nothing, however, precludes other digital data from being stored in place of economic transactions. This storage provided by blockchain technology in the form of decentralized ledgers is secure enough to sustain, even in the presence of cyber attacks. This feature opens a huge scope to a wide range of potential applications, including smart energy and grids, healthcare, and smart devices for smart cities, as well as digital identification schemes [2]. On the other hand, due to their capacity to offer a practical and secure means of authentication, current biometric technologies have grown in popularity in recent years [3]. The unique nature of human biometric traits makes them difficult to copy or steal. For providing improved security mechanism, biometric technologies have been implemented by a number of businesses, including finance, healthcare, and government. Although these systems have made great strides in terms of convenience and security, they

DOI: 10.1201/9781003377818-13

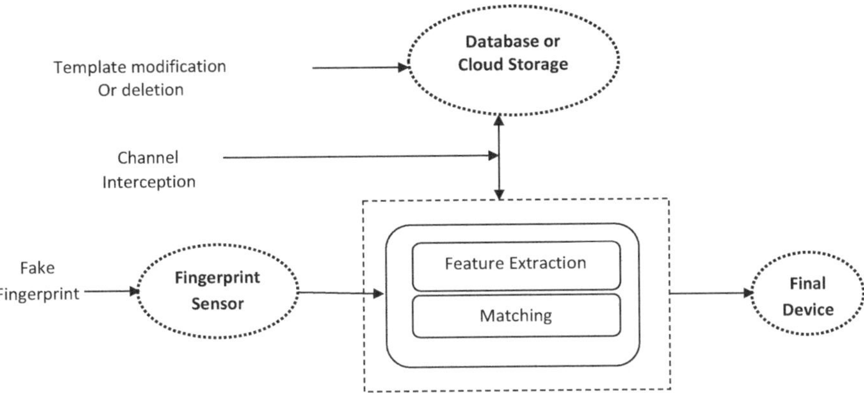

FIGURE 13.1   Traditional Biometric Systems

still have issues with privacy, security, and accessibility. For instance, centralized biometric systems are frequently expensive to run and maintain and are susceptible to attacks and data breaches. Blockchain-based biometric systems provide a potential answer to these problems by offering a decentralized, secure, and open platform for authentication. Biometric data can be kept on a distributed ledger utilizing blockchain technology, which is tamper-proof and accessible to authorized users only. As there is no longer a requirement for a central database, there is less chance of data breaches and unauthorized access. Additionally, blockchain-based systems can be more affordable and accessible than centralized systems. Figure 13.1 shows the working of a traditional biometric system.

1.1 BLOCKCHAIN

Blockchain is a decentralized digital ledger that securely, openly, and impenetrably logs activities. It is a kind of distributed ledger technology where the upkeep is done by a network of computers as opposed to a single hub or middleman [4]. Before being added to the chain, the network of computers, known as nodes, verifies and validates a collection of transactions contained in each block of a blockchain. A block cannot be changed or removed after it has been added to the chain without a network agreement. Blockchain is now a very safe and trustworthy way to store and send info. Cryptographic algorithms are used by blockchain technology to safeguard transactions and guarantee the accuracy of the data on the chain. A consensus method, such as proof of work or proof of stake, which ensures that all nodes on the network concur on the ledger's state, is used to verify the transactions and add them to the chain. The openness and immutability of blockchain technology are two of its main advantages. The complete blockchain is replicated across the network's nodes, making all transactions visible and auditable to anyone with network access. Furthermore, once a transaction is fed to the blocks on the chain, it cannot be altered or removed, ensuring high security and trust in the information stored on the blockchain. [5]

1.2 Genesis Block

The genesis block is the initial block in a blockchain. It serves as the starting point for the complete blockchain and contains data that is distinct from all subsequent blocks in the chain [6]. The blockchain's creator or the project's initial crew typically creates the genesis block. It includes the first transaction, also known as the "coinbase" transaction. The coinbase transaction is a sort of transaction that creates a new cryptocurrency and assigns it to the network's first node. The significance of the genesis block is that it functions as the foundation for the entire blockchain. The genesis block is linked to all subsequent blocks in the chain, resulting in an unbroken sequence of transactions. The data in the genesis block is also used to establish the blockchain's initial parameters, such as the difficulty level of the proof of work algorithm and the maximum number of coins that can be produced. [7]

1.3 Nodes

The individual machines or gadgets that take part in a blockchain network are known as nodes. Together, these nodes validate transactions and add new blocks to the network to preserve the integrity of the blockchain.

A blockchain network is a distributed ledger that records all activities that have taken place on the network, and each node in the network has a copy of the complete blockchain. To keep all copies of the blockchain in sync and exchange information about new transactions and blocks, nodes communicate.

In a blockchain network, there are various node categories, including:

Full nodes: These nodes validate and verify fresh transactions and blocks because they have a complete duplicate of the blockchain on them.

Light nodes: These nodes depend on information about new transactions and blocks from other nodes in the network rather than maintaining a full copy of the blockchain.

Nodes that engage in mining: These nodes help to validate new transactions and add them to the blockchain by resolving challenging mathematical puzzles.

Masternodes: These are specialized nodes for particular blockchain networks, like Dash and PIVX. They offer extra features and services like voting rights and instant transfers.

Nodes are essential to the functioning of a blockchain network because they cooperate to maintain the network's security, openness, and decentralization. Nodes contribute to the ongoing stability of the blockchain and help to keep it secure and reliable by taking part in the validation and verification of fresh transactions and blocks.

1.4 IMMUTABLE LEDGERS

It is a form of digital ledger that, once data has been entered on it, cannot be altered or tampered with. The ledger is referred to as being "immutable" because it is thought to be eternal and unalterable. Every entry made to a ledger in an immutable ledger is permanently documented and cannot be changed, erased, or reversed. Cryptographic algorithms and distributed consensus mechanisms, like those found in blockchain technology, are usually used to accomplish this.

A transaction or piece of information becomes a permanent component of the ledger's history once it is entered into an immutable ledger. As a result, the ledger is very hard to tamper with, cheat, or hack because doing so would require altering the ledger's complete history, which is practically impossible.

In circumstances where there is a need for accountability, transparency, and trust in the data being recorded, immutable ledgers are especially helpful. For instance, the use of immutable ledgers may be advantageous for supply chain management systems, voting systems, and financial transactions as they offer a trustworthy and impenetrable log of transactions.

In conclusion, using immutable ledgers can offer a high level of security and confidence in the data stored on them, which can be advantageous for a variety of applications across various industries.

1.5 CRYPTOGRAPHIC ALGORITHMS

Digital data is secured and protected using cryptographic algorithms, a collection of mathematical rules and procedures, from unauthorized access, alteration, and disclosure [8]. In cryptography, plain text is transformed using codes, ciphers, and other methods into unintelligible and encrypted data that can only be decoded with a hidden key or password. Cryptographic methods come in a wide variety, with each having particular properties and uses. Examples of typical cryptographic methods include:

Symmetric key algorithms: These algorithms encode and decrypt data using the same key. The secret key is used to encrypt and decrypt data or communications.

Public-key encryption: Also known as asymmetric key cryptography, public key encryption employs two different keys: a public key and a private key. The public key encrypts data, and the private key decrypts it.

Hash functions are methods that produce a message's or piece of data's fixed-size digital fingerprint or checksum. Because it is specific to the initial message, the fingerprint can be used to confirm the accuracy of the information.

Applications for cryptographic algorithms include secure contact, digital signatures, and the encryption of confidential data. In blockchain technology, they are also used to protect deals and uphold the accuracy of the ledger. In general, cryptographic methods offer a vital level of security for digital data, assisting in preventing unauthorized access, tampering, and disclosure.

1.6 PROOF OF WORK (PoW)

Blockchain technology uses this method to confirm and validate network transactions. It is a computational riddle that must be solved with some computational work [9]. In PoW, users fight to find solutions to complex mathematical puzzles that demand a lot of processing power. As compensation for their efforts, the first miner to figure out the puzzle receives a new block of transactions and a certain quantity of cryptocurrency [10]. Additionally, the completed puzzle proves that the miner made the required computational effort to validate the transaction. Miners must use their computational power to complete a series of calculations that are challenging but simple to validate to solve the puzzle. Once the puzzle has been solved, the miner broadcasts their answer to the network, where other nodes then confirm the solution's accuracy. The block of transactions is added to the blockchain, and the miner is compensated if the answer is accurate. One of its main advantages is that it makes the network extremely safe because it would take a lot of computational power to try and manipulate or change the transactions in a block. PoW ensures that each block of transactions is validated and certified by the network, maintaining the blockchain's integrity. However, PoW also uses a lot of energy because it takes a lot of computation power for miners to answer the puzzles. Consequently, some blockchain networks are investigating less energy-intensive alternatives to current consensus mechanisms, like proof of stake [11].

1.7 PROOF OF STAKE (PoS)

It is a blockchain network consensus mechanism to validate transactions and generate new blocks. It is an alternative to PoW, the Bitcoin network's consensus method. Validators (also known as "forgers" or "minters") in a PoS blockchain network are chosen based on the amount of cryptocurrency they possess or "stake" in the network. These validators are in charge of validating transactions and generating new blocks. Validators are incentivized to act honestly because they risk losing the cryptocurrency they have staked if they verify invalid transactions.

In a PoS network, the method of validating transactions and creating new blocks differs from that of a PoW network. Miners compete in a PoW network to solve complex mathematical puzzles that demand significant computational power. Validators in a PoS network are selected based on their stake, and generating new blocks is less resource-intensive. Ethereum 2.0, Cardano, and Binance Smart Chain are famous blockchain networks that use PoS. PoS has several advantages, including lower energy usage, lower transaction fees, and increased scalability. However, there are some drawbacks to PoS, such as the potential for network centralization and the chance of a "nothing-at-stake" attack [11].

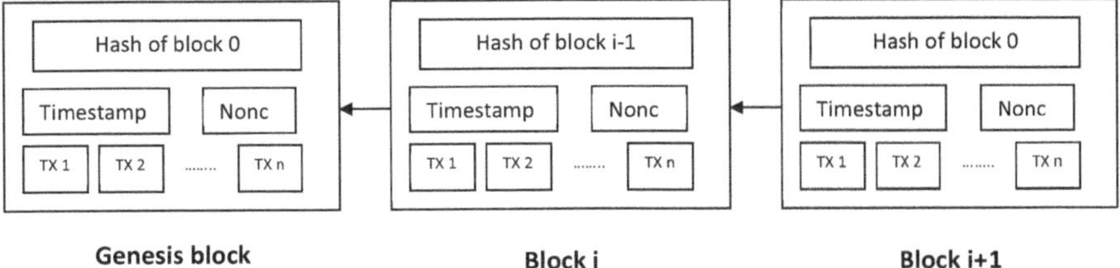

FIGURE 13.2   Sample Blocks of a Typical Blockchain

1.8 SMART CONTRACTS

A smart contract is a digitalized contract that executes automatically if certain terms are met [12], [13]. They are programs that are executed and kept on a blockchain network, enabling the automated, secure, and transparent execution of contracts between parties without the use of middlemen. As they are based on blockchain technology, which offers a tamper-proof and decentralized environment for executing code, smart contracts are made to be highly safe. Typically, they are created using programming languages like Solidity, which were created especially for creating smart contracts on the Ethereum network [14]. Figure 13.2 demonstrates example of a typical blockchain.

For smart contracts to function, a contract's terms and conditions must be written in code and then stored on the blockchain network. The contract's terms are instantly enforced once all of its requirements have been satisfied, at which point the code is automatically run [15]. For instance, once the goods are received and confirmed by a third-party logistics provider, a smart contract could immediately pay a supplier. One of their main advantages is that smart contracts do away with the need for middlemen like lawyers or banks to supervise and implement contracts. Costs can be decreased, efficiency can be raised, and parties' confidence and transparency can all be improved [16]. Several industries, including banking, insurance, supply chain management, and real estate, can benefit from smart contracts. They can be used, for instance, to automate payments, confirm the legitimacy of products, and enable safe and open real estate transactions. Overall, smart contracts offer a highly secure and effective way to automate contract execution, providing several advantages for companies and private individuals.

2 GAP ANALYSIS

Upon literature review, some gaps were found in the already existing literature, which are mentioned in Table 13.1 with their description and potential solution.

3 RELATED WORK

Research on blockchain-based biometric identification systems has been ongoing in recent years, with various studies looking at how this technology might fill in the

TABLE 13.1
Gap Analysis

Gap	Description	Potential Solution
Privacy Concerns	Current biometric systems rely on centralized databases to retain user data, generating privacy and security concerns.	Blockchain-based technologies provide a decentralized platform for user data and privacy protection.
Security Issues	Biometric systems can be hacked, for example, by producing fake biometric data or employing deep fakes to circumvent facial recognition systems.	Blockchain-based solutions can provide a tamper-proof platform, removing the possibility of data modification.
Accessibility	Biometric systems necessitate specialized hardware and software, which can be costly and difficult to obtain for people living in distant places or impoverished countries.	Blockchain-based solutions can provide a low-cost, user-friendly platform that does not require expensive hardware or specialized software.
Integration	It may be challenging to employ biometric systems efficiently if they are not properly integrated into current systems.	Systems built on the blockchain can offer a standard platform that can be combined with various other systems and applications.
Scalability	The scalability of current biometric systems may be limited, especially when dealing with high user densities. Long wait periods and sluggish authentication procedures may arise from this.	Blockchain-based solutions can provide a scalable platform that can support high user numbers without slowing down or sacrificing security.

holes in existing biometric systems. For instance, Wu et al. [17] recently presented a blockchain-based biometric identification system that makes use of a decentralized consensus process to validate biometric data. The system offers a scalable platform that can accommodate high user numbers and has been demonstrated to be more secure and privacy-preserving than conventional biometric systems.

Khan et al.'s paper [18] put forth a blockchain-based biometric authentication system that makes use of smart contracts to handle user authentication and access control. The system was shown to offer a more accessible platform that can be used in locations with limited resources, as well as being more resistant to attacks and data breaches than conventional biometric systems.

A blockchain-based biometric authentication system was proposed in a relevant work by Li et al. [19] that makes use of a distributed ledger to store user data and a zero-knowledge proof mechanism to authenticate biometric data. Comparing the system to standard biometric systems, it was shown to be more safe and private while also providing a more effective platform that may speed up and lower the cost of authentication procedures.

According to a study by Ahad et al. [20], the authors suggested a blockchain-based biometric authentication system that stores user biometric data on a distributed ledger and employs a consensus process to assure the data's accuracy and integrity. The system offers a scalable platform that can accommodate high user numbers and has been demonstrated to be more secure and privacy-preserving than conventional biometric systems.

Using a secure multi-party computation (MPC) technique to safeguard user privacy and prevent unauthorized access to biometric data, Wang et al. [21] suggested a blockchain-based biometric authentication system. In comparison to standard biometric systems, the system was found to be more resistant to attacks and data breaches while also providing a more effective platform that can lower the computational cost of authentication procedures.

A blockchain-based biometric authentication system using smart contracts to govern user authentication and access control was suggested by Liu et al. [22]. The system was proved to be more reliable and effective than conventional biometric systems, and it also provides a more open platform that may be employed in contexts with limited resources.

4   INTEGRATION OF BIOMETRIC SYSTEMS WITH BLOCKCHAIN

To securely store and manage user biometric data, the proposed system will be built utilizing a decentralized architecture that makes use of blockchain technology. These elements will be part of the system:

User Interface: Users will be able to submit their biometric information, such as fingerprint or facial recognition, and identify themselves for access to various applications and services using a user-friendly interface that will be designed.

Biometric Sensor: To record and gather user biometric information, a biometric sensor will be employed. Before being sent to the blockchain network, the data will be safely stored and encrypted.

Blockchain Network: The system will make use of a permissioned blockchain network, which restricts access to and management of data to authorized users only. The network will be built to provide a decentralized platform that can be accessed from anywhere and guarantee the data's integrity and immutability.

Smart Contracts: Smart contracts will be used to automate the execution of many tasks, including managing the authentication process and allowing access to various applications and services.

Decentralized Storage: To store and distribute user biometric data among a number of network nodes, the system will make use of a decentralized storage technique, such as IPFS. In addition to preserving the data's privacy and security, doing this will ensure that it is highly accessible and accessible from anywhere.

4.1   SYSTEM WORKFLOW

Step 1: Users will register their biometric data with the system in the first step by supplying their fingerprints or face recognition data. Before being sent to the blockchain network, the data will be encrypted and collected by a biometric sensor.

Step 2: Biometric Data Storage: Using a decentralized storage system like IPFS, the encrypted biometric data will be kept on the blockchain network. Only authorized individuals will be able to access the data, which will also be securely encrypted.

Step 3: User Authentication: A user enters their biometric information through the user interface to authenticate themselves for access to various applications and services. The information will be sent to the blockchain network for validation and verification.

Step 4: Authentication and Verification: Smart contracts will be used by the system to automate the authentication process and validate the user's identity. The user will be given access to the requested application or service if they are valid.

4.2   SYSTEM DIAGRAM

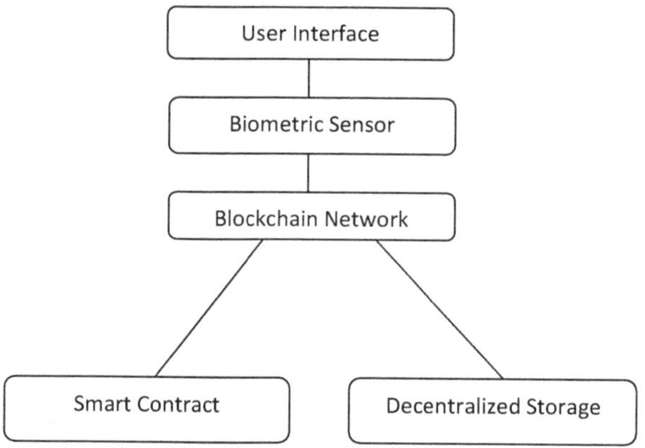

FIGURE 13.3   Flow of the Proposed Architecture

5   PROPOSED SYSTEM

This section introduces a novel blockchain-based biometric authentication system (BDBAS) – a revolutionary concept in futuristic security applications. Figure 13.3 presents the fundamental architecture of the proposed system. This system provides a distributed and decentralized solution for biometric authentication that does not rely on a centralized authentication module by utilizing

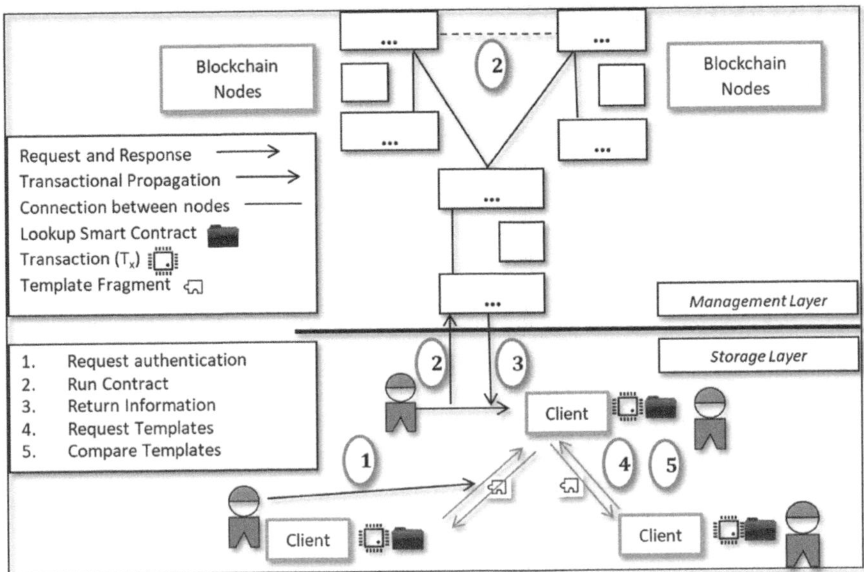

FIGURE 13.4 Operation of the Proposed System

blockchain technology. In the proposed system, the key components are controlled by each client independently and authentication processes are executed without any requirement of central hub. This decentralized approach eliminates the potential of single-point failures and enables well-built authentication. Each template is further subdivided into sections, each of which is managed by a different client. This kind of segmentation allows the scope for secure management of biometric data by lowering the possibility of any artifact or attack. A blockchain-based smart contract implements proposed system fundamentally with features like template maintenance and authentication recording. It is important to mention here that each client in the proposed runs a blockchain node, and the system must be configured with a minimum of three such clients to ensure the security provided by distributed information management. The permissioned blockchain that runs the system is restricted to validating nodes only. There are two prime layers, namely storage layer and management layer that makeup the system as depicted in Figure 13.4. The clients manage user requests in the storage layer, while blockchain nodes create a network of block-chains in the management layer. In contrast to the traditional server-client-based authentication systems, each client independently manages template components and performs authentication. By executing a smart contract, a client can find the correct clients in control of the required fragments. An important feature of the system to be noted is that each authentication process has a blockchain transaction record.

6   OVERVIEW OF BDBAS

The steps that make up the BDBAS enrollment process are as follows:

1. Request Enrollment: A client uses a sensor to gather biometric information from a user, isolates the features, and builds a template;
2. Split Template: A template is split into three sections using a specified segmentation function that is indexed by the template's generation timestamp. Therefore, based on its timestamp, each template is split into several kinds of fragments.
3. Pick Nodes: A client chooses the nodes connected to its corresponding node;
4. Select Clients: Given n clients in the BDBAS, [n/3] copies of each template's component are stored, and a total of [3*(n/3)] clients are selected randomly. For instance, if there are eight clients, each fragment will be saved twice, and six different clients will be randomly selected to manage them.
5. Store Layouts: The determined clients save the given template fragment(s).

The authentication process for the proposed system runs in the following sequence:

1. Request Authentication: A client uses a sensor to gather biometric data from a user and makes an authentication request;
2. Run Contract: A client launches the look-up smart contract to locate the necessary template fragment locations;
3. Information on Return: The client is informed of the pieces' whereabouts;
4. Request Templates: Through different client contacts, a client requests and receives the necessary fragments;
5. Compare Templates: The client assembles the pieces into a whole template and contrasts it with the information needed.

7   IMPLEMENTATION AND EVALUATION

In this section, the summary of the prototype's evaluation and implementation is discussed. The BDBAS Ethereum blockchain is built with Geth (1.9.25) and Solidity (0.6.0), and the blockchain client was built with Python 3.8 with Web3py [23].

We analytically assessed BDBAS' performance in real-world circumstances to verify its dependability. Assume that there are 3n customers in BDBAS (n = 1, 2, 3, etc.), and that these clients are in charge of managing copies of each fragment. The operation of the model can then be ensured as long as fewer than n clients are disabled. However, its authentication would not be possible if more than $3n-2$ clients were disabled [23].

$$P = \frac{s}{e}, \left(s = \sum_{(a,\, b,\, c)\, \in\, X} \frac{(3n - k)!}{a!\,b!\,c!}, \; e = \frac{(3n)!}{n!\,n!\,n!} \right) \qquad (1)$$

$$X = \{(a, b, c) \mid a > 0, b > 0, c > 0 \wedge a + b + c = 3n - k\} \qquad (2)$$

Let P be the likelihood of trustworthy authentication samples and k be the number of disabled customers ($n - 1 < k < 3n - 2$) (see Eq. (1)): The letters a, b, and c stand for the number of clients that are currently available, each containing a different kinds of fragment; s stands for the number of instances with disabled clients but more than one fragment of each template is still accessible to carry out authentication; and e stands for the number of instances where n copies of each fragment are stored across $3n$ clients [23]. In Figure 13.5, the outcome of P with $3n$ ($n = 2, 3, and 4$) is displayed. If two of the six clients in the system are disabled, authentication will most likely proceed normally with a 40% chance. If two of the nine clients in the system are disabled, the regular operation of authentication can be ensured. With a chance of 32%, authentication is still possible even if three of them are disabled. Since this system ensures more reliable authentication operation, it outperforms conventional authentication systems, which cannot guarantee authentication operation if their central server is offline [23]. The authors also established a standard authentication system with one server and one client in order to assess the performance of the proposed system. The difference in execution times between running the prototype and the server-client system on virtual computers was analyzed. Three clients, where each manages a distinct template fragment, are part of the prototype's authentication system. The size of a template was set to 1KB, which is taken as a normal template size (about 0.3KB per fragment) [22]. From process steps (2) to (4) as shown in Section 6, the authors timed the authentication procedure using the prototype model.

According to Table 13.2, obtaining all templets from other clients took 147ms on an average over the system's five loops, whereas receiving the result from the look-up smart contract took approximately 332ms. The time it took for a client to request and gets a template from a server in the server-client system was 281ms. It is clear from the small time difference between the systems that BDBAS assures the dependability of its authentication procedure while imposing little performance overhead. Despite taking a little longer (1806ms) to record an authentication activity, since this did not impair the authentication process itself, the model's performance was unaffected [23].

TABLE 13.2

Variations in the Length of the Authentication Process [23]

Process	BDBAS	Server-Client
Run contract	332ms	–
Request templates	147ms	–
Total elapsed time	680ms	281ms

8   CONCLUSION

In this study, the distributed and decentralized blockchain-based decentralized bio-metric authentication system – which uses blockchain to provide authentication – is introduced. The proposed system improves the security and dependability of the existing biometric authentication systems by breaking a biometric template into pieces and regulating them using a blockchain technique. In particular, this system (1) improves biometric data security through distributed blockchain management, (2) improves authentication operation dependability through decentralized block-chain authentication, and (3) ensures transparency of biometric data flow through a blockchain-based audit mechanism. Using the findings of the evaluation, we successfully implemented the template segmentation storage and authentication client for blockchain-based decentralized biometric authentication system on the Ethereum blockchain. We can confidently affirm that the proposed system delivers trustworthy authentication with a small performance overhead. When compared to current authentication systems, the proposed system always requires a longer authentication procedure. The authentication time may increase in proportion to the size of the system and the number of templates to be managed. This weakness, however, can be mitigated by utilizing optimization approaches for the template segmentation process and inter-node communication.

REFERENCES

[1] Acquah, Moses Arhinful, Na Chen, Jeng-Shyang Pan, Hong-Mei Yang, and Bin Yan. "Securing fingerprint template using blockchain and distributed storage system." *Symmetry* 12, no. 6 (2020): 951.

[2] Delgado-Mohatar, Oscar, Julian Fierrez, Ruben Tolosana, and Ruben Vera-Rodriguez. "Blockchain and biometrics: A first look into opportunities and challenges." In Prieto, J., Das, A., Ferretti, S., Pinto, A., Corchado, J. (eds) *Blockchain and Applications. BLOCKCHAIN 2019. Advances in Intelligent Systems and Computing*, vol 1010. Springer, Cham, pp. 169–177. Springer International Publishing, 2020.

[3] Jain, Anil K., Karthik Nandakumar, and Arun Ross. "50 years of biometric research: Accomplishments, challenges, and opportunities." *Pattern Recognition Letters* 79 (2016): 80–105.

[4] Trivedi, Sonal, and Reena Malik. "Blockchain technology as an emerging technol-ogy in the insurance market. In Sood, Kiran, Rajesh Kumar Dhanaraj, Balamurugan Balusamy, Simon Grima, and R. Uma Maheshwari (eds) *Big Data: A Game Changer for Insurance Industry*, pp. 81–100. Emerald Publishing Limited, Leeds. 2022.

[5] Nofer, Michael, Peter Gomber, Oliver Hinz, and Dirk Schiereck. "Blockchain." *Business & Information Systems Engineering* 59 (2017): 183–187.

[6] Singh, S., and Nirmala Singh. "Blockchain: Future of financial and cyber secu-rity." In *2016 2nd Iinternational Conference on Contemporary Computing and Informatics (IC3I)*, pp. 463–467. IEEE, 2016.

[7] Bhadoria, R.S., Arora, Y., Gautam, K. (2020). Blockchain Hands on for Developing Genesis Block. In: Kim, S., Deka, G. (eds) *Advanced Applications of Blockchain Technology. Studies in Big Data*, vol 60. Springer, Singapore. https://doi.org/10.1007/978-981-13-8775-3_13

[8] Dasgupta, Dipankar, John M. Shrein, and Kishor Datta Gupta. "A survey of blockchain from security perspective." *Journal of Banking and Financial Technology* 3 (2019): 1–17.

[9] Mingxiao, Du, Ma Xiaofeng, Zhang Zhe, Wang Xiangwei, and Chen Qijun. "A review on consensus algorithm of blockchain." In *2017 IEEE international conference on systems, man, and cybernetics (SMC)*, pp. 2567–2572. IEEE, 2017.

[10] Nguyen, G. T., and K. Kim. "A survey about consensus algorithms used in blockchain." *Journal of Information Processing Systems* 14, no. 1 (2018): 101–128.

[11] Zheng, Zibin, Shaoan Xie, Hongning Dai, Xiangping Chen, and Huaimin Wang. "An overview of blockchain technology: Architecture, consensus, and future trends." In *2017 IEEE International Congress on Big Data (BigData congress)*, pp. 557–564. IEEE, 2017.

[12] Kõlvart, M., Poola, M., Rull, A. (2016). Smart Contracts. In: Kerikmäe, T., Rull, A. (eds) *The Future of Law and eTechnologies*. Springer, Cham, pp. 133–147. https://doi.org/10.1007/978-3-319-26896-5_7

[13] Kaur, Amanpreet, Gurpreet Singh, Vinay Kukreja, Sparsh Sharma, Saurabh Singh, and Byungun Yoon. "Adaptation of IoT with blockchain in Food Supply Chain Management: an analysis-based review in development, benefits and potential applications." *Sensors* 22, no. 21 (2022): 8174.

[14] Mohanta, B. K., S. S. Panda, and D. Jena. "An overview of smart contract and use cases in blockchain technology." In *2018 9th international conference on computing, communication and networking technologies (ICCCNT)*, pp. 1–4. IEEE, 2018.

[15] Khan, Shafaq Naheed, Faiza Loukil, Chirine Ghedira-Guegan, Elhadj Benkhelifa, and Anoud Bani-Hani. "Blockchain smart contracts: Applications, challenges, and future trends." *Peer-to-peer Networking and Applications* 14 (2021): 2901–2925.

[16] delberger, Florian, Guido Governatori, Régis Riveret, and Giovanni Sartor. "Evaluation of logic-based smart contracts for blockchain systems." In *Rule Technologies. Research, Tools, and Applications: 10th International Symposium, RuleML 2016, Stony Brook, NY, USA, July 6–9, 2016. Proceedings 10*, pp. 167–183. Springer International Publishing, 2016.

[17] Wu, D., D. Jin, and J. Liu. "A blockchain-based biometric authentication system with consensus mechanism." *Information* 12, no. 3 (2021): 115.

[18] Khan, S., M. Asif, and F. K. Hussain. "Blockchain-based biometric authentication system for secure access control." *Journal of Ambient Intelligence and Humanized Computing* 11, no. 12 (2020): 5567–5582.

[19] Li, Y., S. Li, Y. Li, and L. Dong. "A blockchain-based biometric authentication scheme with zero knowledge proof." *Journal of Ambient Intelligence and Humanized Computing* 11, no. 8 (2020): 3257–3269.

[20] Ahad, M. A., M. M. Islam, M. A. Islam, M. R. Islam, and S. M. Al Mamun. "A blockchain-based biometric authentication system with distributed consensus mechanism." *Journal of Ambient Intelligence and Humanized Computing* 11, no. 9(2020): 3845–3859.

[21] Wang, K., Q. Wu, K. Zhang, and H. Liu. "A blockchain-based biometric authentication scheme with secure multi-party computation." *Journal of Ambient Intelligence and Humanized Computing* 12, no. 3 (2021): 2793–2805.

[22] Liu, J., D. Zou, Z. Zhu, and Y. Zhou. "A blockchain-based biometric authentication system." *Journal of Ambient Intelligence and Humanized Computing* 10, no. 11 (2019): 4271–4282.

[23] Lee, Y. K., and J. Jeong. "Securing biometric authentication system using blockchain." *ICT Express* 7, no. 3 (2021): pp. 322–326. doi:10.1016/j.icte.2021.08.003.

14 Security Issues Related to Cervical Cancer Research
A Bibliometric Analysis

*Pummy Dhiman, Anupam Bonkra,
Amandeep Kaur, and Rupali Gill*

1 INTRODUCTION

Only lung cancer (0.7 million cases) [1], colorectal cancer (0.8 million cases), and breast cancer (2.1 million cases) [2,3] are more frequent among women worldwide than cervical cancer. There were 311,000 fatalities from cervical cancer in 2018 and about 570,000 new cases have cropped up [4]. Women's cervixes can develop cervical cancer, a specific type of cancer. High-risk human papillomaviruses (HPV), which account for 99% of cases, are the main contributor to the development of this malignancy. Cervical cancer claimed 342,000 lives and caused an estimated 604,000 new cases globally in 2020; 90% of these fatalities took place in low- and middle-income nations. While many HPV infections go away without any symptoms, persistent infections can cause women to develop cervical cancer. One of the most treatable types of cancer is cervical cancer, if it is found early and treated well. Even after an advanced cancer diagnosis, the disease can still be managed with the right care and therapy. Cervical cancer rates continue to be high, particularly in low- and middle-income nations, despite the availability of efficient screening programmes [5].

1.1 CAUSE AND TREATMENT

The human papillomavirus (HPV), which is a typical sexually transmitted infection, is the main cause of cervical cancer. As a result of the cervix's cells being infected by this virus, aberrant cell proliferation might eventually result in the onset of cancer. Smoking, a compromised immune system, and a history of STDs are additional risk factors for cervical cancer [6]. Cervical cancer symptoms might include unusual vaginal bleeding, pelvic pain or discomfort, uncomfortable sex, and a bad-smelling vaginal discharge. Regular cervical cancer screening

DOI: 10.1201/9781003377818-14

is essential since the early stages of the disease may not show any signs. The Pap test is frequently used for cervical cancer screening since it is a quick, non-invasive test that can detect abnormal cells in the cervix before they develop into cancer. Additional testing, like a colposcopy or biopsy, may be necessary to confirm the diagnosis if abnormal cells are seen. The stage and location of the illness, as well as the patient's general condition, all influence the cervical cancer treatment approach. Radiation therapy, chemotherapy, surgery, or a combination of these treatments is all possible possibilities for treatment. To treat the malignancy, it may occasionally be necessary to have a hysterectomy, which entails removing the uterus.

1.2 PREVENTION

The majority of occurrences of cervical cancer may be avoided by primary prevention techniques like HPV vaccination and secondary prevention tactics like detecting and treating precancerous lesions [7].

1.2.1 Primary Approach

The HPV vaccine is the main method of cervical cancer prevention and eventual eradication [8]. The lifetime risk of young girls acquiring cervical cancer is considerably reduced by using this evidence-based strategy. Since young cohorts that receive the vaccine won't reach the age where they are most susceptible to the illness until well into adulthood, the effect of vaccination on invasive cervical cancer rates may take some time to become apparent, even though it is very successful in the long term. However, it is essential to act right away to provide HPV vaccine and shield them from potential dangers of cervical cancer in the future.

1.2.2 Secondary Approach

Cervical screening and good precancerous lesion management are established strategies to lower the incidence of invasive cervical cancer and lower mortality rates in adult women who may have already acquired HPV [9].

More advanced screening tests for cervical cancer prevention have been developed as a result of improvements in our understanding of the pathophysiology of cervical cancer and its relationship to HPV infection.

Cervical cancer screening tests come in a few distinct varieties [10]:

1. The Pap test, also known as the Pap smear, involves taking cells from the cervix and analysing them under a microscope to check for abnormal cells. At age 21, it is advised that women begin routine Pap testing.
2. HPV test: This examination checks for the human papillomavirus (HPV), the primary cause of cervical cancer [11]. Pap tests and HPV testing can be done alone or together. Women between the ages of 30 and 65 are advised to get tested for HPV every five years.

3. Co-testing with both a Pap and an HPV test: This procedure comprises both tests. Every five years, both tests are advised for females aged 30 to 65.

4. Cervical cytology, usually referred to as a Pap smear, is a screening procedure that involves taking cells from the cervix and analysing them under a microscope to check for abnormal cells. In order to see the cervix for the test, a speculum is often inserted into the vagina during a pelvic exam. Using a little brush or spatula, the cells are gathered, and they are then sent to a lab for examination.

5. Visual inspection with acetic acid (VIA) is yet another cervical cancer screening technique. In this test, the cervix is exposed to an acetic acid solution that turns aberrant cells white. The medical professional next looks visually for any white patches on the cervix that could be signs of abnormal cells. In low-resource environments, when access to more expensive screening tests may be restricted, VIA is frequently employed.

Remember that your age, medical history, and other variables may affect how frequently you undergo screening tests.

1.3 DATA SECURITY AND PRIVACY CONCERNS

Cervical cancer research faces various security issues including the collection and analysis of private medical data as well as the protection of intellectual property. Rules and regulations are crucial to ensure the security of data and prevent breaches, cyberattacks, and legal and financial penalties. In order to successfully conduct cervical cancer research, it is crucial to use healthcare 5.0 and IoMT technologies as they offer secure and effective ways of gathering, analysing, and protecting sensitive health data [12]. They also help secure physical assets and protect intellectual property. Security is, however, still a top issue in the modern technological age. The following security issues are related to cervical cancer research:

1. Data privacy and confidentiality: Gathering and analysing private health data on individuals is a necessary part of cervical cancer research. The privacy and confidentiality of study participants could be jeopardised by data breaches or unauthorised access to such information.

2. Intellectual property protection: In cervical cancer research, the protection of intellectual property, such as patents or trade secrets, raises additional potential security concerns. Theft or infringement of intellectual property can lead to financial losses and reduce the incentives for innovation in the industry.

3. Cybersecurity: Cervical cancer research, like all other types of research, is susceptible to online crimes including phishing schemes and ransomware attacks that can jeopardise the reliability and accessibility of infrastructure and data [13].

4. Regulatory compliance: Cervical cancer research must adhere to a number of laws and policies, including those that safeguard human subjects and promote ethical research practices. If these rules are broken, institutions and researchers may face legal and financial repercussions as well as reputational harm.
5. Physical security: Protecting research tools and materials, such as biobanks, lab samples, and imaging equipment, from theft, damage, or sabotage is another possible security concern.

1.4 OBJECTIVE

This bibliometric analysis paper's goal is to look at the publications' contributions to research and their effects on publications on cervical cancer. This will be accomplished by examining and quantifying the attributes of the articles, including the quantity of publications, authorship, connections, nations, citation analysis, and keywords employed. Additionally, this study will give a broad overview of the research trends and security concerns and identify the most prolific and prominent authors, institutions, and nations.

1.4.1 Contribution

This bibliometric analysis report on cervical cancer will aid in understanding the research environment in this area and offer perceptions on research trends and effect. It will specifically:

1. Identify the most successful and significant researchers, organisations, and nations in cervical cancer research.
2. Determine highly cited articles and authors by assessing the publications' influence on citations.
3. Give a thorough review of the research output and effect in cervical cancer research during a given time period.
4. Make a contribution to the development of knowledge in the discipline by suggesting potential areas for more study and teamwork.

2 LITERATURE REVIEW

A study by Cynae A. Johnson et al. provides an in-depth analysis of cervical cancer, including information on its pathogenesis, risk factors, screening, diagnosis, therapy, and management [14]. The authors emphasise the significance of early diagnosis through screening and give a summary of the available diagnostic procedures and therapeutic alternatives while highlighting the demand for a multidisciplinary approach. Medical practitioners who are involved in the treatment of cervical cancer patients will find this article to be a useful resource. The purpose of the study [15] was to assess the impact of educational interventions on women's screening behaviour for cervical cancer. The data from 15 researches were examined by the authors, who also did a thorough evaluation of investigations carried out between 2000 and 2020. The findings showed that educational programmes had a favourable effect on women's behaviour about cervical cancer screening. The authors advised healthcare professionals to undertake educational initiatives to raise women's screening rates for cervical cancer. Authors of study [4] conducted a general review of cervical cancer, including its prevalence, inequities in healthcare access, and treatment results. The authors investigate the risk factors, screening guidelines, and epidemiology of cervical cancer. Along with the influence of socioeconomic variables on cervical cancer outcomes, they also talk about differences in cervical cancer incidence and death among various racial and ethnic groups. The authors come to the conclusion that cervical cancer is a disease that can be prevented, and that efforts to widen access to screening and care are essential to lowering inequities and enhancing outcomes. A literature review by 4 authors titled "Cervical cancer control limiting factors and facilitators: a literature review [16]" sought to pinpoint the elements that either hinder or aid cervical cancer control. A total of 43 publications between 2015 and 2020, comprising both qualitative and quantitative investigations, were examined for the study. This study highlighted a number of variables, such as restricted access to screening programmes and healthcare facilities, poor awareness and understanding of cervical cancer, cultural and societal factors, and inadequate healthcare infrastructure and resources, which limit cervical cancer control. The study also discovered that the attitudes and actions of women towards cervical cancer screening and prevention had a big impact on the disease's management. The study comes to the conclusion that a comprehensive approach to cervical cancer control is required, which includes education and awareness-raising, improving access to screening programmes and healthcare services, removing cultural and social barriers, and boosting resources and infrastructure to support efficient prevention and treatment programmes. The article "Recent Advancements in Cervical Cancer Diagnosis for Automated Screening: A Detailed Review [10]" by B. Chitra and S.S. Kumar gives a summary of the most recent advancements in the field of cervical cancer diagnosis using automated screening methods, including the use of liquid-based cytology, computer-aided diagnosis (CAD), and machine learning algorithms. The authors point out the benefits of these techniques, including their improved accuracy, effectiveness, and reduced variability. The scientists contend that by using these fresh methods, early detection rates may be markedly increased, which would ultimately lessen the burden of cervical cancer on women all over the world.

3   RESEARCH METHODOLOGY

Data Gathering: Since Scopus is a well-known bibliographic database with extensive coverage of scientific literature, it was chosen for this study's data collection. It indexes scientific articles in a variety of topics, including cancer and medicine, including journals, books, conference proceedings, and other publications [17]. This bibliometric analysis article on cervical cancer will benefit from using

Scopus in a number of ways. The first benefit of using Scopus is that it gives you access to a wide range of articles that might aid in finding the most current and pertinent research in your area of study. This analysis will be current and thorough as a result of this.

3.1 SEARCH STRING

Here, a search string made up of keywords is created, and the Scopus database is then searched. The search is carried out in the article title, abstract, and keywords by using the Boolean AND, OR operator as demonstrated in the example below.

"Cervical cancer" AND "Prevention" AND ("Deep Learning" OR "Machine Learning" OR "Cloud Computing" OR "Robotics")

3.2 SCREENING

Using the aforementioned search term, the quantity of publications received is preceded for screening. The following list of criteria describes how the articles for this study were bound. As it is not bounded to particular country so this study included all country's publications, but as authors only understand English language so this constraint is put in this study.

TITLE-ABS-KEY ("Cervical cancer" AND "Prevention" AND ("Deep Learning" OR "Machine Learning" OR "Cloud Computing" OR "Robotics")) AND (LIMIT-TO (PUBYEAR, 2006) OR LIMIT-TO (PUBYEAR, 2010) OR LIMIT-TO (PUBYEAR, 2013) OR LIMIT-TO (PUBYEAR, 2015) OR LIMIT-TO (PUBYEAR, 2016) OR LIMIT-TO (PUBYEAR, 2017) OR LIMIT-TO (PUBYEAR, 2018) OR LIMIT-TO (PUBYEAR, 2019) OR LIMIT-TO (PUBYEAR, 2020) OR LIMIT-TO (PUBYEAR, 2021) OR LIMIT-TO (PUBYEAR, 2022) OR LIMIT-TO (PUBYEAR, 2023)) AND (LIMIT-TO (LANGUAGE, "English"))

Study containing undefined authors has been omitted as well as the study containing only cancer. Only the final stage of publications has been selected here. Every publication includes information such as the author, the nation, citations, references, etc.

4 RESULTS AND DISCUSSION

Table 14.1 illustrates the overview of 70 studies that were retrieved and screened for inclusion in this manuscript. Primary data, document contents, and other criteria were used to categorise the information that was retrieved collaborations between writers, document categories, and authors. A total of 2405 references – 55 sources from journals and books – are included in the chosen research. Every paper shows an average annual growth rate of 16.29% and cites 10.33 articles on average. From 402 writers, the publications have 185 keywords. Numerous categories, including book chapters, conference papers, review papers, book chapters, and reviews, are used to categorise the publications.

TABLE 14.1

Visual Representation of Data Used

Description	Results
Main Information about Data	
Timespan	2006:2023
Sources (Journals, Books, etc.)	55
Documents	70
Annual Growth Rate %	16.29
Document Average Age	3.67
Average citations per doc	10.33
References	2405
Document Contents	
Keywords Plus (ID)	993
Author's Keywords (DE)	185
AUTHORS	
Authors	402
Authors of single-authored docs	1
Authors Collaboration	
Single-authored docs	1
Co-Authors per Doc	6.46
International co-authorships %	28.57
Document Types	
Article	44
Book chapter	2
Conference paper	12
Conference review	5
Editorial	2
Erratum	1
Review	4

In order to assess the trends in cervical cancer research, the study has gathered research from various researchers that spans 18 years, from 2006 to 2023. As shown in Figure 14.1, the number of publications has gone up a lot since 2015. The yearly publication trends show how cervical cancer research is changing. There were the most publications (17) on the topic in 2021, which shows that it has recently become more popular. There was a slight drop in the number of publications in the years that followed, but the study activity stayed high compared to earlier times.

Table 14.2 shows the number of publications published annually, the average total number of citations per article, and the citation years. There is no discernible pattern in the citation structure, besides the clear correlation between the frequency of citations and publication age.

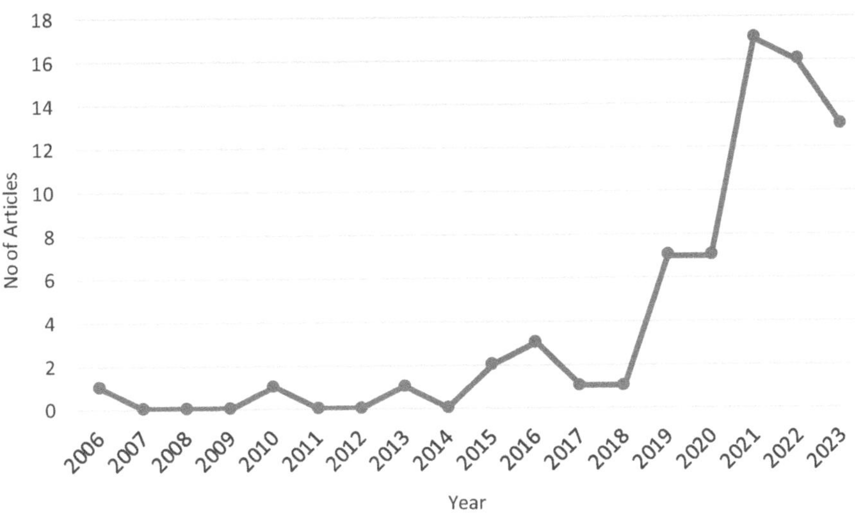

FIGURE 14.1   Annual Publication Trends

TABLE 14.2
Average Citations Per Year

Year	MeanTC per Art	N	MeanTC per Year	Citable Years
2006	6	1	0.32	19
2010	28	1	1.87	15
2013	41	1	3.42	12
2015	29.5	2	2.95	10
2016	25.67	3	2.85	9
2017	1	1	0.12	8
2018	0	1	0	7
2019	14.71	7	2.45	6
2020	15.71	7	3.14	5
2021	12.71	17	3.18	4
2022	4.5	16	1.5	3
2023	0.77	13	0.38	2

4.1 MOST RELEVANT AFFILIATIONS

The use of citations allows for the linking of sources, ideas, principles, and points of view [18]. As a result, by looking at citations, one may determine the impact that various organisations (such as countries, universities, research institutes, or journals) have on the field of scholarship and monitor how their performance evolves over time [19]. The National Cancer Institute has published 20 publications on cervical cancer, making it the foremost source of information

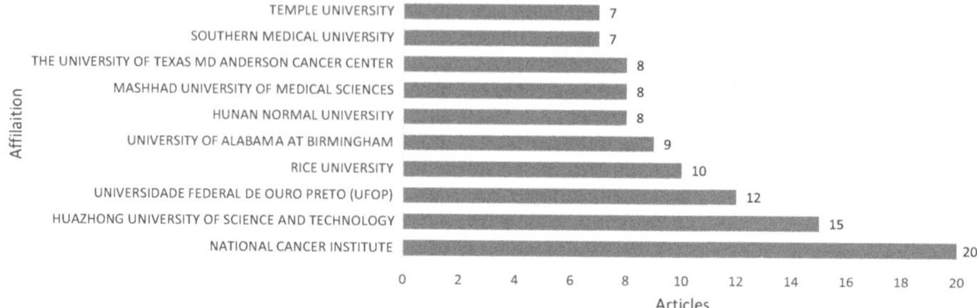

FIGURE 14.2   Most Prominent Affiliation

TABLE 14.3
Top 10 Countries for Scientific Publication

Region	Frequency
USA	118
China	85
South Korea	35
Brazil	30
India	24
Japan	19
Denmark	16
Netherlands	13
Iran	11
Romania	11

on the issue. With 15 articles of its own, Huazhong University of Science and Technology demonstrates its formidable scholarly standing. The University of Texas MD Anderson Cancer Center has eight, and Southern Medical University also has eight. These affiliations collectively serve an important role in promoting cervical cancer research and improving scientific understanding of the disease (Figure 14.2).

4.2   COUNTRIES' SCIENTIFIC PRODUCTION

The United States has led the detection of cervical cancer, as seen in Table 14.3. The 118 articles demonstrated a robust and steady contribution to this field. China also demonstrated significant scientific production. Continuing down the list, other countries that made contributions to this worldwide research scene include Iran, Romania, South Korea, Brazil, India, Japan, Denmark, the Netherlands, and Iran.

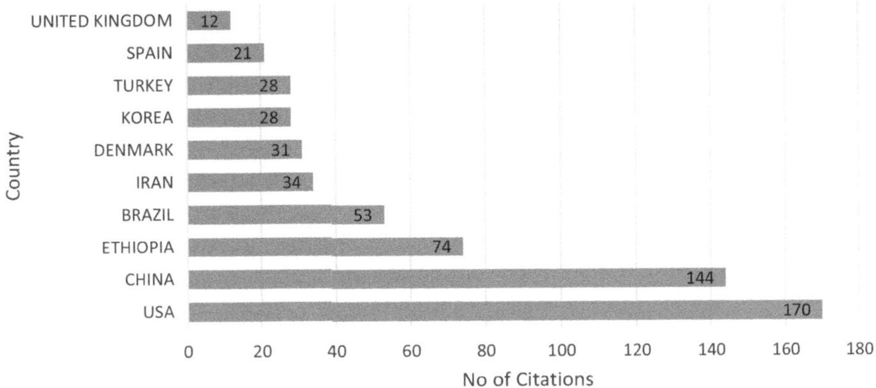

FIGURE 14.3 Citation Wise Most Prominent Countries

4.3 MOST CITED COUNTRY

The country with the greatest number of citations for its research output is referred to as the "most cited country" in bibliometric analysis [20]. This shows that the country has generated a sizeable body of high-quality research that has affected the scientific community and been widely cited by other scholars in their publications. The strength of the nation's research infrastructure, funding, and scientific culture may be reflected in its ranking as the most cited nation.

Figure 14.3 shows with 170 documents citation the USA scores top most position followed by China, Ethiopia, Brazil, Iran, Denmark, Korea, Turkey, and United Kingdom. Table 14.4 shows the top 10 highly cited documents.

4.4 WORD-CLOUD

The most common terms in a document or corpus of papers are displayed visually in a word cloud. Word clouds are frequently used in bibliometrics to show the most frequent terms in a research paper, an article, or a collection of linked materials [21]. In bibliometrics, word clouds may be helpful for rapidly identifying important subjects or themes in a collection of documents as well as for contrasting and comparing the language employed in various texts or from various historical periods. Word clouds should, however, be used in conjunction with other approaches to properly comprehend and interpret the results as they are only one tool in a wider set of bibliometric research tools [22].

The word-cloud based on Keyword Plus and title is shown in Figure 14.4. These keywords are used to define the relationship between a number of specific words, including sensitivity, specificity, uterine cervix cancer, female, colposcopy, artificial intelligence, machine learning [23], deep learning [24], and many more.

TABLE 14.4

Highly Cited Publications

Paper	DOI	Total Citations	TC per Year
CHANDRAN V, 2021, BIOMED RES INT	10.1155/2021/5584004	74	18.50
DOO DW, 2019, GYNECOL ONCOL	10.1016/j.ygyno.2019.03.001	69	11.50
LI X, 2015, EUR J CANCER	10.1016/j.ejca.2015.05.012	47	4.70
SOBAR, 2016, ADV SCI LETT	10.1166/asl.2016.7980	44	4.89
KUMAR S, 2013, GYNECOL ONCOL	10.1016/j.ygyno.2013.04.024	41	3.42
ASADI F, 2020, J BIOMED PHYS ENG	10.31661/jbpe.v0i0.1912-1027	34	6.80
TAN X, 2021, CANCER CELL INT	10.1186/s12935-020-01742-6	32	8.00
JENSEN PT, 2020, EUR J CANCER	10.1016/j.ejca.2019.12.020	31	6.20
ADWEB KMA, 2021, IEEE ACCESS	10.1109/ACCESS.2021.3067195	28	7.00
SUH DH, 2010, J GYNECOL ONCOL	10.3802/jgo.2010.21.3.137	28	1.87

4.5 TREE-MAP

The representation of data in a hierarchical structure using a tree-map is a visualisation approach used in bibliometric analysis [19]. The relative size of various bibliographic units, such as authors, publications, or institutions, can be shown in bibliometrics using a tree-map. A tree-map shows data as a collection of nested rectangles, with each rectangle denoting a distinct bibliographic unit as shown in Figure 14.5. The size of each rectangle relates to a particular characteristic, such as the quantity of publications an institution has contributed to or the quantity of citations an article has received. The rectangles are placed in a hierarchical manner, with the bigger rectangles denoting higher-level categories like a study topic and the smaller rectangles denoting more granular categories like a publication or an author. The tree map in the specified picture shows the top 20 phrases that are most commonly used in publications including the keywords cervical cancer, machine learning, deep learning, Pap test, endometrial cancer [25], colposcopy [26], and other relevant terms.

4.6 BIBLIOGRAPHIC COUPLING – AUTHOR WISE

An approach used in bibliometric analysis to examine the patterns of author collaboration is co-authorship analysis. It entails examining the co-authorship network, a graph that depicts the relationships between writers based on the publications they have co-authored. For the purposes of co-authorship analysis, each

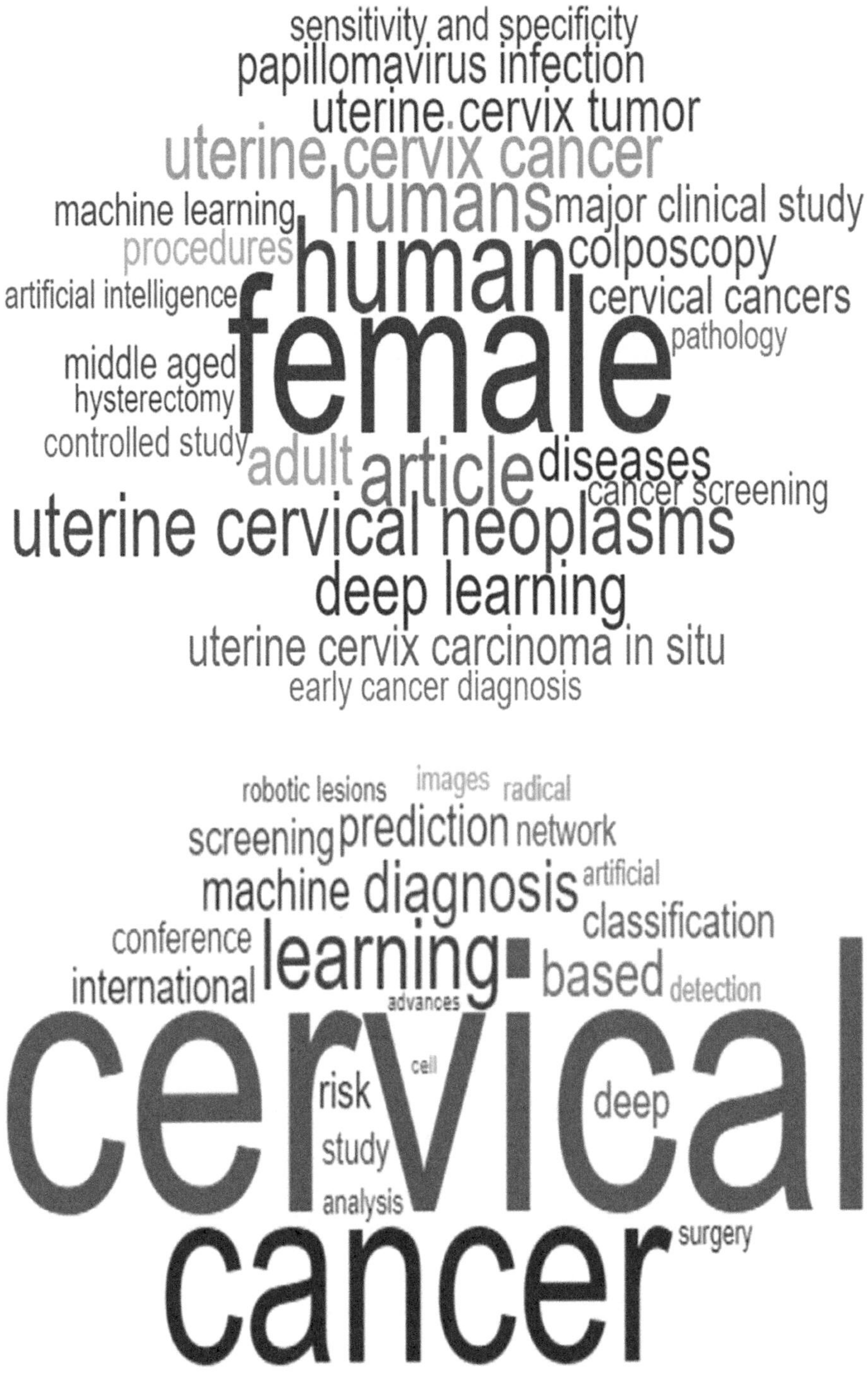

FIGURE 14.4   Word Cloud: (a) Keywords Plus; (b) Article's Title

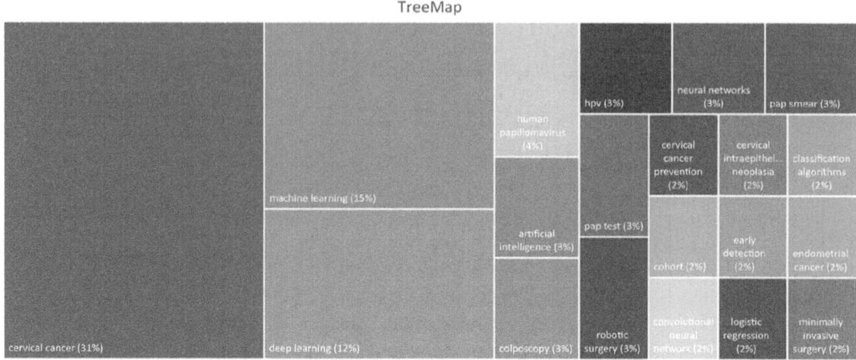

FIGURE 14.5   Tree Map

FIGURE 14.6   Co-authorship Network Based on Collaboration Among Publication Authors

author is represented as a node in a network, and each co-authorship connection is represented as an edge linking the nodes of the writers who have worked together on one or more publications. The resultant network's relationships between writers may be seen by employing network visualisation techniques, including a force-directed layout.

Figure 14.6 shows the relationships between different writers as clusters of colourful bubbles. Only 32 out of 65 authors fulfil the requirements, which are a minimum of 5 documents and 5 citations per author. The authors are grouped into three categories, as depicted in the figure above: red, green, and blue.

4.7   BIBLIOGRAPHIC COUPLING – COUNTRY WISE

When two or more publications share references, a method called bibliographic coupling is employed in bibliometric analysis to determine how closely connected they are. This method is especially effective for examining international research trends and patterns of interdisciplinary collaboration in the sciences. The quantity

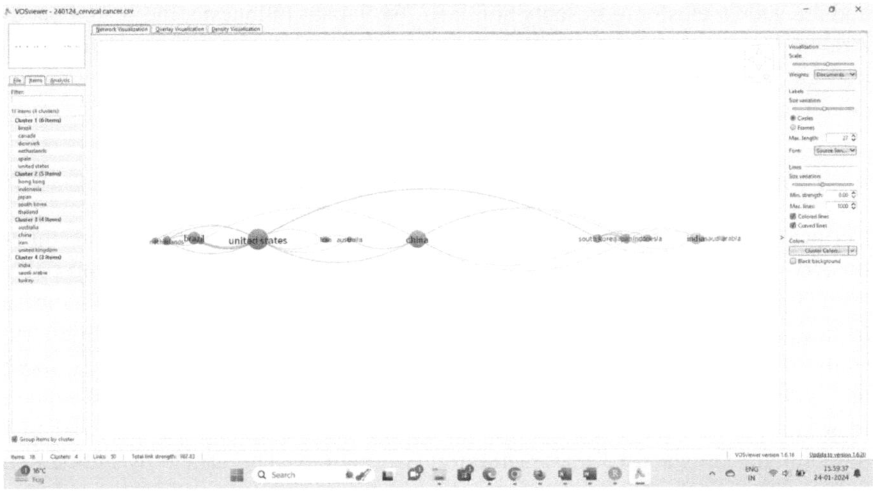

FIGURE 14.7   Bibliographic Coupling by Country

TABLE 14.5
Worldwide Research Collaborations

Country	Documents	Citations
United States	19	236
Brazil	7	74
South Korea	4	44
Japan	3	42
China	14	171
India	7	104
Indonesia	3	72
Netherlands	3	4
Spain	3	24
Romania	3	4

of references those publications from various nations share in common is compared in a process called bibliographic coupling analysis. Each pair of articles receives an individual score called a "bibliographic coupling score" that indicates how many references they have in common. A pair of articles is more connected to one another when their scores on the bibliographic coupling scale are higher (Figure 14.7).

Out of 43 nations, the graph shows that 10 have at least 3 documents and 3 country citations, which is considered to be meeting the standards. Four coloured clusters with bubbles show the path between nodes. The node represented the country, and the path represented the link among them. The red bubbles are used to designate the red cluster, which includes the United States, Brazil, the Netherlands, and Spain. China, Australia, and Iran come under the blue cluster, and the yellow cluster represents South Korea, Japan, Indonesia, India, and Saudi Arabia. Those countries that came under one cluster represented a strong connection among them. Table 14.5 shows the frequency between different countries, documents, and citations with the total link strength.

5 CONCLUSION AND FUTURE DIRECTIONS

Cervical cancer research security issues are complex and multifaceted, but stakeholders must work to improve data privacy, confidentiality, intellectual property protection, cybersecurity measures, regulatory compliance, and physical security to safeguard critical research data and infrastructure. Based on the bibliometric study of Scopus data, it can be said that during the past several decades, there has been a marked rise in the number of publications relating to cervical cancer. In terms of scientific output and citation effect, the research also showed that the United States and China are the top two nations. The article by Schiffman et al. in 2002 with revised recommendations for the treatment of aberrant cervical cytology and histology was found to be the most frequently referenced source of information. According to connections, the investigation uncovered a number of institutions that have significantly aided the fight against cervical cancer, including the National Cancer Institute, the University of Texas, and the Chinese Academy of Medical Sciences. Research on cervical cancer frequently involves worldwide collaboration, according to co-authorship analyses, demonstrating a global effort to combat this illness.

Future study on cervical cancer prevention, early detection, and therapy should address security issues connected to the digitisation of research procedures and the proliferation of sensitive data. It is necessary to improve security measures such as data privacy, cybersecurity, and physical security. There should also be initiatives to increase public understanding of the security dangers and resource limitations in developing countries. Researchers can advance cervical cancer research by proactively addressing these concerns. To increase the precision of cervical cancer screening and diagnosis, the application of artificial intelligence and machine learning algorithms can be studied. Research may also concentrate on finding biomarkers that may be used to predict the likelihood of getting cervical cancer, which can help with early identification and prevention. Finally, initiatives should be taken to raise knowledge about cervical cancer and its preventative methods, particularly in developing nations with poor access to healthcare. Researchers can advance cervical cancer research by proactively addressing these concerns.

REFERENCES

[1] S. Bharathy, R. Pavithra, and B. Akshaya, "Lung Cancer Detection using Machine Learning," *Proc. - Int. Conf. Appl. Artif. Intell. Comput. ICAAIC 2022*, vol. 7, no. 1, pp. 539–543, 2022, doi:10.1109/ICAAIC53929.2022.9793061.

[2] C. Kaushal and A. Singla, "Automated Segmentation Technique with Self-driven Post-processing for Histopathological Breast Cancer Images," *CAAI Trans. Intell. Technol.*, vol. 5, no. 4, pp. 294–300, 2020, doi:10.1049/trit.2019.0077.

[3] D. Koundal, S. Gupta, and S. Singh, "Computer Aided Thyroid Nodule Detection System Using Medical Ultrasound Images," *Biomed. Signal Process. Control*, vol. 40, pp. 117–130, 2018, doi:10.1016/j.bspc.2017.08.025.

[4] A. Buskwofie, G. David-West, and C. A. Clare, "A Review of Cervical Cancer: Incidence and Disparities," *J. Natl. Med. Assoc.*, vol. 112, no. 2, pp. 229–232, 2020, doi:10.1016/j.jnma.2020.03.002.

[5] "Cervical cancer." https://www.who.int/health-topics/cervical-cancer#tab=tab_1 (accessed Apr. 22, 2023).

[6] U. K. Lilhore *et al.*, "Hybrid Model for Detection of Cervical Cancer Using Causal Analysis and Machine Learning Techniques," *Comput. Math. Methods Med.*, vol. 2022, p. 4688327, 2022, doi:10.1155/2022/4688327.

[7] "Home." https://cceirepository.who.int/ (accessed Apr. 22, 2023).

[8] K. Kaarthigeyan, "Cervical Cancer in India and HPV Vaccination," *Indian J. Med. Paediatr. Oncol.*, vol. 33, no. 1, pp. 7–12, 2012, doi:10.4103/0971–5851.96961.

[9] WHO, "DRAFT Strategic Framework for the Comprehensive Prevention and Control of Cervical Cancer in the Western Pacific Region 2023–2030," *Wpr/Rc73/6*, vol. 2, no. 3, pp. 7–65, 2023.

[10] B. Chitra and S. S. Kumar, "Recent Advancement in Cervical Cancer Diagnosis for Automated Screening: A Detailed Review," *J. Ambient Intell. Humaniz. Comput.*, vol. 13, no. 1, pp. 251–269, 2022, doi:10.1007/s12652-021-02899-2.

[11] P. E. Castle, M. Sideri, J. Jeronimo, D. Solomon, and M. Schiffman, "Risk Assessment to Guide the Prevention of Cervical Cancer," *J. Low. Genit. Tract Dis.*, vol. 12, no. 1, pp. 1–7, 2008, doi:10.1097/lgt.0b013e31815ea58b.

[12] A. Bonkra and P. Dhiman, "IoT Security Challenges in Cloud Environment," In *2021 2nd International Conference on Computational Methods in Science & Technology (ICCMST)*, 2021, pp. 30–34. doi:10.1109/ICCMST54943.2021.00018.

[13] J. L. Drummond, M. C. Were, S. Arrossi, and K. Wools-Kaloustian, "Cervical Cancer Data and Data Systems in Limited-resource Settings: Challenges and Opportunities," *Int. J. Gynecol. Obstet.*, vol. 138, pp. 33–40, 2017, doi:10.1002/ijgo.12192.

[14] C. A. Johnson, D. James, A. Marzan, and M. Armaos, "Cervical Cancer: An Overview of Pathophysiology and Management," *Semin. Oncol. Nurs.*, vol. 35, no. 2, pp. 166–174, 2019, doi:10.1016/j.soncn.2019.02.003.

[15] M. S. G. Naz, N. Kariman, A. Ebadi, G. Ozgoli, V. Ghasemi, and F. R. Fakari, "Educational Interventions for Cervical Cancer Screening Behavior of Women: A Systematic Review," *Asian Pacific J. Cancer Prev.*, vol. 19, no. 4, pp. 875–884, 2018, doi:10.22034/APJCP.2018.19.4.875.

[16] V. A. S. Lopes and J. M. Ribeiro, "Cervical Cancer Control Limiting Factors and Facilitators: A Literature Review," *Cienc. e Saude Coletiva*, vol. 24, no. 9, pp. 3431–3442, 2019, doi:10.1590/1413-81232018249.32592017.

[17] J. F. Burnham, "Scopus Database: A Review," *Biomed. Digit. Libr.*, vol. 3, pp. 1–8, 2006, doi:10.1186/1742-5581-3-1.

[18] K. Saluja, A. Bansal, A. Vajpaye, S. Gupta, and A. Anand, "Efficient Bag of Deep Visual Words Based Features to Classify CRC Images for Colorectal Tumor Diagnosis," In *2022 2nd International Conference on Advance Computing and Innovative Technologies in Engineering (ICACITE)*, Greater Noida, India, 2022, pp. 1814–1818, doi:10.1109/ICACITE53722.2022.9823727.

[19] S. Srivastav, K. Guleria, and S. Sharma, "Predictive Machine Learning Approaches for Cervical Cancer Detection: An Analytical Comparison," In *2023 10th International Conference on Computing for Sustainable Global Development (INDIACom)*, pp. 951–956. IEEE, 2023.

[20] A. Bonkra, P. Dhiman, S. Goyal, and N. Gupta, "A Systematic Study: Implication of Deep Learning in Plant Disease Detection," in *2022 IEEE International Conference on Current Development in Engineering and Technology (CCET)*, 2022, pp. 1–6. doi:10.1109/CCET56606.2022.10080181.

[21] A. Bonkra, P. K. Bhatt, A. Kaur, and S. Kamboj, "Scientific Landscape and the Road Ahead for Deep Learning: Apple Leaves Disease Detection," In *2023 International Conference on Artificial Intelligence and Smart Communication (AISC)*, 2023, pp. 869–873. doi:10.1109/AISC56616.2023.10085221.

[22] N. Donthu, S. Kumar, D. Mukherjee, N. Pandey, and W. M. Lim, "How to Conduct a Bibliometric Analysis: An Overview and Guidelines," *J. Bus. Res.*, vol. 133, no. April, pp. 285–296, 2021, doi:10.1016/j.jbusres.2021.04.070.

[23] A. Bonkra, A. Noonia, and A. Kaur, "Apple Leaf Diseases Detection System: A Review of the Different Segmentation and Deep Learning Methods," in *International Conference on Artificial Intelligence and Data Science*, Cham: Springer Nature Switzerland, 2022, pp. 263–278.

[24] ,A. Kaur, et al. "A Mathematical Model of Cervical Cancer Using Causal Analysis," *AIP Conf. Proc.*, vol. 2357, no. 1, AIP Publishing, 2022.

[25] S. Bharti and S. N. Singh, "Analytical Study of Heart Disease Prediction Comparing with Different Algorithms," in *International Conference on Computing, Communication & Automation*, 2015, pp. 78–82. doi:10.1109/CCAA.2015.7148347.

[26] F. Fusco, M. Marsilio, and C. Guglielmetti, "Co-production in Health Policy and Management: A Comprehensive Bibliometric Review," *BMC Health Serv. Res.*, vol. 20, no. 1, pp. 1–17, 2020, doi:10.1186/s12913-020-05241-2.

Index

Note: **Bold** page numbers refer to tables.

accelerometer 55, 90
accessibility 54, 78, 112, 199, 226, 265, 279, 284, 294
accuracy 3, 5, **7–10**, 22, 39, 42, 46, 47, 50, 53–55, 57, 79–83, 95, 97, 99, 101, 102, 147, 167, 182–185, 187, 188, 197, 198, 221, 229, 231, 232, 238, 263, 274, 279, 281, 282, 296
activation function 38, 45, 72, 77, 96
Adaboost 51
adversarial networks 31, 37, 71, 229
alzheimer's disease 30, 70, 115, 151, 214
anomalies 11, 212, 226–28
antibiotics 11, 36
anxiety 107, 114, 214
artificial intelligence 1, **7**, 22, 23, 40, 42, 57, 67, 107, 176, 179, 227, 301, 306
augmented reality 54, 105, 106, 109
autoencoder 37, 71

bacteria 23
Bayes 4, 29, 52, 65, 216
Bayes classifier 29, 52
Bayesian network 11
biases 39, 177, 192, 195
biochemical 150
bioinformatics 188
biological 25, 78, 147, 180, 181, 185, 232
biological traits 232
biopsychosocial 114
biosensors 218
biotechnology 33
Bitcoin 256–58, 265, 278, 282

calibration 191
cancer 5, 10, 11, 25, 30, 31, 42, 43, 48, 51, 77, 78, 80, 112, 138, 183, 184, 189, 214, 292–302, 306
cancerous 44, 183
cardiogram 150
cardiology 180, 184
cardiovascular disease 6, **7**, 16, 19, 26, 64, 83, 89, 138, 183, 209, 241
chemotherapy 293
chronic diseases 9, 25, 53–55, 59, 67, 69, 106, 146, 183, 214, 215
chronic illness 106, 204

classification 4, 5, **7–10**, 29, 37, 38, 42, 44, 45, 47, 51, 52, **61**, 69, 73, 78, 79, 81, 82, 84, 86, 89, 90, 93, 94, 97, 101, 102, 154, 216, 221, 231, 235
classification algorithms 9, 18, 90, 93, 97, 101
classifiers **7**, 47
clock synchronization 162, 165
clustering 51–53, **62**
complexity 25, 78, 95, 122, 196, 259, 270
confidentiality 32, 110, 144, 148, 153, 158, 161, 162, 164, 165, 192, 197, 218, 226, 232, 236, 245, 250, 256, 265, 267, 268, 275, 294, 306
controller 63, 144, 157, 266
convolutional layers 45, 73
convolutional neural network 20, 27, 37, 80, 81, 84, 119, 189, 203, 206, 210
coronavirus 176, 188, 189
cryptocurrency 257, 258, 275, 278, 280, 282
cryptography 110, 142, 155, 157, 158, 165, 167, 255, 259, 281
cyberattacks 198, 219, 224, 233, 234, 270, 271, 294

database 15, 23, 37, **62**, 220, 232, 233, 239, 244, 250, 251, 255, 256, 268, 279, 296, 297
dataset 5, 25, 32, 38, 39, 45–47, 50–52, 60, 78, 81–83, 86, 90–95, 97, 249–51
decoder 37, 71
decryption 152, 157, 158, 221, 250
deep learning 2, 5, 22, 23, 26–28, 30, 31, 33, 36, 37, 39, 40, 42, 67, 68, 72, 82, 84, 179, 183, 186, 228, 246, 252, 297, 301, 302
demographics 36, 59, 188, 191
Denial of services (DoS) 145, 155, 211, 218, 248, 251
deployment 14, 84, 200, 212, 240, 274
diabetes **7**, 9, 10, 29, 46, 47, 51, 69, 88, 110, 183, 198, 214
diabetic 9, 10, 47, 69, 231
diagnose 6, 9, 11, 37, 43, 53, 58, 60, 79, 83, 109, 183, 191, 261
dimension 46, 71, 73, 74, 79, 90
dimensionality 31, 52, 71, 79, 183
disabilities 55, 88, 215
disorders 15, 16, 25, 29, 32, 36, 42, 43, 57, 60, 87, 107, 109, 183, 214